GERIATRIC ORTHOPAEDICS

Rehabilitative Management of Common Problems

Second Edition

Trudy Sandler Goldstein, PT

Founder and Director
Quality Educational Seminars for Therapists
Burlington, Massachusetts

Senior Therapist
Millbrook Physical Therapy
Arlington, Massachusetts

Formerly, Clinical Supervisor
New England Rehabilitation Hospital
Woburn, Massachusetts

AN ASPEN PUBLICATION®
Aspen Publishers, Inc.
Gaithersburg, Maryland
1999

The author has made every effort to ensure the accuracy of the information herein. However, appropriate information sources should be consulted, especially for new or unfamiliar procedures. It is the responsibility of every practitioner to evaluate the appropriateness of a particular opinion in the context of actual clinical situations and with due considerations to new developments. The author, editors, and the publisher cannot be held responsible for any typographical or other errors found in this book.

Library of Congress Cataloging-in-Publication Data

Goldstein, Trudy Sandler.
Geriatric orthopaedics : rehabilitative management of common problems / Trudy Sandler Goldstein.—2nd ed.
p.   cm.
Includes bibliographical references and index.
ISBN 0-8342-1076-2
1. Geriatric orthopedics.   2. Joints—Diseases—Treatment.   3. Physical therapy for the aged.   I. Title.   [DNLM: 1. Joint
Diseases—in old age.   2. Joint Diseases—rehabilitation.   3. Orthopedics—in old age.   WE 304 G624g   1999]
RD732.3.A44G64   1999
618.97′758—dc21
DNLM/DLC
for Library of Congress
98-46715
CIP

Orders: (800) 638-8437
Customer Service: (800) 234-1660

About Aspen Publishers • For more than 35 years, Aspen has been a leading professional publisher in a variety of disciplines. Aspen's vast information resources are available in both print and electronic formats. We are committed to providing the highest quality information available in the most appropriate format for our customers. Visit Aspen's Internet site for more information resources, directories, articles, and a searchable version of Aspen's full catalog, including the most recent publications: **http://www.aspenpublishers.com**
Aspen Publishers, Inc. • The hallmark of quality in publishing
Member of the worldwide Wolters Kluwer group.

Editorial Services: Ruth Bloom
Library of Congress Catalog Card Number: 98-46715
ISBN: 0-8342-1076-2

Printed in the United States of America
1 2 3 4 5

I dedicate this book with love to my parents,

Hyman and Lillian Sandler.

They have taught me to reach beyond the ordinary in order to transform dreams into reality.

This book would not have been possible without their love and support.

Contributor

Jerline Carey, BA, PT
Assistant Professor
Physical Therapy Program
College of St. Scholastica
Duluth, Minnesota

Illustrations by

Mary Fantasia Nuovo, BFA
Woburn, Massachusetts

Table of Contents

Preface to the Second Edition

The fields of geriatrics and orthopaedics continue to gain in importance at the turn of the century. Fractures in the elderly are at epidemic proportions, and rising! Expectations of an improved quality of life in the healthy elderly have fueled a grassroots demand for arthroplasties to replace worn and painful joints. Although there is an increased need for rehabilitation therapy in both the well and frail older populations, there are limited health care dollars with which to pay for the increased services required. This has forced the medical community to accelerate the rehabilitation process in order to "cut costs."

This new edition has been written to help the therapist provide more efficient services while maintaining quality care. All chapters have been updated to include the newest information available. In the treatment chapters, common surgical procedures have been described in greater detail. Soft tissue problems and their rehabilitation have been added. The exercise programs have been changed to reflect current ideas on treatment as well as the need for accelerated recovery time. Many new illustrations, photographs, and tables have been added to augment the text. A "documentation tips" section is now included in all treatment chapters. Although we all despise doing the paperwork, in the end, good documentation will foster improved patient care and will help prove that therapy restores function to our patients. Lastly, a new chapter has been added: Balance Intervention for the Orthopaedic Patient. This chapter provides insight into balance mechanisms and disorders and should give the geriatric therapist the tools to *prevent* some of the devastating falls seen in the elderly population.

Although more topics are covered in greater detail, the text maintains the style of the original edition by emphasizing practical and functional treatment solutions for geriatric patients with orthopaedic problems. The concise format allows the experienced clinician to access treatment ideas quickly for specific problems on a case-by-case basis, while the student and entry-level clinician can find a wealth of information on the aging process, general orthopaedics, and treatment protocols.

Preface

The specialty fields of orthopaedics and geriatrics have grown in importance and popularity over the past 10 years. Many therapy books have been written on orthopaedics that emphasize the problems commonly seen in athletes and adults. This book, however, deals exclusively with the clinical management of the most common orthopaedic problems occurring in the elderly population. The exercise suggestions are based on sound orthopaedic principles and should be used as frameworks for the development of individualized programs. For convenience, I have categorized the problems by joint involvement. A brief anatomical and biomechanical review of each joint is presented in an accompanying chapter. I have also included separately a chapter on the effects of aging, hypokinetics, and disease on the rehabilitation process and a chapter on the principles of the evaluation and treatment of the elderly patient. Each chapter or subject matter can be read independently of the rest of the book.

I have written this book for physical and occupational therapists, assistants, and students who wish to better understand and treat the musculoskeletal problems facing the elderly patient. The student or entry-level clinician can find a wealth of information on the basics of treating general orthopaedic problems in the elderly, while the experienced clinician can refer to this book as problems arise on a case-by-case basis.

I hope that by reading this book you will come to understand and perhaps share my treatment philosophies. Regardless of age, our patients can return to productive lifestyles.

Acknowledgments

I would like to thank my entire family for tolerating my absence while I was burrowed away in "my cave" writing this book, and for encouraging me to complete it. Special thanks go to my father and mother, Hyman and Lillian Sandler, for volunteering to be my models, and to my husband, Alan Goldstein, for taking many of the photographs in the book. Particular thanks go to Mary Fantasia Nuovo, who once again magically transformed my stick figures into wonderful illustrations. I am also grateful to Jeri Carey, PT, who did a fantastic job of summarizing the massive field of balance and fall prevention and of explaining it in clinical terms usable to therapists. I would also like to thank all the people at Aspen Publishers, Inc., who made my job easier and who literally made this book possible.

Trudy Sandler Goldstein

1

The Aging Human

The human body is a remarkable biological machine, and the human mind is a spectacular control center. The human spirit defies description. Together they comprise a living person with the ability to grow in multiple dimensions. Cells mature, horizons expand, dreams are imagined. Together the components of a living person continue to grow until finally they grow old.

Gerontologists have been investigating this phenomenon since man could reason. The mysteries of the aging process are slowly being unraveled, but the work is far from finished. Some known aspects of normal aging are presented here in the hope of helping physical and occupational therapists better treat a growing segment of our population—the elderly. After the year 2010, the first of the Baby Boomer generation will enroll in the ranks of the elderly. By the year 2050, the Bureau of the Census projects that there will be 67 million elderly persons (21.7% of the population) living in the United States.[1(p11)]

THEORIES ON AGING

Why we age is an age-old question to which there is no simple answer. The results of experiments conducted over the years have suggested differing and often contradictory reasons for aging. At present there appears to be no doubt that genetic factors as well as environmental factors play a role. Changes in the immune and endocrine systems may also contribute.[2(pp23,24)]

Waneen Spiraduso, a renowned gerontologist, groups the many aging theories into three main categories: genetic, damage, and gradual imbalance.[3(p17)] The genetic theories have in common the belief that the process of aging is programmed into our genes and include Miguel's theory that DNA mutations of mitochondria build up in cells,[4(pp99–117)] as well as Hayflick's study proving that cells can divide only a limited number of times.[5]

Underlying the damage theories are two concepts: normally occurring chemical reactions in the body begin to produce irreversible deficits in the tissues, and cross-linking occurs in the DNA helix itself. Included in this category is the free-radical theory. A free radical contains an unpaired electron in its outer orbit that can link to other tissues causing damage.[6(pp298–311)]

The gradual imbalance theories are based on the observations that the immune system slowly loses the ability to distinguish foreign antigens from normal body tissues and that the neuroendocrine system slowly fails to function.[3(p20)] Although these theories may be complementary in nature, some gerontologists believe that the concurrence of multiple processes of aging, each under independent control, seems improbable.[7(p1259)] Continued research is needed to resolve this mystery.

Of more immediate concern to the clinician is the recognition that aging varies considerably from individual to individual. There are many elderly persons who simply do not "act" their age or "look" their age. Conversely, there are many middle-aged persons who "act" or "look" old. To help the therapist with treatment planning, many references to chronological age are made in this book; however, the treatment plan must reflect the individual needs of the patient and must not be based solely on the patient's age.

The therapist must also be able to differentiate between dysfunction caused by the normal aging process and that caused by disease or hypokinetics (i.e., decreased activity level). In this chapter the effects of normal aging, hypokinetics, and exercise on the systems of the human body and the resultant effects on function in the elderly are examined. Some common diseases (e.g., arthritis and osteoporosis) and their implications are discussed in later chapters.

EFFECTS OF NORMAL AGING ON HUMAN BODY SYSTEMS

A brief review of some of the major changes in the musculoskeletal, nervous, and cardiopulmonary systems is provided to help the therapist better understand the effects of aging.

The Musculoskeletal System

With aging, there are a number of morphological changes in skeletal muscle. The amount of muscle cytoplasm decreases, while the amounts of connective tissue and fat cells within the muscle increase. The actual number and size of muscle fibers also decrease—mostly in the fast-twitch type II fibers. (The apparent selective loss of type II fibers is still a matter of controversy for both researchers and gerontologists, and requires further study.) There is an increase in the number of obliquely oriented myofibrils, as well as a loss of mitochondrial activity.[8(pp9,20),9(p41)] There is also a loss of the muscle's ability to contract forcibly, owing to a lack of potassium ions.[10(p14)] These declines in muscle function appear related to the decrease in the physical demands placed on the muscles by older persons and may not be inevitable.[11(p247)]

Studies have shown that ligaments and capsular structures lose tensile strength and stiffness. The reasons for these changes remain unknown, but may involve loss of tissue nutrition and changes in cellular matrix composition.[12(pp258–260)]

Articular cartilage also shows changes with maturation with a thinning of cartilage and decrease in cell number. The ability of cartilage to distribute loads efficiently is diminished by a loss of density of the water-binding proteoglycans (chondroitin sulfate) in the cartilage matrix. In addition, older cartilage contains more large-diameter collagen fibrils with an increased number of intermolecular cross-links. The increased rigidity of collagen with decreased water content in the matrix may limit aged cartilage from deforming optimally, but does not seem to limit joint function.[13(pp264–266)]

In the skeletal system, age-related osteoporosis (type II involutional) is characterized by a gradual decrease in density of both trabecular and cortical bone. There is decreased osteoblast activity, which results in decreased formation of new bone. This condition is twice as prevalent in elderly women as in elderly men and can lead to fractures of the vertebrae, humerus, tibia, and femur.[14(pp216,217)] Wedge fractures of the vertebrae, common with this type of osteoporosis, cause the characteristic stooped posture of the elderly. Postmenopausal osteoporosis (type I involutional) is discussed further in Chapter 10.

The Nervous System

With aging, some brain cells atrophy or die with a resultant loss of brain mass. However, there is no relentless deterioration of the cerebral cortex with age.[2(p26)] Nerve conduction velocity decreases by 0.4% per year after approximately 20 years of age, and the conduction of an impulse across a synapse takes longer to occur. There are also decreases in reflex response, reaction time, sensory activities (including the special senses), and alpha waves.[9(p43),15(p71)] There is a mild loss of memory, but intelligence remains the same.[16(pp5,6)]

The Cardiopulmonary System

As the heart ages, it becomes enlarged and functions with less efficiency. Cardiac output decreases from approximately 5 L/min at 20 years of age to 3.5 L/min at 75 years of age. Cardiac reserve also decreases.[9(p42)] Resting heart rate remains the same, but the maximal heart rate achievable declines linearly with age.[17(p45)] Systolic blood pressure rises 10% to 15% and diastolic blood pressure rises 5% to 10%. Hypertensive values in the elderly are considered to be in the range of 160/100 mm Hg and over.[18(pp25–26)] Despite these changes, the National Institute on Aging reports that most heart problems in the elderly are due to disease, not to the normal aging process itself.[2(p26)]

In the respiratory system, the old elderly (over 75 years of age) can suffer a 50% reduction in maximal voluntary ventilation, reflecting an increase in residual volume, or dead space. There is also decreased elasticity in the lung tissue and a loss of alveolar surface area for gas exchange. This results in an increased energy expenditure by the body for the basic survival function of breathing. These changes in the cardiopulmonary system with age reduce the elderly person's tolerance to stress[9(p42)] (Irwin S. 1988. Unpublished lecture notes.)

Other Systems

The aging process affects the entire body. Briefly stated, some of the other changes that occur are

- increased cross-links in collagen macromolecules
- decreased elasticity of the dermis
- decreased ability of lymphocytes to kill tumor cells
- decreased efficiency of neutrophils in combating infection
- decreased regulation of the secretion of hormones
- decreased regulation of body temperature
- decreased efficiency of the renal system[2(pp23–25)]

EFFECTS OF AGING ON FUNCTION

The changes that occur separately in each of the body's systems with age react in different combinations to produce various losses in function in the elderly person. Seemingly small changes can result in major functional loss, whereas an apparently large change can be compensated for by another system. The effects of aging vary so greatly from individual to individual that one elderly person can continue to run marathons while another of the same chronological age is institutionalized.

Strength and Endurance

Isometric strength and dynamic strength increase in humans up to the age of 30 years, stay the same up to the age of 50 years, and then begin to decline. This age-related decline in strength is widely reported to be between 16.5% and 37%. There is a greater loss of strength in the lower extremities (LEs) and trunk. In the LEs, the loss of strength is greater proximally than distally and is not accompanied by a reduction in girth, perhaps because fat cells replace the atrophied muscle cells.[19(p2)]

Declining strength is attributed in part to the following factors:

- decreased amount of excitable muscle tissue
- increased fat and connective tissue within the muscles
- hormonal changes
- decreased number of neurons
- altered neurotransmissions
- diminished capacity of the cardiopulmonary system to deliver the raw materials required.[10(p14),19(p2),20(pp61,62)]

Endurance does not diminish as dramatically as strength in the elderly. Slow-twitch type I fibers remain steady in number, probably because they are stimulated more often— even in sedentary individuals.

Flexibility

Increased joint stiffness and loss of normal range of motion (ROM) are common complaints in the elderly population. This loss of flexibility is thought to be caused by the changes in collagen that occur with normal aging.[10(p12)] Age-related joint stiffness has been documented in the ankles, knees, fingers, and spine.[21(p374),22(pM17)]

At present there are no normal ROM values specifically for the elderly population. The normative data found in the Handbook of the American Academy of Orthopaedic Surgeons (AAOS) differ from those in a 1984 study by Walker et al[23(pp921,922)] on the elderly person's ROM (Table 1–1). These ROM values for the elderly are provided in later chapters to show the general motions available by joint. Until true normative data for ROM in the elderly are established, this information along with AAOS normative ROM for the general population can be used in combination to set reasonable treatment goals for the elderly patient. In general, the therapist can expect to find decreased ROM in the geriatric population, but aging alone may not be responsible for the losses found.

Balance

The ability to maintain one's center of gravity over the base of support diminishes with age. Balancing requires the integration of data from different sensory systems: visual, exteroceptive, vestibular, and proprioceptive.[15(p73)] The age-related changes that contribute to the elderly person's loss of balance include:

- decreased proprioception in the feet
- increased lateral postural sway (greater in women than in men)
- decreased vibratory sensation in the distal LEs
- decreased visual acuity
- increased reaction time
- decreased strength
- decreased ROM

Table 1–1 Comparison of Sample Mean Values with American Academy of Orthopaedic Surgeons (AAOS) Handbook Values Where the Difference Exceeded 1 SD and Intertester Error

Motion	Present Study $\overline{X}$	s	AAOS Average	Difference(°)
Sexes combined				
Hip				
Abduction	23	7	48	−25
Adduction	14	5	31	−17
Medial rotation	29	10	45	−16
Lateral rotation	31	7	45	−14
Ankle plantar flexion	34	8	48	−14
First metatarsophalangeal flexion	6	8	37	−31
Men only				
Shoulder extension	38	11	53	−19
Wrist extension	61	6	71	−10
Women only				
Shoulder flexion	169	9	158	+11
Radioulnar supination	65	11	84	−19

Source: Reprinted from J.M. Walker, D. Sue, N. Miles-Elkovsy, G. Ford, and H. Trevelyan, *Physical Therapy*, Alexandria, Virginia, American Physical Therapy Association, 1984, Vol. 64, No. 6, p. 922, with permission of the American Physical Therapy Association.

Bohannon et al[24(pp1068,1069)] found that healthy elderly persons can maintain bilateral standing balance for 30 seconds with eyes open or closed. The tendency to sway or fall when the eyes are closed and the feet are approximated (Romberg sign) is therefore an abnormal state in persons aged 79 years and younger. Panzer et al[25(pp156,157)] also found no postural instability in older subjects in quiet standing, despite an increased variability in the displacement of their centers of gravity. Apparently, older persons adopt a postural control strategy that provides a comparable stability to younger subjects during quiet standing.

During more advanced balancing activities, Bohannon et al found that elderly persons aged 60 to 69 years maintained one-legged standing balance for an average of 22.5 seconds with eyes open and for an average of 10.2 seconds with eyes closed. Older persons (aged 70 to 79 years) maintained their balance for 14.2 seconds with eyes open and for 4.3 seconds with eyes closed.[24(pp1068,1069)]

Chapter 17 provides more information on balance and fall prevention.

Gait

Ambulation is usually an automatic activity requiring minimal energy expenditure. However, the mechanics of normal walking are so complex that any change in the musculoskeletal or cardiopulmonary system can drastically affect the quality of ambulation.

A healthy elderly person may display the following gait deviations as compared with a younger person of the same body type and leg length (Table 1–2):

- smaller step length
- smaller stride length
- slower ambulation velocity
- decreased ankle motion[26(ppl385,1386)]

Although the gait patterns of elderly persons are significantly different from those of younger persons, they do not necessarily limit everyday function. Many researchers have studied the changes in gait speed associated with aging.[26(p1385),27(pp163–165),28(p88)] Healthy women over age 65 walked at a velocity ranging from 175 to 260 ft/min, whereas younger women 20 to 64 years old walked at a slightly higher velocity of 244 to 270 ft/min. Men generally walked an additional 10 to 20 ft/min than women at comparable ages. Most of these walking speeds are over the 208 ft/min speed required to safely cross a large city street.[29(p1373)] During free walking, a healthy older woman will take only 2 minutes more to walk a mile than her 20-year-old counterpart.

Activities of Daily Living

The human body requires complex interactions of its systems to achieve movement and to survive. Losses of strength, ROM, cardiopulmonary function, coordination, or balance can greatly affect the elderly person's ability to perform activities of daily living (ADL). In a survey by the National Institute on Aging, more than 90% of the elderly performed their ADL independently or with minimal assistance. Table 1–3 shows the percentage of the elderly population that was unable to perform selected ADL tasks without help. Most of the participants in the survey had more difficulty with activities involving the LEs than with those involving the upper extremities (UEs).[30(pp56,57)]

Sexual function also changes with aging due to reduction in the hormones testosterone, estrogen, and progesterone. The vaginal wall thickens and loses elasticity and lubrication. The sexual organs of both sexes get smaller. Both sexes also take longer to become excited and have shorter orgasms.[31(p13)]

Table 1–2 Comparison of Gait Characteristics Measured from the Side-View Camera

Variable	Elderly Women (n = 13)		Young Women (n = 13)		
	$\overline{X}$	s	$\overline{X}$	s	t*
Step length (cm)	66.34	6.77	80.68	5.43	7.10[†]
Stride length (cm)	134.92	14.71	162.70	10.84	6.47[†]
Ankle range of motion (°)	24.62	4.61	31.31	5.22	–3.93[†]
Velocity (cm/s)	131.94	23.85	153.53	16.39	–4.90[†]
Vertical center-of-gravity excursion (cm)	2.87	1.34	3.51	1.77	–1.33

*df = 12.
†P <.01.

Source: Reprinted from P. Hageman and D.J. Blanke, *Physical Therapy*, Alexandria, Virginia, American Physical Therapy Association, 1986, Vol. 66, No. 9, p.1385, with permission of the American Physical Therapy Association.

Table 1–3 Percentage of Elderly Population Unable To Perform Activities of Daily Living Tasks

Activity of Daily Living	Percentage of Elderly Population Unable To Perform Task without Help
Heavy housework	38.0%
Walk ½ mile	23.8%
Push/pull large objects	15.0%
Stoop, crouch, or kneel	12.2%
Negotiate stairs	12.1%
Walk (under ½ mile)	9.3%
Bath/shower	8.6%
Dress	5.6%
Transfer (bed-to-chair)	5.1%
Toilet	3.7%
Groom	2.7%
Eat	2.0%

Source: Reprinted from *Established Populations for Epidemiologic Studies of the Elderly*, National Institute on Aging, U.S. Department of Health and Human Services.

EFFECTS OF HYPOKINETICS

Hypokinetics, or decreased activity, is a frequent characteristic of the elderly. Whether originally caused by an injury, a fall, or increased fatigue, an elderly person begins to "slow down." A vicious cycle ensues that affects all systems of the body and eventually results in loss of function and possible injury.

The Musculoskeletal System

During any immobilization (e.g., for fracture healing or for bed rest), selective atrophy of the slow-twitch type I muscle fibers begins immediately.[19(p9)] Complete immobilization results in a 2% to 3% loss of strength per day.[9(p44)] Flexor muscles kept in shortened positions for long periods of time (as in sitting) develop collagenous adhesions more easily, resulting in loss of extensor ROM,[10(p12)] which has detrimental effects on posture and balance control.

Complete unloading of bone resulting from bed rest or weightlessness induces the most rapid loss of bone mass.[32(p25)] Months or years may be required for complete restitution of bone mass.[33(pp22–23)] The loss of normal activity also causes demineralization of bone, which can lead to vertebral fractures and changes in posture (Figure 1–1).

The Cardiopulmonary System

When the activity level of a person decreases, the metabolic requirements of the body remain the same or decline. The cardiovascular system efficiently responds by decreasing its functional output; however, over time the system loses the ability to increase its output when stressed.[18(p25)]

Other adverse effects of hypokinetics on the cardiopulmonary system include:

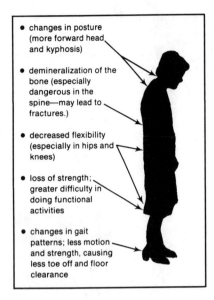

- changes in posture (more forward head and kyphosis)

- demineralization of the bone (especially dangerous in the spine—may lead to fractures.)

- decreased flexibility (especially in hips and knees)

- loss of strength; greater difficulty in doing functional activities

- changes in gait patterns; less motion and strength, causing less toe off and floor clearance

Figure 1–1 Hypokinetic changes in the older person. *Source:* Reprinted from C.B. Lewis, *Clinical Management in Physical Therapy* Alexandria, Virginia, American Physical Therapy Association, 1984, Vol. 4, No. 4, p. 12, with permission of the American Physical Therapy Association.

- thrombus formation
- edema
- hydrostatic pneumonia
- slower and more shallow respirations
  34(p12),3(p112)

Diminished cardiopulmonary function has a direct impact on the body's capacity to maintain homeostasis. The body is less able to respond to environmental and internal stresses, and endurance for functional activities—even walking—is compromised.

NORMAL AGING, HYPOKINETICS, AND DISEASE

Many of the symptoms of old age are really due to a combination of normal aging, disuse, and accumulated disease processes.

Present research cannot yet determine exactly which age-related changes are caused only by physiological aging. It is becoming clearer that many of the changes originally thought of as inevitable are in actuality quite preventable. One thing is certain: disuse exacerbates the changes that occur during the aging process. Disease further complicates the picture.

An elderly man who fractures his hip develops muscle atrophy of both type I and type II fibers, with resultant loss of strength and endurance. If he is a smoker or has heart disease, his cardiopulmonary system will be taxed during minimal exertions. Any other neurological or metabolic diseases further complicate his ability to survive. Even the pharmaceuticals prescribed to control his pain or regulate his metabolism can make him more tired or even confused. How does the geriatrician treat this "typical" patient?

EFFECTS OF EXERCISE IN THE ELDERLY

The body as a biological entity continues to change in response to stress, even as it ages. The supporters of activity and exercise have long espoused the virtues of "doing." Research has confirmed the positive impact of exercise on the musculoskeletal, nervous, and cardiopulmonary systems for all ages.

Theoretically, exercising should affect only the bodily changes that occur as a result of injury, disuse, or disease. The changes that occur strictly as a result of physiological aging should, by definition, be irreversible.

Musculoskeletal Changes

During resistive exercise training, older subjects gain strength at a rate equal to or higher than that of younger subjects. Studies involving low-intensity strength training in older adults show strength increases of 20% and less, while high-intensity strength training can result in strength increases over 200%.[20(p63)] There is reversal of muscle atrophy (mostly in fast-twitch fibers) and an increased ability to recruit motor units. In a yearlong study, Cress found an increase in the myofibrils of the vastus lateralis muscles of a 65–83-year-old female exercise group that correlated with a 48% increase in muscle strength, as well as increased ability to climb stairs.[35(pp4,9)] Since there is insufficient muscle hypertrophy to cause such a marked increase in static and dynamic strength, there must also be a significant neural factor involved in strength acquisition in the elderly.[19(pp5–8)] Strength gains from participation in an exercise training program appear to last for at least 5 weeks before slowly reverting to old norms.[36(p209),37(p311)]

Gentle, active exercise can decrease complaints of joint stiffness and improve ROM. Exercise that causes repetitive loading of ligaments and joint capsules up to a critical level increases cell synthetic function and matrix organization, thereby increasing ligament strength. If the exercises are too demanding, they will cause an overuse syndrome with tissue degradation.[12(pp256,257)]

Exercise can also be beneficial to articular cartilage. Intermittent loading improves chondrocyte nutrition; however, static loading has a negative effect on the cartilage matrix. Moderate joint use seems to increase chondrocyte metabolism and proteoglycan synthesis.[13(pp269,270)] More research is needed to determine the exact type of exercise that promotes cartilage health rather than causes cartilage destruction, which leads to osteoarthritis.

Weight-bearing and high-intensity exercises result in maintained or increased bone mass in most postmenopausal women.[32(p32),38(pp1911–1913)] However, the exercises must be specific to the bone site. For example, walking or standing exercises may improve the bone density of the femur, but they will have no effect on the UEs.

Cardiopulmonary Changes

Improved aerobic capacity and increased oxygen transport result from exercising. Other changes in the cardiopulmonary system that result from exercising include the following:

- decreased resting and exercise heart rates
- decreased systolic blood pressure
- increased VO_2 max
- increased cardiopulmonary efficiency[3(p117),39(p205)]

Immunity Changes

Theoretically, moderate exercise should have a beneficial effect on the immune system by increasing endocrine hormone production and enhancing the resting natural killer cells. There is even some evidence that circulating T cell function is better maintained in the elderly who exercise.[40(p42)] However, the exact amount of exercise that is beneficial has not yet been determined. A study by Rincon et al on exercise and the frail elderly shows decreased activity of the natural killer cells with only mild overexertion.[41(p109)] Further research is needed in this area.

Functional Changes

Implementing an exercise program can reverse some of the above-mentioned physical impairments caused by aging, disuse, and disease. By initially improving strength, ROM, and balance, the patient will be better able to participate in functional training activities such as developmental sequence, tub and toilet transfers, reaching and carrying, dressing and grooming, and gait training. By increasing cardiopulmonary function, endurance for ADL tasks can be achieved. Most studies on exercise training in the elderly support the hypothesis that increasing strength and endurance will cause an improvement in functional ability, including gait.[42(ppM161–M168),43(pp568–572),44(pp648–652),45(pp46–57)] Therefore, exercise and increased activity levels can reduce some of the functional limitations seen in the elderly population.

SUMMARY

- Aging varies considerably from individual to individual.
- Three categories of theories on aging include
  1. genetic
  2. damage
  3. gradual imbalance

- Some of the effects of normal aging include
  1. decreased strength
  2. osteoporosis (type II involutional)
  3. loss of flexibility
  4. decreased balance
  5. altered gait pattern
  6. decreased efficiency of cardiopulmonary, immune, and endocrine systems
- Some of the effects of disuse (hypokinetics) include
  1. decreased strength with selective atrophy of slow-twitch muscle fibers
  2. demineralization of bone
  3. loss of flexibility
  4. diminished cardiopulmonary function
- Some of the effects of exercise include
  1. increased strength
  2. increased flexibility
  3. maintained or increased bone mass
  4. improved cardiopulmonary function
  5. improved mobility and function

REFERENCES

1. Brock DB, Wineland T, Freeman DH, et al. Demographic characteristics. In: Established Populations for Epidemiologic Studies of the Elderly. Bethesda, MD: National Institute on Aging. US Dept of Health and Human Services; 1986:11–32. NIH publication 86-2443.

2. Bethesda, MD: National Institute on Aging. US Dept of Health and Human Services; July 1983:23–24. NIH publication 83-1129.

3. Spiraduso W. Physical Dimensions of Aging. Champaign, IL: Human Kinetics; 1995.

4. Miguel J. An integrated theory of aging as the result of mitochondrial-DNA mutation in differentiated cells. Arch Gerontol and Geriatr. 1991;12:99–117.

5. Hayflick L. The cellular basis for biological aging. In: Fitch CE, Hayflick L, eds. The Handbook of the Biology of Aging. New York: Van Nostrand Reinhold; 1977.

6. Harmon D. Aging: A theory based on free radical and radiation chemistry. J Gerontol. 1956;11:298–311.

7. Miller RA. When will the biology of aging become useful? Future landmarks in biomedical gerontology. J Amer Geriatr Soc. 1997;45:1258–1267.

8. Kauffman T. Skeletal muscle and the aging process: Implications for physical therapy. Clin Manage Phys Ther. January–February 1986;6:18–21.

9. Payton OD, Poland JL. Aging process implications for clinical practice. Phys Ther. January 1983; 63:41–47.

10. Lewis CB. Musculoskeletal changes with age. Clin Manage Phys Ther. September–October 1984; 4:12–15.

11. Kirkendall DT, Garrett WE. Effects of aging and physical training on skeletal muscle. Sports Med and Arthroscopy Rev. 1996;4(3):243–249.

12. Buckwalter JA, Woo SL. Age-related changes in ligament and joint capsules: Implications for participa-

tion in sports. *Sports Med and Arthoscopy Rev.* 1996; 4(3):250–262.

13. Martin JA, Buckwalter JA. Articular cartilage aging and degeneration. *Sports Med and Arthroscopy Rev.* 1996;4(3):263–275.

14. Netter FH. *The CIBA Collection of Medical Illustrations. The Musculoskeletal System, Part 1.* Summit, NJ: CIBA-GEIGY Corp. 1987;8:195–239.

15. Brown M. Selected physical performance changes with aging. *Top Geriatr Rehabil.* July 1987; 2:68–76.

16. Felsenthal G, Garrison SJ, Steinberg FU, eds. *Rehabilitation of the Aging and Elderly Patient.* Baltimore: Williams & Wilkins; 1994.

17. Lewis CB, Bottomley JM, eds. *Geriatric Physical Therapy: A Clinical Approach.* Norwalk, CT: Appleton & Lange; 1994.

18. Lewis CB. Effects of aging on the cardiovascular system. *Clin Manage Phys Ther.* July–August 1984;4:24–29.

19. Knortz KA. Muscle physiology applied to geriatric rehabilitation. *Top Geriatr Rehabil.* July 1987; 2:1–9.

20. Porter MM, Vandervoort AA. High-intensity strength training for the older adult: A review. *Top Geriatr Rehabil.* March 1995;10(3):61–74.

21. Einkauf DK, Gohdes ML, Jensen GM, et al. Changes in spinal mobility with increasing age in women. *Phys Ther.* 1989;67:370–375.

22. Vandervoort AA, et al. Age and sex effects on mobility of the human ankle. *J Geront. (Med Sci.)* 1992;47:M17–M21.

23. Walker JM, Sue D, Miles-Elkovsy N, et al. Active mobility of the extremities in older subjects. *Phys Ther.* June 1984;64:919–923.

24. Bohannon RW, Larkin PA, Cook AC, et al. Decrease in timed balance test scores with aging. *Phys Ther.* July 1984;64:1067–1070.

25. Panzer VP, Bandinelli S, Hallett M. Biomechanical assessment of quiet standing and changes associated with aging. *Arch Phys Med Rehabil.* 1995; 76(2):151–157.

26. Hageman P, Blanke DJ. Comparison of gait of young women and elderly women. *Phys Ther.* September 1986;66:1382–1387.

27. Himann JE, Cunningham DA, Rechnitzer PA, et al. Age-related changes in speed of walking. *Med Sci Sports Exerc.* 1988;20:161–166.

28. Bohannon RW, Andrews AW, Thomas MW.

Walking speed: Reference values and correlates for older adults. *J Orthop Sports Phys Ther.* 1996;24(2): 86–90.

29. Robinett CS, Vondran MA. Functional ambulation velocity and distance requirements in rural and urban communities. *Phys Ther.* 1988;68(9):1371–1373.

30. Foley DJ, Berkman LF, Branch LG. Physical functioning. In: *Established Populations for Epidemiologic Studies of the Elderly.* Bethesda, MD: National Institute on Aging. US Dept of Health and Human Services; 1986:56–94. NIH publication 86-2443.

31. Zeiss AM. Sexuality and aging: Normal changes and clinical problems. *Top Geriatr Rehabil.* 1997; 12(4):11–27.

32. Martin AD, Brown E. The effect of physical activity on the human skeleton. *Top Geriatr Rehabil.* January 1989;4:25–35.

33. Lanyon LE. Strain-related bone modeling and remodeling. *Top Geriatr Rehabil.* January 1989;4:13–23.

34. Lewis CB. What's so different about rehabilitating the older person? *Clin Manage Phys Ther.* May–June 1984;4:10–15.

35. Cress ME. Functional training: Muscle structure, function, and performance in older women. *J Orthop Sports Phys Ther.* 1996;24(1):4–10.

36. Sforzo GA, McManis BG, Black D. Resilience to exercise detraining in healthy older adults. *J Amer Geriatr Soc.* 1995;43(3):209–215.

37. Taafe DR, Marcus R. Dynamic muscle strength alterations to detraining and retraining in elderly men. *Clin Physiol.* 1997;17(3):311–324.

38. Nelson ME, Fiatrone MA, Morganti CM. Effects of high-intensity strength training on multiple risk factors for osteoporotic fractures: A randomized controlled trial. *JAMA.* 1994;272(24):1909–1914.

39. Brown M, Kohrt WM. Endurance training of the older adult. In: *Geriatric Physical Therapy,* Guccione AA, ed. St. Louis, MO: Mosby-Yearbook, Inc, 1993.

40. Venkatramen JT, Fernandes G. Exercise, immunity and aging. *Aging—Clin and Exper Res.* 1997; 9(1–2):42–56.

41. Rincon HG, Solomon GF, Benton D, et al. Exercise in frail elderly men decreases natural-killer-cell activity. *Aging—Clin and Exper Res.* 1996;8(2): 109–112.

42. Rooks DS, Kiel DP, Parsons C, Hayes WC. Self-paced resistance training and walking exercise in community-dwelling older adults: Effects on neuro-

motor performance. *J Gerontol. (Med Sci.)* 1997; 52(3):M161–M168.

43. Ades PA, Ballor DL, Ashikaga T, et al. Weight training improves walking endurance in healthy elderly persons. *Ann Intern Med.* 1996;124(6): 568–572.

44. Lord SR, Castell S, Dip RG. Physical activity program for older persons: Effect on balance, strength, neuromuscular control, and reaction time. *Arch Phys Med Rehabil.* 1994;75(6):648–652.

45. Shumway-Cook A, Gruber W, Baldwin M, Liao S. The effect of multidimensional exercises on balance, mobility, and fall risk in community-dwelling older adults. *Phys Ther.* 1997;77(1):46–57.

2

Evaluation and Treatment of the Geriatric Patient

The first step in the treatment of any patient is to perform a thorough evaluation to determine the patient's physical impairments and functional limitations and to determine the extent of the musculoskeletal injury or disease process. The second step is to enter into a partnership with the patient to determine common treatment goals. This step has also been called "establishing rapport." The third step is to create an individualized practical treatment program to achieve the rehabilitation goals.

THE EVALUATION

Without a comprehensive evaluation, the therapist cannot design an effective treatment plan for the patient. The examiner is akin to a murder mystery detective, who must seek out all possible leads and collect all available data. In the beginning the sleuth does not know which clue is irrelevant or is the key to solving the murder: neither does the examiner. But the evaluation must be comprehensive lest the key to solving the mystery of how best to treat the patient be lost because of sloppy detective work.

In the case of the elderly patient, a thorough evaluation usually takes several sessions to complete. The therapist must efficiently "work around" the patient's endurance level by assessing the most important areas first, such as mobility status. For example, a newly admitted patient is half asleep on a chair next to her bed. After introductions, the therapist can take her medical history and vital signs, assess sitting posture, and begin a partial assessment of her motion and strength. If she is agreeable, they can "go for a short walk," allowing the therapist to evaluate her sit-to-stand transfer as well as her ambulation ability. If she complains of extreme fatigue, the therapist can offer to help her into bed, thereby assessing her chair-to-bed transfer along with her bed mobility. Either way, the therapist has initiated the evaluation process while establishing a platform of trust for the next session. In general, the evaluation should include, but not necessarily be limited to, the following areas. (For more detailed information on how to perform the various assessments discussed, the reader is referred to the texts at the end of this chapter.)

Inspection

When the therapist and patient meet and introduce themselves, subconscious and conscious observations are made that create what are commonly called first impressions. During this informal session of getting to know one another, the therapist should observe the patient's normal posturing, body language, gait pattern, pain behavior, and general mobility status. This golden opportunity for casual observation is very brief. As soon as the therapist begins taking the patient's medical history, the patient cannot help changing his or her mannerisms. To detect any major discrepancies, the therapist must compare the patient's initial behavior with the behavior exhibited during the remainder of the evaluation procedure. In the younger patient, the therapist is often on the lookout for the "malingerer," the patient that is displaying worse symptoms than actually exist for secondary gain. In the geriatric patient, the exact opposite is often the case. Patient sometimes portray themselves as having higher function or symptoms than they really have.

Medical History

The therapist must obtain a detailed history from the patient even in the hospital setting, where the patient's medical record is readily available. Many examiners consider this to be the most important part of the total examination. With increasing time constraints, the therapist must resist the temptation to take only a cursory medical history of the patient.

Although the taking of a patient's medical history appears to be simply a matter of asking questions and getting answers, the reality of the situation is altogether different. There is a definite art to asking questions in a manner that does not bias the answers given. Perhaps an even greater art is the art of asking questions that force the patient to quantify vague answers. Some of the major areas addressed in the history are

- present complaint or symptoms
- onset of symptoms
- mechanism of injury
- past medical problems (e.g., old surgeries, allergies, illnesses, fractures)
- secondary diagnoses
- surgical corrections
- results of any medical tests (e.g., roentgenography, computed tomography scanning, magnetic resonance imaging)
- medications
- age
- occupation or avocation interests
- prior level of function

In many instances, the patient cannot provide the therapist with the information desired. This often happens in the home care or nursing home setting, where the patient may not even know the operative procedure performed to stabilize a fracture. When the hospital referral summary finally arrives, the home care therapist may find it full of useless information (strength and range of motion [ROM] measurements 3 weeks old) and lacking in vital information (type and location of fracture, type of internal fixation, weight-bearing orders, and exercise/weight-bearing precautions). The acute care therapist must include this necessary orthopaedic information in the referral or discharge summary in order to fill in the gaps in the patient's medical history. (See Documentation Tips.)

Cardiopulmonary Screening

Many elderly patients have compromised cardiopulmonary function due to normal aging, disuse, or disease. At a minimum, the therapist should take the patient's vital signs: heart rate, respiration rate, and blood pressure. The therapist should also be aware of any cardiopulmonary symptoms the patient may be experiencing, such as angina, light-headedness, or shortness of breath.

Posture

The therapist should assess the patient's normal posture for vertebral alignment (e.g., increased thoracic kyphosis, scoliosis) and peripheral joint alignment (e.g., anteriorly displaced humeral head, laterally displaced patella). Postural faults can be the cause or the result of muscle imbalances accumulated through the years. Both joint malalignment and muscle imbalance are major causes of impairments in the musculoskeletal, myofascial, and respiratory systems of the elderly patient.

Bony Palpation

The therapist should systematically check the integrity of the skeletal system by comparing the injured site with the (hopefully) uninvolved counterpart. The therapist feels for discrepancies between the two, such as tenderness, breaks in the continuity of the bone, formation of callus, deformities, and malalignment.

Soft Tissue Palpation

The therapist next should explore the various soft tissue structures for signs of damage. Again, the therapist attempts to ascertain normalcy for the patient through bilateral comparison. For example, many ligamentous insertions normally are quite tender when palpated. The patient must subjectively feel that one side is more painful than

the other for the therapist to suspect ligament damage. Some of the signs of injury to soft tissue structures include

- localized warm skin temperature
- tenderness or pain
- edema
- muscle atrophy
- muscle spasm
- loss of normal muscular contour or shape
- tender ligaments
- capsular thickening
- palpable bursa or synovium
- fascial restrictions

Range of Motion

The therapist evaluates normal ROM for two basic reasons: (1) to determine baseline data from which to prove patient progress and (2) to help differentially diagnose a mechanical problem. To establish a database, the therapist measures the patient's motion with a goniometer (bilaterally) and notes any pain associated with movement. Areas of hypomobility and hypermobility are noted. Unaffected areas are also investigated, but in a less precise manner.

To help discover the mechanical origin of the patient's problem, the therapist also needs to look for

- any differences in active versus passive ROM
- specific movements that are painful
- a painful arc
- a capsular pattern
- restricted accessory motion
- the type of end-feel present (e.g., bone-to-bone, capsular, empty)

Strength and Endurance

Strength and endurance can be assessed in a variety of ways, depending on the patient's individual needs. The manual muscle test is not as objective or as accurate as a dynamometer, but it is reliable, practical, and readily available. The therapist can also assess the uninvolved limbs quickly and easily with this method.

The therapist should also determine the ability of muscles to stabilize surrounding joints. Many postural muscles act to maintain joint integrity. The stability required to prevent motion in an unwanted direction is as important as the strength required to move the bones.

The therapist must also resist the muscles isometrically with the joint protected in neutral, not necessarily to assess strength per se, but to collect information on the integrity of the musculotendinous unit. In this instance, the therapist can determine whether an isometric contraction reproduces the patient's pain, which would implicate the muscle or tendon as the injured site.

Endurance can also be measured by many parameters. Depending on the individual situation, the therapist can measure exercise, sitting, walking, cardiovascular, and functional endurance levels.

Motor Control

The clinician needs to assess the quality of the patient's movement. Injuries, swelling, sensation loss, and muscle imbalances can contribute to alterations in muscle recruitment, disrupting optimal timing and coordination of movement. The therapist should determine if the patient's movement patterns are

- jerky
- nonfluid
- inefficient
- painful

Mobility Status

The therapist needs to evaluate the quality and level of dependence of the patient's mobility. This is one of the major areas of the therapist's expertise and should be addressed in detail. Among the mobility areas to assess are

- bed mobility: rolling, scooting, sit-to-supine, etc.
- wheelchair mobility: propelling, braking, etc.
- transfer: bed-to-chair, chair-to-toilet, wheelchair-to-car, etc.
- gait: device, distance, velocity, gait deviations, etc.
- advanced gait: uneven surfaces, stairs, sidestepping, etc.

Neurological Status

Because neurological function becomes impaired with age, it is important to screen the patient for dysfunctions that can affect the rehabilitation process. The therapist must also be alert to nerve findings that are not associated with normal aging, such as shooting pains, paresthesias, and tingling sensations. Depending on the individual, some of the neurological functions to be assessed are the patient's

- sensation
- proprioception
- reflexes
- neural tension
- tone
- balance (see Chapter 17)
- coordination

Specialty Tests

Because some orthopaedic injuries have similar signs and symptoms associated with them, different physicians have devised special tests to stress certain tissues selectively (e.g., Trendelenburg test for evaluating the strength of the gluteus medius). These special tests aid in the differential diagnosis and should be used by physician and therapist alike.

Functional Status

The therapist must also determine the patient's ability to perform life tasks to fulfill societal roles. The assessment should include the patient's ability to perform

- activities of daily living (ADL): grooming, eating, dressing, toileting, etc.
- instrumental ADL: shopping, driving, preparing meals, having sex, etc.
- work activities: pushing, pulling, carrying, lifting, manipulating objects, etc.
- recreation: walking, throwing, swimming, knitting, woodworking, etc.

Functional limitations can be determined by observing the patient perform simulated tasks or by having the patient do a self-report through a disability questionnaire. (A therapist observing a patient perform selected functional tasks does not necessarily provide a more accurate indication of the patient's actual functional level.)

Cognitive Status

Clearly, the patient's cognitive status is one of the most important factors considered in the planning of a treatment program. Although the therapist does not possess the expertise to diagnose any of the dementias that affect the elderly, the therapist can refer the patient to a specialist if cognitive impairment is suspected. After completing the physical assessment, the therapist should determine the patient's

- orientation to person, place, and time
- memory
- safety awareness
- judgment

Emotional Status

During the evaluation process, the therapist must be aware of the patient's emotional state. Once again, the clinician is not sufficiently trained in this area to evaluate it properly; yet how the patient feels has a profound effect on the ability to perform a rehabilitation program. As the mind controls the body, the human spirit powers the physical recovery. The therapist should assess whether the patient appears to be pleasant, cooperative, depressed, etc. Problems in this area must be referred to another team member, such as a psychiatrist, a psychologist, or a social worker, for resolution.

Other Considerations

To project long-term goals properly, the therapist must know the extent of the patient's family or community support. It is also important to know the structural layout of the patient's home, including the location of any bathrooms and bedrooms, the number of stairs, availability of guardrails, and the type of flooring. For a detailed, efficient home evaluation tool, the reader is referred to SAFE AT HOME (Securing a Functional Environment with the Anemaet-Trotter Home Observation and Modification Evaluation) in Appendix 1-A at the end of this chapter.

Patient Goals

The identification of the patient's priorities, desires, and long-term goals is of vital importance. The therapist should also know from the onset whether the patient personally wishes to attend therapy. Surprisingly few therapists formally request and obtain this crucial information.

Assessment

The therapist now analyzes all the numbers and words. Proficiencies, deficiencies, inconsistencies, and meaningful patterns should emerge from the data. Armed with this information, the therapist can determine the patient's problems (i.e., make a physical therapy or occupational therapy diagnosis), project the patient's potential, estimate the duration of treatment, and create an individualized plan of care based on specific long-term goals. Hopefully these goals are similar to the patient's own long-term goals.

THE PARTNERSHIP

After the evaluation is complete, the patient and the therapist enter into a working partnership. This unspoken contract imparts certain duties and responsibilities to both parties. The therapist creates a rehabilitation program to correct any physical impairment present and to help restore the patient to normal function. The therapist must also explain to the patient the rationale for the treatment, as well as how to do the exercises and activities. However, only the patient can actually perform the program. Therefore, the responsibility for the success of the rehabilitation program rests primarily with the patient.

In this era of managed care, the amount of therapy visits covered by insurance is limited. Faster discharges from the acute care hospital force patients into rehabilitation settings sooner. Some geriatric patients find it difficult to participate in the rigors of an intensive program in spite of the fact that the health care system expects them to become the leading players on the rehabilitation team. The therapist often becomes the patient's guide on the journey back to health, acting as both motivator and teacher. In a society where everyone looks for the quick fix, the therapist must encourage the patient to accept the challenge of working hard in order to return to normal function.

THE PROGRESSIVE EXERCISE PROGRAM

The importance of creating a specific, individual, and doable exercise program cannot be overemphasized. Without reasonable patient participation, the rehabilitation process will fail. Prescribing an exercise regimen is an art based on scientific principles. Along with an in-depth knowledge of anatomy, biomechanics, and the aging process, the therapist must also understand how the pathology or disorder affecting the patient resulted in the observed physical impairments and functional limitations. Of equal importance, the therapist must know the patient's goals, plans, priorities, and desires in order to individualize the exercise program. Only the most self-motivated patient will be able to successfully complete a rehabilitation program derived from a preprinted sheet of standardized exercises.

The progressive exercise program consists of three parts: the injury-specific program, the reconditioning program, and the home program. An important challenge facing the physical or occupational therapist is the creation of a dynamic exercise program that constantly changes as the patient improves.

The Injury-Specific Program

The type of injury, disease process, or surgery defines the actual exercises, precautions, and contraindications needed to implement the rehabilitation program. Initially the patient requires intensive therapist input and assistance with the basic exercise program. The therapist spends a lot of treatment time teaching and physically helping the patient learn these exercises. These core exercises, usually geared to the patient's greatest weaknesses, must be performed properly. The therapist must emphasize the quality, not the quantity, of the exercise program by ensuring that the desired muscle groups are being trained and that the patient is breathing correctly. The need for good oxygenation of tissues for healing is commonly overlooked in this population. Once the patient is independent in this basic exercise program, the responsibility for carrying it out rests with the patient.

New Activities in the Exercise Program

In the available "one-on-one" time, the therapist teaches and assists the patient in new areas. Each treatment session should include at least one different activity to offset the necessary but often tedious independent program. Depending on the therapist's creativity, this interaction with the patient can be fun as well as therapeutic. Unfortunately, the game playing and creativity associated with pediatric rehabilitation are all too often missing from geriatric programs. The elderly patient is considered too old to have fun during treatment sessions. The benefits of laughter and a good mental attitude during the healing process cannot be overstated. The therapist who incorporates different kinds of interesting exercises into the rehabilitation program rarely reports problems with patient motivation and compliance.

Consider the hypothetical case of a 75-year-old man whose stated goal is to return to golfing in 1 month. An excellent balance and coordination retraining program for him would include the sport skill of "putting" a golf ball in the therapy gym. The therapist could provide manual assistance for safety if needed. Upper extremity (UE) strengthening could be achieved by using one of his golf clubs as a dowel and attaching cuff weights to it. Although such modifications of an exercise program are minor, they can make a big difference in patient compliance.

If a patient is cognitively impaired, the therapist should intentionally prescribe a repetitive exercise program. Performing the same exercises in a specific sequence helps the patient with memory loss through the rehabilitation process. Of course, even an exercise program such as this must change to reflect improvements in the patient's physical status as well as cognitive status.

In following chapters, detailed rehabilitation guidelines for common injuries or diseases of the musculoskeletal system in the elderly patient are presented by joint involvement.

Intensity Level of the Exercise Program

If people were machines, the intensity level of the progressive exercise program would rely only on the nature of the injury to the mechanism, as well as its general condition. But people are people, and the human factor plays a large role in determining the frequency and duration of treatment sessions.

Exercises for the elderly generally should be performed with moderate intensity (light resistance), for short duration (low repetitions), and at high frequency (throughout the day). In reality, the intensity, duration, and frequency of treatment sessions correlate directly with these patients' premorbid lifestyles and general conditioning levels.

The Reconditioning Program

In addition to a specific exercise program to rehabilitate the injured or diseased site, the geriatric patient often requires a reconditioning program to offset the effects of prolonged bed rest or an inactive lifestyle. The patient evaluation should clearly reveal these cardiopulmonary and musculoskeletal impairments.

Cardiopulmonary Reconditioning

The therapist initially should instruct the geriatric patient in proper breathing techniques. Tactile cues help the patient learn to breathe diaphragmatically and to expand both lungs fully. The classic kyphotic and round-shouldered posture of the elderly patient physically impairs inhalation. The patient should be encouraged to sit up straight before practicing deep breathing. Combining the phases of respiration with bilateral elevation and depression of the UEs (e.g., as in chopping and lifting types of exercise, yoga, or Tai Chi) can open up the chest area to allow easier inspiration.

The exercise prescription to improve aerobic function in elderly patients is very similar to the prescription for younger adults. For the majority of patients, walking will have an aerobic training effect. Bicycle riding, dancing, and swimming are also excellent ways to improve cardiopulmonary functioning in the elderly. In addition, regular practice of Tai Chi has improved the cardiorespiratory function of older individuals.[1(p1222),2(p612)] Table 2–1 shows the cardiac training ranges for active and sedentary elderly patients.

Optimally, the patient should undergo a stress test before an aerobic program is initiated, but often this is not done. It is imperative to monitor the patient's response to both aerobic and general exercises. Carole Lewis has listed seven signs and interventions by which the therapist can monitor the cardiopulmonary condition of the elderly patient (Exhibit 2–1). In addition, the therapist must not allow the patient to exercise under temperature conditions that are too hot or too cold. The additional stress of maintaining homeostasis under severe weather conditions can be life threatening for the geriatric patient.

General Musculoskeletal Reconditioning

One efficient method of reconditioning uninvolved extremities is through the use of proprioceptive neuromuscular facilitation (PNF) techniques. With these hands-on tech-

Table 2–1 Aerobic Training Parameters for Active and Sedentary Elderly Patients

Aerobic Training Range	Active Elderly	Sedentary Elderly
Maximal heart rate*	60–80%	40–60%
Duration	20 min	10 min
Frequency	3× /wk	5× /wk
Training Period	14 wk	14 wk

*Maximal heart rate equals 220 beats per minute minus age.

Source: Data from Clinical Management in Physical Therapy Vol. 4, No. 4, p. 26, © 1984, American Physical Therapy Association.

Exhibit 2–1 Cardiac Warning Signs and Interventions

Monitoring Interventions

1. **Pulse rate.** Before beginning to exercise, the pulse rate should be 60–100 beats per minute. The pulse rate increases as work increases. If it decreases, *stop* the exercise. It is also *not* good to have large increases early in the exercise session.

2. **Blood pressure.** Systolic blood pressure increases with exercise. If measurement exceeds 225–230 mm Hg—*stop*. During lower extremity rhythmic exercise, diastolic blood pressure will change very little—if it increases more than 20 or increases suddenly, this may indicate the patient has exceeded cardiac reserve. If diastolic blood pressure increases over 130, the person may be shunting blood from organs. Also, blood pressure *should not drop* during exercise; this could indicate cardiac failure.

3. **Respiration.** Depth and rate increase with exercise. Breathing should not be labored. The patient should be able to speak.

4. **Skin.** The cheeks, nose, and earlobes should be pink and warm. If they are pale and cool, *stop* or *decrease* the exercise. There may be insufficient cardiac output.

5. **Fatigue.** This may be a result of depression, inactivity, or decreased sensory input. Exercise may help. Fatigue from exercise can be an indication that exercise should be decreased or stopped.

6. **Pain.** *Stop* if the person experiences pain in the chest, jaw, or upper extremity during exercise. These may be symptoms of myocardial ischemia.

7. **Coordination and equilibrium.** Decreases in coordination and equilibrium may be a sign of cerebral ischemia or hypoglycemia. *Stop* or decrease exercise.

Source: Reprinted from C.B. Lewis, *Clinical Management in Physical Therapy*, Alexandria, Virginia, American Physical Therapy Association, 1984, Vol. 4, No. 4, p. 29, with permission of the American Physical Therapy Association.

---

niques, the therapist can improve the patient's strength, endurance, ROM, or coordination in functional patterns. The patient can also be instructed in an independent PNF program with or without resistance.

For strength training, progressive resistive exercise can be initiated. High intensity resistive training has been well tolerated by the elderly.[3(pp69–71)] To help maintain function in the elderly, Judge has developed a moderate-to high-intensity training program performed three times per week, with emphasis on strengthening the following muscles:

- gluteus medius
- gluteus maximus
- hamstrings
- quadriceps femoris
- ankle dorsiflexors
- finger flexors
- biceps
- triceps
- muscles involved in combined shoulder/elbow motions.[4(pp45–48)]

Dumbbells, cuff weights, Theraband™, and rubber tubing can provide graded resistance as needed. An isotonic exercise program should emphasize eccentric (lengthening) as well as concentric (shortening) contractions. The program should include both open-chain and closed-chain (also called weight-bearing) exercises. Isokinetic exercise (e.g., with Kinetron or Cybex) is another efficient method of exercising that should not be denied the geriatric patient on the basis of age alone. The appropriate speed for isokinetic training the elderly is not yet known. However, initiating a training program at moderate velocities that are similar to the angular velocities for function (60° to 100°/s) makes intuitive sense.[4(p41)] Isometric training (e.g., with quadriceps sets or gluteal sets) can be effective as an adjunct to the isotonic or isokinetic program.

Stretching is an important component of the reconditioning program as many older patients have a loss of ROM of the spine and the joints of the lower extremity.[4(p45)] Prolonged static stretching, preceded by a heat modality, is often needed to restore flexibility, due to the changes in collagen that occur with aging.

Depending on the circumstances, bringing the elderly patient through the developmental sequence or a modified developmental sequence is extremely beneficial in retraining function and should not be saved for the "neurological" patient. Rolling and attaining a prone or a prone-on-elbows position improves bed mobility and cocontraction at the shoulders. Exercising in quadruped promotes weight bearing through the UEs and increases strength and stability in the shoulder girdle; it also provides a stimulus for bone growth in the radius and humerus. Trunk mobility, coordination, and strength can improve if the patient performs other exercises such as the "angry cat" or rocking forward and backward. Although many elderly patients do not wish to lie prone ("I haven't been on my stomach in 40 years!") or attain quadruped ("This is for a baby, not someone like me who's 83 years old!"), the therapist should encourage this type of exercise for older patients who are willing to try it ("You know, I always used to sleep on my stomach. This feels great!").

Incorporating yoga or martial arts training into the reconditioning program is a pleasant and fun alternative for the elderly patient. Tai Chi has been effective in decreasing falls[5(p489)] and maintaining strength gains.[6(p505)] These disciplines involve mental as well as physical reconditioning and can be superior to "mindless" repetitive exercising.

The Home Program

The home program is an important offshoot of the independent program. The therapist determines the patient's greatest needs and prescribes a program for the patient to perform in addition to the formal therapy session. "Home" becomes the patient's hospital room, a lounge, a waiting room, or a car at a stoplight.

The most glaring error made in home program prescription is in the length and frequency of the program. The amount of exercise prescribed is prohibitive to many patients, especially sedentary patients. Many therapists forget the amount of energy expended by their clients in the performance of everyday activities and saddle them with unreasonable amounts of exercise. As a result, they fail to comply with the home program. The number of home exercise programs found tucked away in bedpans gives some insight to the patient's thoughts on the matter.

To be effective, the home program must be specific, practical, and short. The great excuse of all patients, "I didn't have the time," is rendered ridiculous by a program that takes only 2 to 3 minutes to perform.

The Hospital Home Program

The patient should leave each therapy session in the hospital with a new home program. Even after the initial evaluation session, the therapist should select one or two simple exercises for the patient to perform later in the day or night. For example, a 74-year-old woman with a cemented total knee arthroplasty (TKA) may be given respiratory exercises to perform every hour while she is on the continuous passive motion machine. The patient may be instructed to breathe diaphragmatically five times in a row before returning to her normal breathing pattern. This home program will take only 1 or 2 minutes of her free time. It cannot interfere with the visits of friends or relatives or with other activities such as watching television, making phone calls, or reading; yet her respiratory function may improve and she may attain some relaxation benefits as well. Her initial experience with therapy will not be associated with horror stories of pain and torture but will be calm and positive. At the very least, she will have begun to accept responsibility for her own rehabilitation by exercising as prescribed.

After each session, the therapist selects a new area on which to work. In the case of the woman with the TKA, the therapist might now wish to focus on strengthening the uninvolved side. The patient is asked to perform ten repetitions each of sitting hip flexion (marching) and sitting knee extension (kicking) during every advertisement of a 1-hour television show. Once again, the patient's free-time activity is not interrupted with exercises. As a matter of fact, the activity itself (watching television) acts as a reminder to exercise.

During each subsequent treatment session, the therapist prescribes a new home program. The program can be expanded easily if necessary. When appropriate, the patient can select which exercises to include in the home program from the growing independent program. This gives the patient more responsibility and control of the therapy process.

The Outpatient Home Program

The outpatient home program will be more effective if the outpatient therapist incorporates the exercise program into a functional activity. For example, a 69-year-old woman with recent cast removal following a Colles' fracture of the right wrist has weak intrinsics and grasp, along with some edema, incoordination, and loss of motion. Her functional home program could consist of writing checks or a letter to a friend or any activity that requires fine motor use of her right hand (e.g., knitting, model building, or light housekeeping). As the patient progresses and becomes more acclimated to the home environment, a more intensive program can be prescribed for the UEs. It should be short (3 to 5 minutes), but it should be done throughout the day (five to eight times).

The Homebound Home Program

Many patients are discharged to home quite ill and debilitated with no access to outpatient services. The community care therapist may attend to such a patient's needs two or three times per week. This home program must be intensive enough to return the patient quickly to basic functioning capabilities, but concise enough that the patient will do it. The program should include specific strengthening and flexibility exercises, along with a lot of walking. A 10-minute program done five times per day usually is effective.

The Doable Home Program

The therapist somehow finds the doable home program incomplete. It seems too short to benefit the patient at all. But a 10-minute program done five times per day will yield almost an hour of quality exercising. A 4-minute program done every 2 hours will yield about a half-hour of exercise. Additionally, there are approximately 15 minutes of advertising during every television hour, in which the patient can exercise. As the patient progresses, an aerobic activity can be added to round out the program. The important thing to remember is that the home program is usually only an adjunct to the treatment sessions. Viewed in that light, the home program can be "incomplete" and still be beneficial to the patient's recovery.

Outside the formal therapy treatment sessions, a patient will do only a short program, because he or she will be too busy being a person the rest of the time. The 74-year-old woman with a TKA is the proud grandmother of four children and has been a wife for 53 years. The 69-year-old patient with a Colles' fracture is the proprietor of the corner store in town. When the therapist goes home at night, these elderly people just might want to do a little normal living, too.

DOCUMENTATION TIPS

There are many reasons why therapists need to document what occurs in therapy. Although most clinicians dread doing "the paperwork," the primary reason to document is for the therapist's own benefit. As Bernstein et al. state,

> It is our clinical memory and guidance system. It establishes what our patient's goals are, what we intend to do to meet them, and what the patient's response is to treatment. We use this system to help us make clinical decisions as to whether our treatment approach is appropriate and effective.[7(p28)]

Documentation is also done to provide legal evidence as to exactly what took place during each therapy session, to communicate with other health professionals, and to justify to insurers that proper care was provided and deserves to be reimbursed. Good documentation is an essential part of patient care. The documentation tips sections included in this chapter and upcoming treatment chapters help clinicians document the skilled care they provide, but do not always describe in their evaluations, progress notes, and discharge summaries. For more detailed information on proper documentation, refer to appropriate texts on this topic.

The Dos of Good Documentation

- Write notes in a timely fashion, preferably during or at the conclusion of each treatment session.
- Stick to the facts without editorializing or judging.
- Be accurate.
- Be brief but informative. (Longer is not necessarily better.)
- Be professional: use standard abbreviations and correct spelling.
- Whenever possible, use the newer disablement model in documentation. Documenting physical impairments (decreased strength, impaired balance, etc.) and functional limitations (assisted transfers, inability to drive a car, etc.) focuses the treatment on the patient's ability to function.

continues

- Document any incidences in detail, including patient status, and any actions taken.

The Evaluation of the Geriatric Patient

- Include detailed diagnosis (e.g., right subcapital hip fracture).
- Include onset of injury and patient age.
- Include detailed medical history.
- Include description of surgery performed, specifying the type of orthopaedic repair (e.g., left cemented, unconstrained total condylar TKA).
- Include prior level of function as well as present level of function.
- Add a separate piece of paper to the standard evaluation form, if space available is insufficient to write all your findings. (This happens commonly when trying to document posture, motor control, and skin integrity.)

- Be accurate in your objective findings of patient status without extrapolation. For example, if a patient can transfer independently from the *plinth* to the wheelchair, simply state that. Do not write that the patient is independent in *bed* to wheelchair transfers.
- Avoid vague terminology such as "functional strength." It is better to write actual strength findings $(3+/5)$ under the "objective section" describing patient status. Use the "assessment/clinical impression section" to render your professional opinion as to whether that particular strength is functional for that particular patient.
- Whenever possible, use standard assessment tools and tests.
- Document all doctor orders, precautions, and contraindications.
- Include rehabilitation goals, treatment plan, and estimated length of stay.

SUMMARY

- A thorough evaluation of the patient is a prerequisite to an effective rehabilitation program.
- The orthopaedic evaluation may take several sessions to complete in the elderly patient and should include:
  1. an inspection
  2. a detailed medical history
  3. the patient's vital signs (or cardiopulmonary screening)
  4. a description of posture and joint alignment
  5. bony and soft tissues palpation findings
  6. an assessment of ROM
  7. a manual muscle test or dynamometric assessment of strength
  8. a description of the quality of movement
  9. a detailed assessment of all mobility skills
  10. a neurological screening
  11. a functional assessment or questionnaire
  12. observations of cognitive and emotional states
- The establishment of good rapport assists in the implementation of the exercise program.
- The progressive exercise program consists of

1. the injury-specific program
2. the reconditioning program
3. the home program
- Patient education is necessary to ensure that the exercises are done properly and without undue exertion.

- The patient must take responsibility for the success of the rehabilitation program by doing the prescribed exercises and activities.
- Good documentation is an essential part of the geriatric evaluation.

REFERENCES

1. Lai JS, Lan C, Wong MK, et al. Two-year trends in cardiorespiratory function among older Tai Chi Chuan practitioners and sedentary subjects. *J Amer Geriatr Soc.* 1995;43:1222–1227.

2. Lan C, Lai JS, Wong M, et al. Cardiorespiratory function, flexibility, and body-composition among geriatric Tai Chi Chuan practitioners. *Arch Phys Med and Rehabil.* 1996;77(6):612–616.

3. Porter MM, Vandervoort AA. High-intensity strength training for the older adult: A review. *Top Geriatr Rehabil.* 1995;10(3):61–74.

4. Judge JO. Resistance training. *Top Geriatr Rehabil.* 1993;8(3):38–50.

5. Wolf SL, Barnhart H, Kutner NG, et al. Reducing frailty and falls in older persons: An investigation of Tai Chi and computerized balance training. *J Amer Geriatr Soc.* 1996;44(5):489–497.

6. Wolfson L, Whipple R, Derby C, et al. Balance and strength training in older adults: Intervention gains and Tai Chi maintenance. *J Amer Geriatr Soc.* 1996; 44(5):498–506.

7. Bernstein F, Eguchi K, Messer S, et al. Documentation for outpatient physical therapy. *Clinical Manage.* 1987;7(2):28–33.

SUGGESTED READING

Cress ME. Age-related changes: A scientific basis for exercise programming. *Top Geriatr Rehabil.* 1993; 8(3):22–37.

"Guide to Physical Therapy Practice." *Phys Ther.* 1997;77(11):1163–1636.

Johnson JH, Searles LB, McNamara S. In-home geriatric rehabilitation: Improving strength and function. *Top Geriatr Rehabil.* 1993;8(3):51–64.

Knott M, Voss DE. *Proprioceptive Neuromuscular Facilitation.* 2nd ed. New York: Harper & Row Publishers; 1968.

Mennell J McM. *Joint Pain.* Boston: Little Brown & Co Inc; 1964.

RECOMMENDED ASSESSMENT TEXTS

Cyriax J. *Textbook of Orthopaedic Medicine. Diagnosis of Soft Tissue Lesions.* 7th ed. London: Bailliere Tindall; 1978.

Emlet CA, Crabtree JL, Condon VA, et al. *In-Home Assessment of Older Adults: An Interdisciplinary Approach.* Gaithersburg, MD: Aspen Publishers, Inc; 1996.

Goldstein TS. *Functional Rehabilitation in Orthopaedics.* Gaithersburg, MD: Aspen Publishers, Inc; 1995.

Hoppenfeld S. *Physical Examination of the Spine and Extremities.* New York: Appleton & Lange; 1976.

Kane RA, Kane RL. *Assessing the Elderly.* Lexington, MA: Lexington Books; 1981.

Magee DJ. *Orthopedic Physical Assessment.* 3rd ed. Philadelphia: WB Saunders Co; 1997.

Winkel D, Matthijs O, Phelps V. *Diagnosis and Treatment of the Lower Extremities.* Gaithersburg, MD: Aspen Publishers, Inc; 1997.

Winkel D, Matthijs O, Phelps V. *Diagnosis and Treatment of the Upper Extremities.* Gaithersburg, MD: Aspen Publishers, Inc; 1997.

Appendix 2-A

Securing a Functional Environment with the Anemaet-Trotter Home Observation and Modification Evaluation

SAFE AT HOME

HOME DESCRIPTION

☐ yes ☐ no Windows Open Easily
☐ yes ☐ no Stairs in Residence   Number_____ Location(s) _____ Stair Surface Type_____
_____ Number of Floors
_____ Residence Type: Mobile Home/Condominium/Apartment/ALF

ENVIRONMENTAL

Driveway
☐ yes ☐ no Paved
☐ yes ☐ no Level Surface
☐ yes ☐ no Adequate Walking Space
_____ Feet to Home Entrance

Access to Mailbox
☐ yes ☐ no Paved
☐ yes ☐ no Level Surface
☐ yes ☐ no Can Patient Open Box?
☐ yes ☐ no Steps number _____
_____ Feet from Home Entrance

Primary Path to Home Entrance   Other Safety Concerns
☐ yes ☐ no Paved
☐ yes ☐ no Level Surface
☐ yes ☐ no Adequate Walking Space
☐ yes ☐ no Steps   Number_____
☐ yes ☐ no Rails Number_____
☐ yes ☐ no Secure Rails
☐ yes ☐ no Doormat
☐ yes ☐ no Nonskid Mat

Home Entrance Doorway
☐ yes ☐ no Door Opens In to Home
☐ yes ☐ no Threshold Present
☐ yes ☐ no Self-Closing Door
☐ yes ☐ no Door Closes Securely

GARAGE

Negotiation
☐ yes ☐ no Scatter Rugs
☐ yes ☐ no Nonskid Rugs
☐ yes ☐ no Adequate Lighting
☐ yes ☐ no Obstructed Path

Negotiation   Other Safety Concerns
☐ yes ☐ no Automatic Door Opener
☐ yes ☐ no Steps Number_____
_____ Flooring Type

Source: Reprinted from M.E. Moffa-Trotter and W.K. Anemaet, Home Care for Hip Fracture Survivors and Fallers: The "Be HIP!" Program, *Topics in Geriatric Rehabilitation,* Vol. 12, No. 1, pp. 55–58, © 1996, Aspen Publishers, Inc.

HALLWAYS

Negotiation
❑ yes ❑ no Scatter Rugs
❑ yes ❑ no Nonskid Rugs

Negotiation
❑ yes ❑ no Adequate Lighting
❑ yes ❑ no Obstructed Path
_____ Flooring Type

Other Safety Concerns

ELECTRICAL

Light Switches
❑ yes ❑ no Accessible Locations
❑ yes ❑ no In Working Order
Outlets
❑ yes ❑ no Accessible Locations
❑ yes ❑ no In Working Order
❑ yes ❑ no Electrical Hazards Present
Phones
❑ yes ❑ no Accessible Phone Locations
❑ yes ❑ no Emergency # Posted Nearby

Smoke Detectors
❑ yes ❑ no Appropriate Locations
❑ yes ❑ no In Working Order
_____ Type: Battery/Electrical/None
_____ Number of Detectors
Electrical Cords
❑ yes ❑ no Obstructive Cords
❑ yes ❑ no Cords Used Appropriately
❑ yes ❑ no Cords Secured with Tape

Other Safety Concerns

OTHER

LIVING ROOM

Negotiation
❑ yes ❑ no Scatter Rugs
❑ yes ❑ no Nonskid Rugs
❑ yes ❑ no Adequate Lighting
❑ yes ❑ no Obstructed Path
_____ Flooring Type

Patient's Preferred Seating
❑ yes ❑ no Seat Height Adequate
❑ yes ❑ no Arm Rests Present
❑ yes ❑ no Arm Rests Proper Height
❑ yes ❑ no Proper Seat Depth
❑ yes ❑ no Stable Seating
_____ Type of Furniture

Other Safety Concerns

EATING AREA

Negotiation
❑ yes ❑ no Scatter Rugs
❑ yes ❑ no Nonskid Rugs
❑ yes ❑ no Adequate Lighting
❑ yes ❑ no Obstructed Path
_____ Flooring Type

Table
❑ yes ❑ no Appropriate Location
❑ yes ❑ no Adequate Height
❑ yes ❑ no Adequate Leg Clearance
❑ yes ❑ no Stable Table
Chair
❑ yes ❑ no Adequate Height
❑ yes ❑ no Has Arm Rests
❑ yes ❑ no Chair Is Stable
_____ Swivel/Gliders/Rollers

Other Safety Concerns

KITCHEN

Negotiation
- ❏ yes ❏ no   Scatter Rugs
- ❏ yes ❏ no   Nonskid Rugs
- ❏ yes ❏ no   Adequate Lighting
- ❏ yes ❏ no   Obstructed Path
- _____ Flooring Type

Refrigerator
- ❏ yes ❏ no   In Working Order
- ❏ yes ❏ no   Door Opens Easily
- ❏ yes ❏ no   Necessary Items Accessible
- _____ Door Handle on Left/Right
- _____ Type

Sink
- ❏ yes ❏ no   Appropriate Height
- ❏ yes ❏ no   Appropriate Depth
- ❏ yes ❏ no   Faucet in Working Order

Dishwasher
- ❏ yes ❏ no   In Working Order
- ❏ yes ❏ no   Appropriate Height
- ❏ yes ❏ no   Door Opens Easily

Stove
- ❏ yes ❏ no   In Working Order
- ❏ yes ❏ no   Door Opens Easily
- ❏ yes ❏ no   Adequate Height
- ❏ yes ❏ no   Flammable Items out of Range

Microwave
- ❏ yes ❏ no   In Working Order
- ❏ yes ❏ no   Appropriate Height
- ❏ yes ❏ no   Location Appropriate
- ❏ yes ❏ no   Door Opens Easily

Cupboards and Drawers
- ❏ yes ❏ no   Appropriate Height
- ❏ yes ❏ no   Doors Open Easily
- ❏ yes ❏ no   Necessary Items Accessible

Counters
- ❏ yes ❏ no   Appropriate Height
- ❏ yes ❏ no   Rough Edges
- ❏ yes ❏ no   Overly Cluttered

Water
- ❏ yes ❏ no   Temperature <120° F

Other Safety Concerns

LAUNDRY AREA

Negotiation
- ❏ yes ❏ no   Scatter Rugs
- ❏ yes ❏ no   Nonskid Rugs
- ❏ yes ❏ no   Adequate Lighting
- ❏ yes ❏ no   Obstructed Path
- _____ Flooring Type

Washer/Dryer
- ❏ yes ❏ no   Controls Accessible
- ❏ yes ❏ no   Necessary Items Accessible
- _____ Front Load/Top Load

Other Safety Concerns

BATHROOM

Negotiation
- ❏ yes ❏ no   Scatter Rugs
- ❏ yes ❏ no   Nonskid Rugs
- ❏ yes ❏ no   Adequate Lighting
- ❏ yes ❏ no   Obstructed Path
- _____ Flooring Type

Toilet
- ❏ yes ❏ no   Adequate Height
- ❏ yes ❏ no   Easily Accessible
- ❏ yes ❏ no   Accessible Toilet Paper
- ❏ yes ❏ no   Grab Bars Present
- _____ Type: Riser/3 in 1/Hi-John

Shower/Tub
- ❏ yes ❏ no   Shower Bench Present
- ❏ yes ❏ no   Hand Held Shower Head
- ❏ yes ❏ no   Grab Bars Present
- ❏ yes ❏ no   Accessible Toiletries
- ❏ yes ❏ no   Accessible Faucets
- ❏ yes ❏ no   Accessible Towel Bars
- ❏ yes ❏ no   Nonskid Surface
- _____ Type: Tub/Walk-in Shower
- _____ L × W × H of Step/Tub Wall

Other Safety Concerns

Sink

❏ yes ❏ no   Appropriate Height
❏ yes ❏ no   Water Temperature <120° F
❏ yes ❏ no   Accessible Faucets
❏ yes ❏ no   Accessible Toiletries
❏ yes ❏ no   Accessible Towel Bars

BEDROOM

Negotiation

❏ yes ❏ no   Scatter Rugs
❏ yes ❏ no   Nonskid Rugs
❏ yes ❏ no   Adequate Lighting
❏ yes ❏ no   Obstructed Path
_____ Flooring Type

Dresser

❏ yes ❏ no   Opens with Ease
❏ yes ❏ no   Appropriate Height
❏ yes ❏ no   Necessary Items Accessible
_____ 1 or 2 Hands to Open Drawer

Bed

❏ yes ❏ no   Adequate Height
❏ yes ❏ no   Firm Mattress
❏ yes ❏ no   Appropriate Location
❏ yes ❏ no   Bed Rails Present
❏ yes ❏ no   Electric Blanket in Use
_____ Size

Closet

❏ yes ❏ no   Opens with Ease
❏ yes ❏ no   Necessary Items Accessible
❏ yes ❏ no   Appropriate Rod/Shelf Height
_____ 1 or 2 Hands to Open Drawers
_____ Size

Other Safety Concerns

3

The Hip Joint

More than 300,000 hip fractures occur annually in the United States, primarily in elderly patients.[1(p871)] In addition, approximately 150,000 total hip replacements and hemiarthroplasties are performed each year.[2(p2)] To provide proper care to this growing patient population, the therapist must understand the anatomy and biomechanics of the hip joint, as well as the physical parameters required at the hip for normal function.

ANATOMY OF THE HIP JOINT

The hip is a ball-and-socket joint that offers good stability and a wide range of motion (ROM) in all planes. The femoral head is covered with articular cartilage, except at the insertion of the ligament of the femoral head (ligamentum teres). An incomplete cartilaginous ring occupies the lunate surface of the acetabulum and is widest and thickest superiorly to withstand the upward pressure of the weight-bearing force. The acetabular labrum is a fibrocartilaginous rim that deepens the acetabular cup and provides additional stability.[3(p446)] In the superficial layer of the labrum, collagen fiber is sparse and sensory nerve endings have been observed, suggesting the labrum is involved in both nociceptive and proprioceptive function.[4(p181)]

Ligaments

The ligamentous structures around the hip are strong and further protect this inherently secure joint. The stout joint capsule attaches circumferentially around the acetabulum and inserts around the base of the femoral neck—except posteriorly, where it inserts into the midneck.[2(p2)] The longitudinal bands of the capsule, the retinacula, contain the blood vessels that supply the head and neck of the femur. The synovial membrane lines the inner walls of the capsule and is involved in nutrition, maintenance, and lubrication of the joint structures.[3(p396)] The iliofemoral ligament, or Y ligament, provides strong anterior protection for the hip joint. It is taut in symmetrical standing and also controls excessive hip abduction, adduction, and external rotation (Figure 3–1). The pubofemoral ligament provides more anterior support and functions primarily to limit hip abduction (Figure 3–1). The ischiofemoral ligament attaches posteriorly from the neck of the femur to the ischium and limits internal rotation of the hip. All three ligaments blend intimately with the joint capsule. The ligament of the head of the femur is inconsistent in strength and appearance and may be deduced to limit hip adduction.[3(p447)]

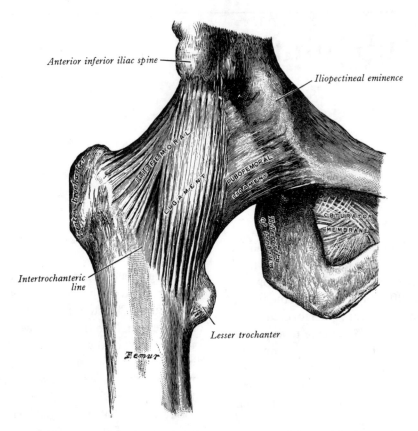

Figure 3–1 Anterior aspect of the right hip joint. *Source:* Reprinted from *Gray's Anatomy*, 35th ed, p. 448, 1973, by permission of the publisher Churchill Livingstone.

Bursae

The bursae help reduce the frictional forces that occur when muscles contract over bony prominences. Bursae are usually highly innervated and cause great discomfort when inflamed. There are four clinically important bursae around the hip (Figure 3–2):

1. The iliopectineal bursa is located under the iliopsoas muscle on the anterior surface of the joint capsule.
2. The deep trochanteric bursa is found just posterior to the greater trochanter of the femur near the insertion of the gluteus maximus.
3. The superficial trochanteric bursa is located between the greater trochanter and the skin.
4. The ischiogluteal bursa is found at the ischial tuberosity.[5](pp350,351)

Muscles and Motion

The hip moves freely through all planes of movement. The exact amount of motion available varies with the individual, but approximate norms for the elderly are depicted in Table 3–1. Although the shaft of the femur moves into what is commonly termed flexion, extension, abduction, adduction, rota-

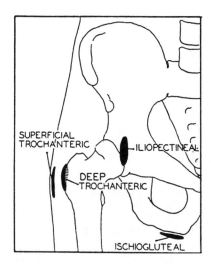

Figure 3–2 The most commonly affected bursae about the hip. *Source:* Reprinted with permission from R.B. Raney and H.R. Brashear, *Shands' Handbook of Orthopaedic Surgery*, 10 ed., p. 399, © 1986, Mosby-Year Book, Inc.

tion, and circumduction, the head of the femur is actually rotating within the acetabulum around different axes. The close-packed position of the hip is full extension, some abduction, and some internal rotation. In this stable position, the joint surfaces are congruent, all the ligaments are taut, and no further motion is possible.[3(pp448,449)]

The amount of hip motion necessary to perform everyday activities is generally much less than the parameters for normal ROM. The patient with minor hip dysfunction is thus able to maintain a fairly active lifestyle. Functional ROM of the hip consists of flexion of 120°, abduction of 20°, and external rotation of 20°.[6(p156)] Full hip extension is also needed for a normal gait pattern. Table 3–2 shows the necessary ROM at the hip to perform some of the activities of daily living.

An in-depth description of all the musculature surrounding the hip joint and their ac-

tions is not within the scope of this book. Table 3–1 provides a brief review of the available hip motions, the primary and secondary muscle movers, and their innervations. The therapist should remember that these muscles do not act alone but in concert with one another to achieve normal hip function. (For more information on hip musculature, refer to the texts at the end of this chapter.)

Innervation

The hip receives its nerve supply from the femoral, obturator, sciatic, and superior gluteal nerves. Specific muscle innervations are described in Table 3–1. Because the hip joint is formed largely from the third lumbar segment, pain can be referred from the groin, down the front of the thigh to the knee, and down the front of the leg to just above the ankle.[7(p602)]

Blood Supply

One major determinant when selecting an appropriate fixation device for a hip fracture is whether the blood supply to the fracture site is intact. Without proper circulation to the femoral head, avascular necrosis will occur.

The blood supply to the femoral head varies with age. In adults the circulation comes from three sources:

1. the retinacular arteries, which arise from the medial circumflex artery
2. the artery of the ligamentum teres, which arises from the obturator artery
3. the nutrient artery of the femoral shaft, which arises from the deep femoral artery (Figure 3–3)[5(pp332,333)]

At first glance, the blood supply to the femoral head seems redundant and therefore sufficient to withstand a disruption of one of its sources. However, the blood supply

Table 3–1 Geriatric Hip Motions, Muscles, and Innervations

Motion	Primary Muscles*	Secondary Muscles*	Innervation*
Flexion[†] 0°–115°	Psoas major		Femoral: L1-3
	Iliacus		Femoral: L-2, L-3
		Pectineus	Femoral: L-2, L-3
		Sartorius	Femoral: L-2, L-3
		Rectus femoris	Femoral: L2-4
Extension 0°–15°	Gluteus maximus		Inferior gluteal: L-5, S-1, S-2
	Semitendinosus		Sciatic (tibial): L-4, L-5, S-1, S-2
	Semimembranosus		Sciatic (tibial): L-5, S-1, S-2
	Biceps femoris		Sciatic (tibial): L-5, S-1, S-2
Abduction[‡] 0°–30°	Gluteus medius		Superior gluteal: L-5, S-1
	Gluteus minimus		Superior gluteal: L-5, S-1
		Tensor fasciae latae	Superior gluteal: L4-L5
		Sartorius	Femoral: L2-3
Adduction[†] 0°–15°	Adductor longus		Obturator: L2-4
	Adductor brevis		Obturator: L2-4
	Adductor magnus		Obturator: L2-4 and Sciatic (tibial): L2-4
		Pectineus	Femoral: L-2, L-3
		Gracilis	Obturator: L-2, L-3
Internal rotation[†] 0°–30°	Tensor fasciae latae		Superior gluteal: L-4, L-5
	Gluteus minimus		Superior gluteal: L-5, S-1
	Gluteus medius		Superior gluteal: L-5, S-1
External rotation[†] 0°–30°	Gemellus superior		L-5, S-1
	Gemellus inferior		L-5, S-1
	Obturator externus		Obturator: L-3, L-4
	Obturator internus		L-5, S-1
	Quadratus femoris		L-5, S-1
		Piriformis	L-5, S-1, S-2
		Gluteus maximus	Inferior gluteal: L-5, S-1, S-2
		Sartorius	Femoral: L-2, L-3

Sources: *Gray's Anatomy*, ed 35 (pp 449, 560–570), by R Warwick and PL Williams (eds), Churchill Livingstone, © 1973.
[†]*Physical Therapy* (1984;64[6]:922), Copyright © 1984, American Physical Therapy Association.
[‡]*American Journal of Physical Medicine and Rehabilitation* (1989;68[4]:164), Copyright © 1989, Williams & Wilkins Co.

Table 3–2 Mean Hip Motions Necessary for Activities of Daily Living

Task	Flexion	Extension	Abduction	Adduction	Internal Rotation	External Rotation
Walking*	37°	15°	7°	5°	4°	9°
Stair climbing (7-inch rise)						
Up	67°	7°	8°			10°
Down	36°		7°			5°
Standing up from a chair (18-inch seat height)	112°		20°			17°
Squatting	114°		27°		19°	5°
Shoe tying						
Foot on floor	129°		18°			13°
Foot across thigh	115°		24°			28°

Sources: Clinical Orthopedia (1970;72:205–215), Copyright © 1970, JB Lippincott Co.
Archives of Surgery (1973;107:411), Copyright © 1973, American Medical Association.

through the ligamentum teres is usually diminished or nonexistent in elderly patients, and the nutrient artery supplements the blood supply of the femoral head only in some cases. The one reliable source of blood to the femoral head is the posterior branch of the retinacular arteries.[5(pp332,333)] Unfortunately, this source can be disrupted during an intracapsular fracture, necessitating the insertion of a prosthesis to replace the femoral head and neck.

KINETICS OF THE HIP JOINT

To treat the hip joint properly, the therapist needs to appreciate how the distribution and absorption of forces affect the rehabilitation process. In particular, the therapist should understand the relationship of body weight, muscular force, gait pattern, and ambulation devices to the joint reaction force at the hip (hip joint pressure). To illustrate these concepts, a very simplified hip model is used. The force diagram in Figure 3–4 shows the hip as the fulcrum in a lever system. Similar force diagrams can be presented for all of the joints in the body, but that is not within the scope of this book; therefore, only the kinetic information necessary for the clinical management of the joints is considered in subsequent chapters. The reader is referred to the biomechanical texts listed at the end of this chapter for more information on this fascinating subject.

The hip joint acts as the fulcrum of the lever system shown in Figure 3–4. The four factors that alter the hip joint pressure are

1. the supported body weight (approximately five-sixths of the body weight

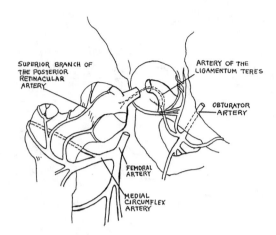

Figure 3–3 Blood supply to the adult femoral head. The superior branch of the posterior retinacular artery, which arises from the medial circumflex artery, provides the main blood supply to the femoral head. The blood supply from the artery of the ligamentum teres diminishes with age and often is absent in the elderly population. A fracture of the femoral neck can disrupt the circulation to the femoral head, resulting in avascular necrosis.

in a one-legged stance or two-thirds of the body weight in a bilateral stance)

2. the distance between the line of supported body weight and the hip joint, which is controlled by
   (a) the obliquity of the pelvis
   (b) the position of the head and trunk
   (c) the position of the limbs
3. the vertical component of gluteal tension
4. the distance between the insertion of the gluteal muscles and the hip[8(p552)]

In order for the lever system to be balanced, the turning moments about the fulcrum (hip joint) must be equal ($Wy = Xz$). In the example shown in Figure 3–4, a 120-lb woman is standing on one leg. The supported body weight (W) equals 100 lb, the distance y equals 4 inches, and the distance z equals

2 inches. In this case, the force of the gluteal muscles (X) would have to equal 200 lb ($X = Wy/z$). If the distance z were shortened as the result of an impacted subcapital fracture to a new distance of only 1 inch, the gluteal muscles would have to exert 400 lb of pressure to keep the system in equilibrium.

The weight supported by the fulcrum (hip joint pressure) is the sum of the weights acting at each end of the lever bar ($F = W + X$). In the first example, the weight supported by the woman's hip (F) equals 300 lb (100 + 200), or two and one-half times her body weight; in the second example, the forces acting through her hip (F) equal 500 lb (100 + 400), or four times her body weight. These examples demonstrate that seemingly small changes in any of the four factors listed above can cause significant alterations in hip joint pressure. Because the hip joint is part of a biological system rather than a

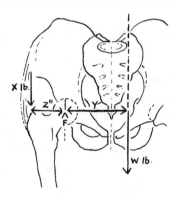

Figure 3–4 The hip as a fulcrum. The four factors that alter hip joint pressure (F) are the supported body weight (W) acting at a distance (y) and the vertical component of gluteal tension (X) acting at a distance (z). In this simple lever system, the hip joint pressure (F) is equal to the sum of the weights acting at each end of the lever bar $W + X$. *Source:* Adapted with permission from *Journal of Bone and Joint Surgery,* Vol. 41B, No. 3, p. 552, © 1959, Journal of Bone and Joint Surgery, Inc.

simple lever system as given in the examples, exact calculations are more complicated.

Research studies of hip reaction forces during dynamic activities have been conducted with a variety of methods using (e.g., force plate systems, instrumented prostheses, and instrumented nail plates).[6(pp168,169),9(p65)] Both research data and calculations based on physical principles confirm that forces far greater than the body weight act on the hip joint during normal activities. Table 3–3 summarizes some of the hip joint reaction forces encountered in activities common to elderly patients.

Research has also been performed on acetabular contact pressures that occur during rehabilitation programs following hip surgery.[10(pp1378–1386),11(pp691–699),12(pp700–710),13(pp51–59)] Although it is not known how these pressures correlate with hip joint reaction forces, higher acetabular pressures logically infer higher forces.[11(p11)] Table 3–4 summarizes some of

the acetabular pressures found in a case study of one 73-year-old woman with an instrumented endoprosthesis performing a physical therapy strengthening program.

SUMMARY

- The hip joint is an inherently stable ball-and-socket joint.
- The hip joint is further stabilized by the acetabular labrum, strong capsular and ligamentous structures, and massive musculature.
- The hip is innervated by the femoral, obturator, sciatic, and superior gluteal nerves.
- The primary blood supply to the femoral head in the elderly patient is the posterior branch of the retinacular artery.
- The hip moves freely through all planes of movement. Its functional ROM is

Table 3–3 Approximate Hip Joint Pressures during Activities of Daily Living

Activity of Daily Living	Pressure on a Single Hip Joint (Units of Body Weight)
Bridging (getting on a bedpan)	4
Bridging with a trapeze	1⅓
Bilateral standing	⅓
Unilateral standing	2¾
Gait	
Stance phase	
Full weight bearing	2¾–7
Partial weight bearing	⅘*
Swing phase, non-weight bearing	1
Ascending stairs	3–6†
Running	4½–5†

Sources: Basic Biomechanics of the Skeletal System (pp 160–171) by VH Frankel and M Nordin, Lea & Febiger, © 1980.

**Journal of Bone and Joint Surgery* (1959;41B[3]:556), Copyright © 1959, Journal of Bone and Joint Surgery.

†*Kinesiology: Application to Pathological Motion* (p 188) by GL Soderberg, Williams & Wilkins Co, © 1986.

Table 3–4 Acetabular Pressures during a Rehabilitation Program

Rehabilitation Activities	Acetabular Pressure in MPa (1 MPa = 144 psi)
Bed rest (supine lying)	1.4
Riding a stationary bicycle	1.6
TDWB gait with crutches (10 lbs on foot)	2.0*
NWB gait with crutches	2.4
Isometric quadriceps (quad set)	3.4*
PWB gait with crutches	3.5
Active hip abduction in supine lying	3.8*
Resisted isometric hip abduction	4.2
Active antigravity hip flexion	4.8*
Isometric hip extension (gluteal set)	4.9
FWB gait unsupported	5.5
Jogging	7.7
Stair climbing	10.2
Rising from a chair	18.0

Sources: Data from *Journal of Bone and Joint Surgery* (1989;71-A[9]:1381–1383), Copyright © 1989, Journal of Bone and Joint Surgery.
Physical Therapy (1992;72[10]:695), Copyright © 1992, American Physical Therapy Association.

120° of flexion and 20° of both abduction and external rotation. Extension is vital to normal gait.

- The hip joint acts as a fulcrum in a lever system. As such, the hip joint forces greatly exceed the body weight during most activities of daily living. In addition, some rehabilitation exercises, such as isometrics, cause hip joint forces in the vicinity of those recorded for normal walking.

REFERENCES

1. Jacobsen SJ, Goldberg J, Milest TP, et al. Hip fracture incidence among the old and very old: A population-based study of 745,435 cases. *Amer J Public Health.* 1990;80:871–873.

2. Kozinn SC, Wilson PD Jr. Adult hip disease and total hip replacement. *Clin Symp.* 1987;39(5):2–32.

3. Warwick R, Williams PL, eds. *Gray's Anatomy.* 35th ed. Edinburgh, Scotland: Churchill Livingstone; 1973.

4. Kim YT, Azuma H. The nerve endings of the acetabular labrum. *Clin Orthop.* 1995;320:175–181.

5. Raney RB, Brashear HR. *Shands' Handbook of Orthopaedic Surgery.* 8th ed. St. Louis, MO: CV Mosby Co; 1971.

6. Frankel VH, Nordin M. *Basic Biomechanics of the Skeletal System.* 2nd ed. Philadelphia: Lea & Febiger; 1989.

7. Cyriax J. *Textbook of Orthopaedic Medicine.* 7th ed. London: Bailliere Tindall; 1978.

8. Denham RA. Hip mechanics. *J Bone Joint Surg.* 1959;41-B(3):550–557.

9. Shelley FJ, Anderson DD, Kolar MJ, et al. Physical modeling of hip-joint forces in stair climbing. *J Engin Med.* 1996;210(1):65–68.

10. Hodge WA, Carlson KL, Fijan RS, et al. Contact pressures from an instrumented hip endoprosthesis. *J Bone Joint Surg.* 1989;71-A(9):1378–1386.

11. Strickland EM, Fares M, Krebs DE, et al. In vivo acetabular contact pressures during rehabilitation, Part I: Acute phase. *Phys Ther.* 1992;72(10):691–699.

12. Givens-Heiss DL, Krebs DE, Riley PO, et al. In vivo acetabular contact pressures during rehabilitation, Part II: Postacute phase. *Phys Ther.* 1992;72(10):700–710.

13. Krebs DE, Robbins CE, Laine L, et al. Hip biomechanics during gait. *J Orthop Sports Phys Ther.* 1998;28(1):51–59.

SUGGESTED READING

Frankel VH, Nordin M, eds. *Basic Biomechanics of the Skeletal System.* 2nd ed. Philadelphia: Lea & Febiger; 1989.

Gowitzke BA, Milner M. *Scientific Bases of Human Movement.* 3rd ed. Baltimore: Williams & Wilkins; 1988.

Kendall FP, McCreary EK, Provance PG. *Muscles: Testing and Function.* 4th ed. Baltimore: Williams & Wilkins; 1993.

4

Treatment of Common Problems of the Hip Joint

The hip joint of the elderly patient is well protected from outside trauma. The greatest danger to the integrity of the hip comes from within: osteoporosis. The loss of bone mass that occurs with this condition is described in Chapters 1 and 10. Osteoporosis makes the femur more susceptible to one of the older person's greatest fears—hip fracture.

HIP FRACTURES

The incidence of hip fractures is at epidemic proportions. Hip fracture is a devastating injury to a frail population, causing major losses in functional ability and high incidences of death. Approximately 300,000 hip fractures occurred in the United States in 1990[1] and 18,000 hip fractures occurred in Canada in 1987.[2(p111)] In North America and Europe, the rate of proximal femoral fractures is greater than can be explained by demographic changes alone. Because this increased rate affects both genders equally, the etiological factor probably responsible is an increased sedentary lifestyle.[2(pp114–117)] Much research has been conducted on the population at risk for hip fracture. A summary of some of the research findings is presented next.

- In the United States, the overall rate of hip fracture increases with age, is greater in women than in men, and is higher in the South.[3]
- Hip fracture is associated with reduced muscle strength rather than reduced body mass.[4]
- Hip fracture rates are lower in rural areas than in urban areas.[5]
- The risk of hip fracture is doubled among patients with rheumatoid arthritis who have functional impairments. The risk is also doubled among patients on steroid medication.[6]
- The risk of hip fracture in women 5'8" or taller is twice as great as women under 5'2".[7]
- In patients who have a hip fracture:
  50% have arthritis
  39% have hypertension
  38% have fallen in the preceding 3 months
  36% have cataracts
  31% have heart disease
  31% have difficulty walking or rising from a chair
  27% are on psychotropic drugs
  20% have had a previous stroke[8]
- Circumstances of a hip fracture are:

76% occur indoors, mostly in the bed-
room, living room, or kitchen
60% occur in the daytime
42% occur when not wearing prescribed
eyeglasses[8]

Types of Hip Fracture

There is a tendency among therapists to
treat all patients with hip fractures in the
same way. Hip fractures are described by
their severity (i.e., simple, comminuted, displaced) and by their location on the femur
(i.e., subcapital, intertrochanteric). A simple
fracture in an elderly patient usually heals in
6 to 8 weeks. However, a severely comminuted or shattered fracture may take 3 months
or more to heal completely. The actual fracture site influences the type of surgical intervention and subsequent physical rehabilitation. Hip fractures are classified as either
intracapsular or extracapsular (Figure 4–1).

Intracapsular Fractures

Intracapsular fractures are synonymous
with femoral neck fractures and include all
breaks within the confines of the hip capsule,
such as subcapital, transcervical, and basilar
fractures. This fracture is further categorized
as displaced or nondisplaced. It is usually
caused by direct trauma, as in a fall. However, in the severely osteoporotic patient, it
can also be caused by an indirect rotational
force and is considered a spontaneous fracture. The incidence of spontaneous fractures
is low, ranging from 1 to 5%.[8(p129),9(p325)]

A displaced intracapsular fracture can disrupt the retinacular arteries, thereby compro-
mising the blood supply to the femoral head.
Without an intact blood supply, the fracture
will not heal, or avascular necrosis of the

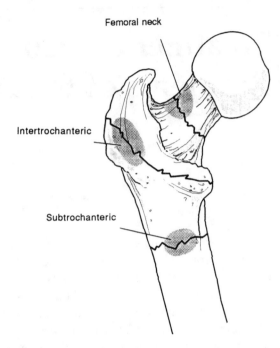

Figure 4–1 Different types of hip fracture by location. *Source:* Adapted from S. Gitelis, "The
Treatment of Pathological Hip Fractures," *Techniques in Orthopaedics* Vol. 4, No. 2, p. 74, ©
1989 Aspen Publishers, Inc.

femoral head will occur. Because of this, the
orthopaedic surgeon usually opts for removing the femoral head and replacing it with a
prosthesis in the older patient. However,
many surgeons prefer internal fixation for
the young elderly patient (under 75 years of
age.)[10(p271)] Occasionally, the fracture impacts
on itself or is only minimally displaced. In
this instance, the treatment of choice is open
reduction and internal fixation (ORIF) with
insertion of multiple 6.5 mm cancellous lag
screws (Figure 4–2).[11(p179)] Surgical complications from ORIF include a 10 to 20%
nonunion rate and a 26% rate of avascular
necrosis.[12(pp197–199)] Hemiarthroplasty compli-

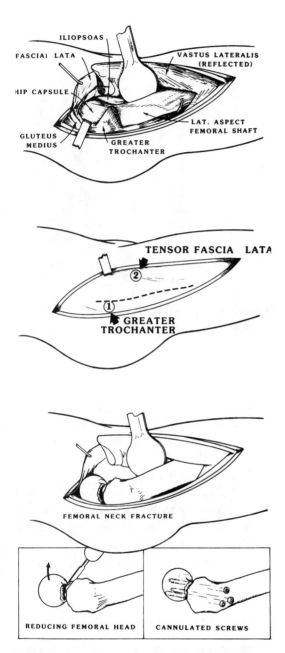

Figure 4–2 Cannulated screw fixation for femoral neck fracture. *Source:* Reprinted from R. Kyle, "Operative Techniques of Fixation for Femoral Neck Fractures in Young Adults," *Techniques in Orthopaedics* Vol. 1, No. 1, p. 36, © 1986, Lippincott-Williams & Wilkins.

cations mostly consist of a prosthetic dislocation rate of 1 to 7%.[13(p35)]

Extracapsular Fractures

Extracapsular fractures include breaks just outside the insertion of the hip capsule and are often described as trochanteric or intertrochanteric fractures; they are further categorized as stable or unstable. They are almost always caused by trauma. There can be significant blood loss requiring transfusion. Depending on the nature of the break, a patient with an extracapsular fracture may need to be put into traction to help align the bony segments. By the time such a patient attends therapy, it is common to see huge bruises encompassing the thigh region. In spite of all this, the blood supply to the femoral head remains intact with the rate of postoperative avascular necrosis at only 0.4%.[14(p182)] The fixation of choice for this injury is a compression screw and plate.

Subtrochanteric fractures are rare in the elderly population and are usually the result of severe trauma (e.g., as sustained in a car accident). Because the break occurs outside the capsule, blood flow to the femoral head remains intact. A patient with a subtrochanteric fracture undergoes ORIF with an interlocking nail or sliding hip screw.[11(p187)]

Common complications for both intracapsular and extracapsular hip fractures include:

- deep vein thrombosis
- pulmonary embolism
- infection
- nonunion or delayed union
- aseptic necrosis
- mortality[15(p63)]

Types of Internal Fixation Devices

It is important for the therapist to know which of the many types of internal fixation devices is stabilizing the patient's fracture. Each of the devices has inherent strengths and weaknesses that can affect the rehabilitation process.

Knowles Pin

The Knowles pin (Figure 4–3A) is used primarily in reducing noncomminuted intracapsular fractures. It is a thin (3 to 4 mm in diameter) stainless steel rod with one threaded end, culminating in a very sharp point.[16(pB103)] To the untrained eye, it looks akin to a stiletto. For proper fixation, at least three pins need to be inserted within 0.6 cm of the subchondral bone.[12(p196)] The average operation time is very short, averaging only 20 minutes.[17(p90)] If the danger of open surgery is too great for the patient, the Knowles pin can also be inserted percutaneously.

If too much weight bearing (WB) is allowed, the fracture may impact further, causing the pin to pierce through the femoral head or snap under the load. In general, the patient begins touch-down weight bearing (TDWB) on postoperative (PO) Day 2 to 5 and progresses slowly to full weight bearing (FWB) when the fracture is completely healed. However, some physicians allow WB as tolerated with crutches or walker by PO Day 3.[12(p196)]

Nails

Jewett and Smith-Petersen nails are now rarely used to stabilize hip fractures. The tri-flanged nail-plate construction proved to carry high incidences of fixation failure and

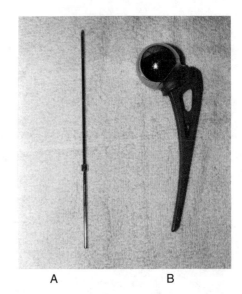

A   B

Figure 4–3 Surgical fixation devices for hip fracture. (A) Knowles Pin, (B) Moore-type prosthesis.

malunion.[18(p41)] The Massie sliding nail allows a controlled collapse of the unstable fracture and prevents medial migration of the femoral shaft.[16(pB97),18(p42)]

Depending on the severity of the fracture, TDWB usually begins PO Day 2 to 5 and progresses to FWB when the fracture is completely healed. If too much weight is placed on the limb prior to complete bony union, the nail can pierce the femoral head.

Sliding and Intermedullary Hip Screws

The sliding hip screw (e.g., Richards compression screw) is the internal fixation device of choice for most intertrochanteric fractures. It consists of two stainless steel pieces, a lag screw and a tube plate assembly (Figure 4–4).[16(pB74)] By tightening the screw, the surgeon can approximate the bony seg-

The patient may begin partial weight bearing (PWB) on PO Day 2 and progress quickly to FWB as tolerated by PO Week 6 to 8.

Enders Rods

Enders rods are prebent, flexible, stainless steel rods 4.5 mm in diameter. Approximately three to six rods are needed to stabilize a fracture.[19] The therapist needs to be aware that these intermedullary rods are inserted at the medial femoral condyle of the knee joint. The fixation itself may cause an external malrotation of the hip joint (i.e., a severe toeing-out of the foot). This condition generally cannot be corrected by strengthening or gait training. Although the hip need not be opened surgically for this fixation device to be inserted, the therapist will discover that now two joints, the hip and the knee, will need to be rehabilitated. Due to persistent knee pain, 15% of patients will require removal of the rod within one year of surgery.[18(p47)]

Because of the length of the fixation device (i.e., the length of the patient's femur, approximately 400 mm), the Enders rod can withstand large amounts of force. As a result, the WB progression for a patient with an Enders rod is rapid. The patient may begin PWB on PO Day 2 and progress to FWB in 6 weeks.

Uncemented Prostheses

The Austin Moore prosthesis (Figure 4–3B) is in the first generation of uncemented prostheses. It is cast of a strong cobalt-chromium-molybdenum alloy (Vitallium). The Austin Moore prosthesis has a large femoral head (approximately the size of

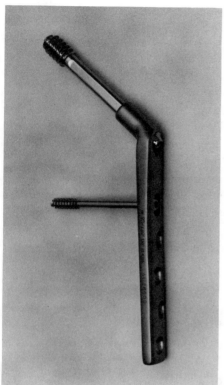

Figure 4–4 Richards compression screw and plate. This fixation device is commonly used to stabilize an intertrochanteric hip fracture. Courtesy of Richards Medical Co., Memphis, Tennessee.

ments and promote the healing process. As the fracture site impacts, the lag screw collapses into the tube plate, maintaining alignment of the femur and preventing protrusion into the acetabulum.

The intermedullary hip screw has a similar lag screw to the sliding hip screw, but the side plate is replaced with an intermedullary rod that is usually fixed distally with locking bolts. Although similar results have been attained with both fixations, the intermedullary hip screw has higher rates of fracture complications.[5(p183)]

the human femoral head) and a fenestrated stem for bony fixation.[16(pA74)]

The second generation of uncemented prostheses includes the porous-coated prostheses. The porous surface is created by a fine mesh of titanium wires or by small metal beads sintered onto the femoral stem.[20(p6)] The porous surface allows bony ingrowth to occur, stabilizing the implant. New implant surfaces such as calcium-phosphate ceramic coating (e.g., hydroxyapatite) are biocompatible and may have osteoconductive properties that promote bone fixation to the metal implant.[21(p1439)]

In both the Austin Moore and coated prostheses, the large metallic head causes extensive wear on the acetabulum over time and cannot be used on patients with severely osteoporotic acetabula.[16(pA74)] Another type of fixation device, the bipolar prosthesis (e.g., Bateman's, Omnifit, and Intermedics 1.0.1. Bipolar), is designed to cause less wear on the acetabulum (Figure 4–5).[20(p7)] This type of prosthesis has a large metallic cap lined with ultrahigh-molecular-weight polyethylene. A standard total hip arthroplasty (THA) femoral head snap-fits into the cap. Thus this prosthesis has two articulations (bipoles), each one contributing to the total hip motion. The average operation time for this procedure is 88 minutes.[22(p77)] The bipolar prosthesis can also be converted to a THA by exchanging the large metallic cap for an acetabular component.

To prevent prosthetic dislocation, the patient usually is placed on total hip precautions (THPs) for the first 3 weeks after surgery. THPs are explained in more detail later in this chapter. Generally, a patient with an uncemented prosthesis begins TDWB on PO Day 2 and progresses to FWB in 6 to 8 weeks.

Cemented Prostheses

Cemented prostheses (monopolar or bipolar) are the fixation devices of choice for intracapsular hip fractures in "old" geriatric patients (over the age of 75 years). The different types of prostheses have solid Vitallium stems that are stabilized in the femoral shaft with acrylic cement, allowing the elderly patient the luxury of early ambulation and mobility. (See acrylic cement section in this chapter.) Patients with cemented prostheses report significantly less thigh pain than patients with uncemented prostheses.[22(p75)] The surgical time for ce-

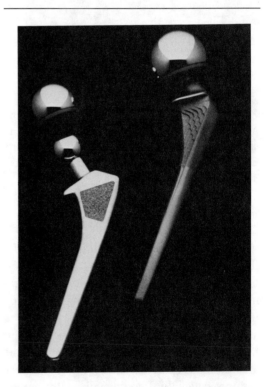

Figure 4–5 Intermedics I.O.I. Bipolar prosthesis. The small femoral head snap-fits into a larger cap. This design causes less acetabular erosion. Courtesy of Intermedics Orthopedics, Inc., Austin, Texas.

mented prostheses is approximately 20 minutes longer than for uncemented prostheses.[22(p77)]

PWB begins on PO Day 2 and immediately progresses to FWB (as tolerated)
on PO Day 3 to 14, depending on the
orthopaedic surgeon's personal preference.
As with uncemented prostheses, THPs
should be enforced for the first 3 weeks
postoperatively.

Revisions

Hip surgery can fail immediately because
of infection or avascular necrosis, or over
time because of loosening of the fixation device. If avascular necrosis occurs, the fixation hardware (i.e., pins, nail, or screw) can
be removed along with the femoral head and
a prosthesis can be inserted. If a prosthesis
fails, it must be removed along with part of
the femoral shaft. Long-stemmed prostheses
can be inserted with or without bone grafts.
The patient with a revision undergoes a
slower, more conservative rehabilitation
process.[23(p257)] In general, FWB commences 3
to 6 months after the revision.

Sometimes due to persistent infection, a
prosthetic component cannot be reimplanted.
The surgeon must resect the femoral head,
removing the infected prosthesis or fixation
device. This is called a Girdlestone procedure and results in a makeshift "hip joint"
consisting of the acetabulum articulating
with the beveled shaft of the femur. Not
surprisingly, a Girdlestone resection causes
a significant leg length discrepancy and
pain. In general, the less bone removed,
the better the patient's functional outcome
(Figure 4–6). Many patients can ambulate with a walker or crutches, but some remain wheelchair-bound because of severe
pain on WB.

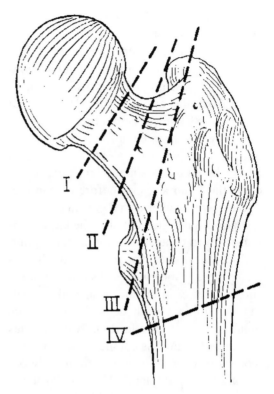

Figure 4–6 The anatomical levels of Girdlestone
resections. Type I—a substantial portion of the
femoral neck remains, type II—a small portion
(less than 1.5 cm) of the femoral neck remains,
type III—an intertrochanteric resection, and type
IV—a subtrochanteric resection. *Source:* Reprinted with permission from J.D. Grauer et al.,
The Journal of Bone and Joint Surgery, Vol. 71-A,
No. 5, p. 671, © 1989 Journal of Bone and Joint
Surgery, Inc.

Acrylic Cement

In 1960 Sir John Charnley of England
used polymethyl methacrylate (PMMA), a
well-known dental cement, to stabilize a
THA.[23(p1)] His work revolutionized the surgical treatment of intracapsular fractures and
THAs. The immediate stable fixation of the

prosthesis or THA allowed patients the benefits of early mobility.

Unfortunately, it later became apparent that the original cementing techniques contributed to loosening of the prostheses in 30 to 45% of the cases within 10 years of surgery.[24(p983)] Newer cementing techniques (second generation femoral cementing) were developed to prevent cement fragmentation and included using a medullary plug to occlude the femoral canal before cementing, injecting the cement with a gun, and improving the design of the implant. The latest techniques (third generation femoral cementing) include decreasing the porosity of the cement (thereby increasing its strength), pressurizing the cement in the canal, and precoating the implant with cement to promote bonding.[25(pp2–3)] In addition, research has proven that PMMA is not the cause of the osteolysis or bone destruction commonly occurring around implants. The periprosthetic bone softening is now called "particle disease" and is caused by an immune reaction to particles of metal or polyethylene that have been abraded off the prostheses.

The advantages to continued use of PMMA in the fixation of prostheses in the elderly patient are:

1. Within hours of application, PMMA provides a stable fixation that allows immediate WB.
2. By shaping the PMMA putty, the surgeon can correct any incongruities between the implant and the bone bed.
3. By shaping the PMMA putty, the surgeon can orient the prosthesis independently of the shape of the bone bed.[23(p32)]

The disadvantages of using PMMA are:

1. The cement can become defective over time (15–20 years), causing the prosthesis to loosen.[23(p14)]

2. PMMA can sometimes cause local tissue or systemic toxicity.[23(p32)]

Much controversy still remains in orthopaedics as to the use of cement in hemiarthroplasty and joint replacement. In general, the patient will ultimately receive what the individual orthopaedic surgeon prefers.

Weight-Bearing Considerations

Most therapy prescriptions for a patient with a fractured hip include WB orders. These orders take into account the severity and location of the fracture, the patient's weight, the integrity of the patient's bone, the ability of the fixation device to withstand stress, and the patient's cognitive state. Descriptions of the varying WB orders are provided in Table 4–1. The therapist is responsible for teaching the patient how to limit weight on the affected limb while ambulating and transferring, thereby promoting the healing process. The therapist must understand how each of the parameters, individually and collectively, affects the WB orders, in order to discuss treatment possibilities intelligently with the physician.

Consider the theoretical case of a 79-year-old woman with a comminuted intertrochanteric fracture of her left hip. She has undergone ORIF with a Richards compression screw and plate and comes to therapy on PO Day 2 for evaluation and treatment while maintaining PWB on the left leg. After the initial evaluation, some of the significant findings are

- pain: an ache in the groin region and tenderness over the suture site
- left hip strength: Poor (2/5)
- left hip range of motion (ROM): minimally to moderately limited
- right lower extremity (LE) strength and ROM: Good minus (4–/5)

Table 4–1 Weight-Bearing Considerations

Weight-Bearing Order	Percentage of Body Weight Placed on Limb	Ambulation Device Needed	Hip Joint Reaction Force
Non-WB	0	Walker/crutches	1 × Body wt*
TDWB	10–15	Walker/crutches	Neutralized
PWB	30	Walker/crutches	⅚ × Body wt†
50% WB	50	Cane	1 × Body wt*
FWB	75–100	Cane/no device	2¾ × Body wt*

Sources: Data from *Basic Biomechanics of the Skeletal System*, 2nd ed (pp 135–151), by VH Frankel and M Nordin, Lea & Febiger, © 1989.
†*Journal of Bone and Joint Surgery* (1959;41B[3]:556), Copyright © 1959, Journal of Bone and Joint Surgery, Inc.

- body weight: 145 lb
- general conditioning: fair to good
- cognitive status: pleasant but impaired

With verbal and tactile cues, the rehabilitation process commences. It soon becomes obvious, however, that no amount of cuing will prevent this elderly woman from placing her weight onto her affected left hip. The therapist's song, "walker, left, right, walker, left, right . . .," goes unheeded. This woman persists in carrying her walker like a bag of groceries instead of using it to unload her hip. Not only is she FWB on her hip, but she is carrying an additional 5-lb burden. Interestingly, she does not complain of any pain on WB. The therapist obviously must contact the orthopaedic surgeon.

What can the therapist reasonably ask the orthopaedic surgeon? The known facts follow:

- The patient cannot learn PWB.
- The patient is ambulating FWB without pain.
- The internal fixation device can absorb large amounts of stress.

- The blood supply to the fracture site should be intact.

The therapist does not know the bone consistency, fracture severity, fixation device alignment, or any problems that occurred during surgery. In addition, the fracture site must be stabilized and protected. When the therapist contacts the physician, a reasonable request might be to increase the WB status to WB as tolerated with a rolling walker for a limited distance. The final decision obviously rests with the orthopaedic surgeon.

Many elderly patients have difficulty maintaining their prescribed WB orders. Some recent studies have suggested that failure to properly bear weight after a hip fracture may not result in the catastrophe originally thought. Shih and Wang report a study of 121 cases allowing WB as tolerated with crutches or a walker on PO Day 3 for a Knowles pin fixation of a femoral neck fracture. They had a high bony union rate and only a 1% incidence of the pin penetrating the acetabulum.[12(p196)] Koval et al report on 596 elderly patients who were allowed immediate unrestricted WB after surgical fixation for any type of hip fracture.[26(p526)] The revision rate was only 3.4%. They believe the results of their study support the use of unrestricted WB in the elderly population, because the benefits of early mobility outweigh the potential complications.

The therapist must recognize that there is still great controversy in orthopaedic medicine concerning the rate of progression of WB versus fracture healing versus mobility. Philosophies vary within different regions of the United States and among physicians in the same hospital. Close communication with each physician is a must in order to provide the patient with quality care.

Prevention of Hip Fractures

The epidemic incidence of hip fractures comes with a high cost in human anguish and health care dollars. As such, enormous research has been performed on hip fracture with the hope that the information obtained will someday help prevent this devastating injury. One of the most discussed methods of reducing hip fractures is by reducing the falls that contribute to the fracture. As such, the reader is referred to Chapter 17 for a more in-depth discussion on balance and fall prevention.

The likelihood of preventing falls completely seems improbable; therefore, another approach would be to limit the damage from the falls. This could be accomplished through the use of protective padding for the hip. In a study by Lauritzen, Petersen, and Lund, wearing hip protectors over the greater trochanters conferred a 53% protection against hip fractures. No one fractured a hip while wearing the pads;[27(p13)] however, the protectors only work if they are worn. Cameron and Quine investigated whether elderly women would actually wear hip protec-

tors. Most participants indicated that they would not use the protectors because of perceived lack of comfort as well as the belief that they were not at high risk.[28(pp276,277)] The evolution of hip protectors continues with the pads becoming smaller, less cumbersome, and reasonably priced. The HipSaver (Canton, MA) retails for under $20 (Figure 4–7). For more information on hip protectors, contact the company listed at the end of this chapter.

Another way to approach hip fracture prevention is to change the elderly person's intrinsic qualities that specifically contribute to fractures. To decrease risk of hip fracture, an individual should increase bone density and muscle strength by minimizing caffeine intake, not smoking, and walking for exercise.[29(pp771,772)]

Treatment of Hip Fractures

During the initial evaluation, the therapist should ascertain the following information in addition to the standard assessment pre-

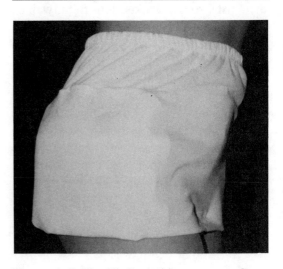

Figure 4–7 The HipSaver hip protector. Courtesy of HipSaver Inc., Canton, Massachusetts.

sented in Chapter 2: The therapist needs to know the type of fracture (intracapsular or extracapsular), the method of internal fixation if any, the WB orders, special precautions, and the mechanism of injury. (It is important to discover whether the patient had had several falls or whether the patient had slipped on a patch of ice while shoveling snow from the front walk.) In addition, the therapist needs to determine the patient's premorbid status of function and gait. Many studies have determined that poor prior functional level in either basic activities of daily living (ADL) (eating, dressing, grooming, toileting, etc.), instrumental ADL (shopping, preparing meals, using the telephone, etc.), poor prefracture gait, or dementia lead to longer hospital stays and discharges to nursing homes.[30(p293),31(pp570,571)]

Phase I (PO Days 2 to 14)

During the initial recovery phase, it is imperative to protect the fracture site from external and internal forces. The strength of the involved hip is generally in the Poor (2/5) range. The patient usually complains of an ache in the groin region and tenderness over the suture line. Passive ROM is minimally impaired and active ROM is moderately decreased. Depending on the type of fracture and other preexisting conditions, edema commonly is present.

Exercise Program. During Phase I, straight-plane exercising provides the best strength and ROM recovery at the hip (Figure 4–8). The combination movements (i.e., proprioceptive neuromuscular facilitation [PNF] skill patterns) prevalent in everyday life may cause too much torque at the fracture site or cause prosthetic dislocation. Active-assisted sitting and mat exercises create a caring, educational, and pain-free experience. Less force is applied to the hip joint while the mat supports the patient, and the patient requires less strength to complete the tasks successfully. The therapist can easily switch to active or even manually resisted exercise without altering hand contact on the patient's LE. During this phase, the exercises should be performed slowly with emphasis on both concentric and eccentric control. The repetitions can be increased as tolerated, but they should not be overwhelming (i.e., 5 to 15 repetitions). Low resistance (1 to 3 lb) can also be added as needed. Two exercises that should not be included at this stage are bridging and active straight leg raising (SLR). The power generated by the massive hip muscles is so great during these exercises that there is a danger of displacing the fractured segments. In addition to the basic hip program, the therapist must prescribe a reconditioning program (see Chapter 2) based on the evaluation results.

Mobility Program. The patient performs the mobility portion of the program concurrently with the exercise and reconditioning programs. The patient with prosthetic insertion is instructed in the THPs of rolling to the unaffected side with pillows between the legs and generally avoiding contorted positions, such as crossing the legs. The patient with pins, nail, or screw fixation can simply try to avoid contorted positions. The patient should use a trapeze during bed activities, if possible, as this has been shown to decrease hip joint pressure by as much as two-thirds.[32(p173)] Bed-to-chair and chair-to-mat transfers should be performed toward the unaffected side to prevent excessive hip abduction on the fractured side.[33(p401)] Because enormous hip joint reaction forces occur during sit-to-stand transfers, the patient should be encouraged to use both hands on the armrests to

Sitting

1. Knee extension (kicking)

Slowly extend knee fully, hold for 1 second, and return slowly to flexed position under control.

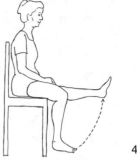

4–8A

2. Hip flexion (marching)

Lift alternate knees to chest, as if slowly marching in place while sitting.

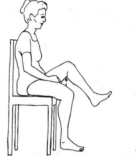

4–8B

3. Forward bending of trunk

Slowly reach hands down along the insides of the legs. Stop at the first pulling sensation. Return slowly to erect posture.

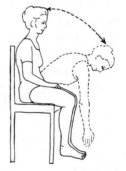

4–8C

4. Armchair push-ups

Place hands on armrests (or push-up blocks) and extend both elbows, lifting torso from chair seat. Feet should be placed on floor for balance, support, and assist.

Figure 4–8 Basic hip exercise program in straight planes

continues

Figure 4–8 continued

Supine Lying
 5. **Hip rotations**
    With hips slightly abducted and knees extended, slowly roll legs in and out.

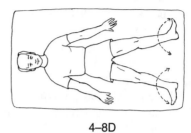

4–8D

 6. **Heel slides**
    Slide heel along mat toward the buttocks and slowly return to original position.

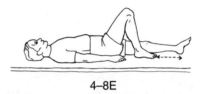

4–8E

 7. **Knee to chest**
    Flex hip, bringing knee toward the chest, and slowly return limb to extended position.

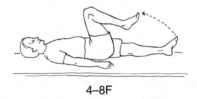

4–8F

 8. **Hip abduction/adduction**
    Slowly spread legs apart and pull them together, keeping the knees extended and the toes pointed upward.

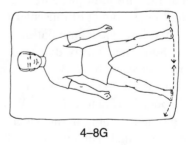

4–8G

 9. **Terminal knee extension** (see Figure 6–6 in Chapter 6)

Prone Lying
10. **Hip flexor stretch**
    Lie prone for up to 20 minutes daily. Place pillow or bolster under ankles for comfort.

continues

Figure 4–8 continued

11. Knee flexion

Flex knee and bring heel toward buttocks.
Return to extended position.

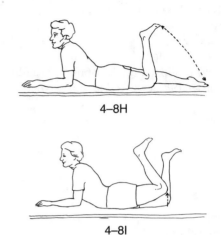

4–8H

12. Hip extension

With knee flexed to 90°, lift knee slightly off
mat without rotating pelvis and slowly lower
knee to mat.

4–8I

push off during transfers. The ability to perform the three functional milestone activities
of supine-to-sit transfer, sit-to-supine transfer, and sit-to-stand transfer independently
(along with ambulation) increases the odds
of being discharged directly to home from
the acute care hospital.[34(p824)]

Ambulation Program. Ambulation activities are limited by WB orders and the patient's tolerance. The therapist should remember that hip joint pressure increases in
relation to the amount of muscular force applied; therefore, slow ambulation is prefer-
able. (The patient rarely disagrees on this
matter.) Patients with PWB orders can ambulate with a device on level surfaces. If a therapeutic pool is available, the TDWB patient
can begin gait training in the water after the
sutures are healed. The buoyancy of the water prevents excessive hip joint pressure during normal ambulation. TDWB (10% WB)
can be performed with the patient submerged
to neck level and PWB (25% WB) can be
performed in chest-high water.[35] Depending
on physician preference, many patients are
allowed unrestricted WB at this time. The

therapist should be alert for any increases in
symptoms during stance phase for this patient. All patients should begin to learn basic
maneuvering skills (walking forwards, backwards, sideways, around furniture, etc.) with
appropriate device and assistance for short
distances.

Activities of Daily Living Program. ADL
are also dependent on WB orders. If the patient is TDWB, most activities are better
learned while sitting. If the patient is PWB,
most grooming activities can be performed
safely in a bilateral standing position with a
chair nearby for safety. The therapist needs to
guard the patient closely during these activities until the patient achieves independence.
For patients with hemiarthroplasties, care
should be taken to avoid excessive hip flexion, adduction, and internal rotation (IR)
during dressing activities. In addition, excessive trunk flexion (when putting on shoes
and socks) can also place too much stress on
the prosthesis, increasing the risk of dislocation. The patient should be taught to use
dressing sticks and stocking aids as needed.
(See THPs later in this chapter.) A raised toi-

let seat or grab bars may also be needed for safe toileting and should be evaluated by the therapist.

Phase II (PO Weeks 2 to 6)

After the initial two weeks of rehabilitation, sufficient soft and bony tissue healing has occurred to allow for more intensive exercise, ambulation, and ADL programs. By now, the patient's hip strength should be approaching the Fair/Fair plus (3+/5) range, the ache in the groin and over the suture line should be disappearing, ROM should be within functional limits, and general conditioning should be good. At PO Week 3, the physician may request radiographs to confirm the healing process. If all is proceeding satisfactorily, the physician usually orders increased WB for the patient and discontinues the THPs for patients with prostheses.

Exercise Program. The patient can now perform most of the mat exercise program independently or as part of the home program. At this time, the patient continues to work on any remaining strength or ROM deficits and begins to exercise with more emphasis on speed.

Since the hip is a WB joint, it should be reeducated in its position of function; therefore, the majority of the one-on-one exercise program should now be performed in the upright position. The patient begins the standing exercise program shown in Figure 4–9, while the therapist provides contact guard as needed for balance and safety. If the patient is PWB on the affected limb, external support (e.g., a walker, a table, or parallel bars) must be provided during the exercises.

The therapist must also start to customize the program to the patient's interests. For example, a 71-year-old artist could sketch while standing at an easel, thereby improving her standing balance and endurance. In addition, therapy can be made fun by transforming aluminum walkers into soccer goals or straight canes into hockey sticks or baseball bats. Balloons and Nerf balls make the safest soccer balls, pucks, and baseballs. With a healthy imagination, home situations can also be simulated easily in the therapy gym.

If a therapeutic pool is available (or even a hotel pool), additional conditioning exercises can be performed along with the pool ambulation program. Woolfenden[36(p216)] recommends the following exercises for elderly patients recovering from femoral neck fractures: begin with shallow-water ambulation activities and progress to the deep-water exercises of walking with breast stroke, sidelying scissor kicks, and T-exercises as described in Exhibit 4–1.

Mobility Program. The mobility retraining program focuses on normalizing motion. If a trapeze has been used, it can now be discontinued. With the THPs lifted, the patient can move around freely with minimal fear of dislocation. However, common sense dictates that contorted positions still should be avoided as much as possible. All transfers can now safely be performed to both sides. A major goal of therapy should be independence in sit-to-stand and stand-to-sit transfers since one of the major reasons for nursing home placement is the inability to transfer independently.

Ambulation Program. The ambulation training program begins in earnest. High-level gait skills must be started now, even though the patient might still need a walker or physical assistance. The patient continues to work on maneuverability as well as balance activities. The patient's ambulation ve-

1. **Bilateral standing balance**
   Stand unsupported with weight distributed evenly between both legs (must be at least 50% weight bearing). Progress from static to dynamic balance training through functional activity or game playing (e.g., shooting Velcro darts). Progress to heel-offs (ankle plantarflexion) and toe-offs (ankle dorsiflexion) if sufficient ankle ROM is present.

2. **Marching in place**
   With external support for balance, alternately lift knees as high as possible.

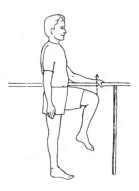

3. **Slight knee bends**
   Bend knees slightly (20°) and straighten, maintaining erect posture. Do not squat.

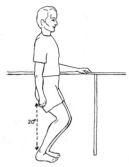

4. **Hip abduction**
   While holding onto a table or chair, lift leg out to side, keeping knee straight; return to bilateral standing.

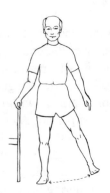

Figure 4–9 Basic standing hip exercise program

continues

Figure 4–9 continued

5. Hip extension
While holding onto a table or chair, lift leg backward and return to bilateral standing. The knee can be straight or bent.

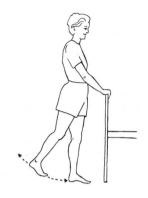

6. Transfer training
Scoot to the edge of the chair and stand. Maintain standing balance for at least 5 seconds, then slowly return to sitting.

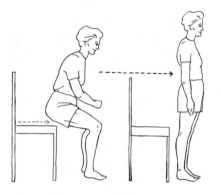

locity (distance/time) and ambulation endurance should be measured and trained. To ambulate safely in the community (e.g., cross streets, shop, bank), the patient should be able to walk at a velocity of 150 to 208 ft/min (44.5 to 63.5 m/min) and be able to traverse a distance of about 1,000 ft.[37(pp1372,1373)] (Because of reimbursement problems, many patients do not achieve these ambulation goals before discharge.) The patient should also begin to negotiate uneven surfaces such as ramps, curbs, and stairs, even for limited distances.

Activities of Daily Living Program. When the THPs are discontinued, the thera-pist should wean the patient off the assistive devices for dressing (i.e., stocking aids, dressing sticks). The patient should be independent in most grooming and toileting activities, preferably while standing. Showers should be taken on a tub seat for obvious safety reasons. Meal preparation should be attempted (or simulated) as should other kitchen activities such as reaching into a cupboard or carrying a cup of tea while also managing the proper ambulation device.

Phase III (PO Week 6 on)

During Phase III, the therapist concentrates on bringing the patient to the highest

Exhibit 4–1 Aquatic Exercises for Elderly Patients with Femoral Neck Fractures

---

Aquatic Exercise Tips

- Exercises are performed without pain or without increasing pain.
- Whenever possible, treat decreases in range of motion (ROM) and weakness simultaneously. The supportive and resistive nature of water permits this more easily than on land.
- Any exercise may be made more difficult by increasing the speed of performance, the surface area or length of the resistance arm, or the amount of buoyant resistance.
- Initially the time spent in shallow water is short, and is used to familiarize the patient with control of movement in the aquatic environment.
- It is important to train and develop spinal stability and postural alignment. Do not let lumbar movements substitute for hip or other lower extremity (LE) motions.

Deep-Water Exercises for Patients with Femoral Neck Fractures

1. **Walking with breast stroke arms forward and backward.** Start by moving the arms in a symmetrical motion of breast stroke and the legs in a bicycling motion. Gradually change the bicycling motion of the legs to a striding motion.
2. **Side-lying scissors.** Perform while holding barbells or instructional swim bars or doing upper extremity sidestroke motion. The legs are moved in a scissoring motion in an anteroposterior plane. In the stretch position, the anterior LE is positioned with hip flexed, knee extended, and ankle dorsiflexed. The posterior LE is positioned with hip extended, knee flexed, and ankle plantarflexed or relaxed. During the push phase, the back knee is extended, and then the two extremities switch positions.
3. **T-exercises:** Perform in vertical, while lightly holding onto two instructional swim bars for support. Maintain neutral spine position.
   a. *Scissors:* Asymmetrically flex and extend at the hips with knees extended. When lower extremity is in front of the body, dorsiflex the foot.
   b. *Hip abduction and adduction:* Abduct and adduct the hips bilaterally and dorsiflex the ankles in the abducted position.
   c. *Hip circles:* Perform hip circles with straight legs by first flexing the hips, then abducting them, then simultaneously extend and adduct the hips and then return to the starting position. Repeat in opposite direction. When the legs are in the forward position, dorsiflex the ankles.

Source: Adapted with permission from J.T. Woolfenden, Aquatic Physical Therapy Approaches for the Extremities, *Orthopaedic Physical Therapy Clinics of North America*, Vol. 3, No. 2, pp. 209–230, © 1994, W.B. Saunders Company.

---

functional level possible. Exercises per se are limited to the patient's home program. The therapist can now safely add bridging and SLR to the exercise regimen. As the patient approaches complete fracture healing and FWB, gait training consists of eliminating gait deviations, progressing ambulation devices, increasing ambulation velocity, increasing ambulation endurance, and improving the patient's maneuvering ability on all surfaces (including stairs). Treadmill training with handrails can be initiated to improve gait pattern and gait speed, but care should be taken as many elderly patients have vestibular problems. If FWB, the active patient should strive for one-legged standing balance (with eyes open) of 5 to 10 seconds, but this is extremely difficult. In a study by Jarnlo and Thorngren, patients perceived that their balance was impaired up to 2 years after they fractured their hips. This was confirmed by an observed increased postural sway on a computerized platform. The investigators recommended that rehabilitation include more emphasis on balance retraining.[38(p422)] Depending on the patient's personality, many therapeutic games or avocational simulations can be performed at this time to hone high-level ambulation, coordination, proprioception, and balancing skills.

If a patient continues to complain of high levels of pain, the patient should be rechecked by the physician. If the medical results are negative, the therapist should reevaluate the patient for possible pelvic dysfunction. The impact of the fall that caused the hip fracture can also alter pelvic alignment. In a study by Scotece et al., manual therapy (consisting of muscle energy and strain-counterstrain techniques) and stabilization exercises for the lumbar spine and sacroiliac joint decreased pain and increased function in 32 elderly patients who had hip surgery.[39]

The performance of ADL tasks should be approaching independence with an ambulation device. For a patient with balance impairment, a walker basket or pouch may be a necessary addition for independent functional ambulation. Dressing and toileting aids also should be prescribed as needed, as well as railings, grab bars, raised toilet seats,

bedside commodes, and shower/tub seats for the home.

Exercising after Discharge from Therapy

Continuing the exercise program after the patient is discharged from therapy is crucial to patient improvement. Functional outcomes (see below) have been poor after hip fracture. Sherrington and Lord developed a simple strengthening exercise for patients living at home, which they implemented approximately 7 months after the fracture.[40(pp210,211)] The exercise consisted of performing an increasing number of step-ups and step-downs on a 5 or 10 cm step (made out of telephone books wrapped in packing tape). The therapist evaluated the appropriate size step and the number of repetitions (between 5 and 50) to be performed daily by each patient. Patients could hold onto furniture for support. After 1 month of independent exercising, they found the exercise had a high compliance rate, was safe, and significantly increased lower limb strength and walking velocity. Theoretically, this simple exercise should reduce the risk of future falls and subsequent fractures. Further studies need to be done to see if this is actually the case in this high-risk group.

Functional Outcomes of Hip Fracture

Functional outcome studies are only now becoming available for patients with hip fracture. Some older studies mention the ability to ambulate on a flat level surface, but not under functional conditions. For survivors of hip fracture, major disability commonly occurs and lasts for months to years after the incident. Some of the functional outcomes measured 1-year postfracture are:

- 55.4% of patients return to independent ADL.[41]

- 41% of patients return to prefracture ambulatory ability.[42]
- 16.7% of institutionalized patients regain prior functional ability and only 12.9% return to their prior ambulation ability.[43]
- 21% of patients over 75 years return to prefracture instrumental ADL.[44]

Few studies have indicated what is the best rehabilitation program for patients with hip fracture. An interdisciplinary approach with emphasis on functional goals has been successful in decreasing hospitalization and improving independence. The amount of therapy received has also had a positive effect on functional outcome. In a study by Guccione et al, the odds of being discharged to home directly from the acute care hospital were 5.7 times greater for those patients receiving one or more physical therapy sessions a day.[34(p824)] However, further research into the type of therapeutic treatment that will optimize functional recovery for patients with hip fractures still needs to be done.

Summary of Treatment of Hip Fractures

- Know the type of fracture and internal fixation, as well as the WB order and any movement precautions ordered.
- *During the first 2 weeks postoperatively*
  1. protect the fracture site from unnecessary WB or rotational forces
  2. begin active-assisted exercises in sitting, supine, and prone positions, progressing to active exercise in straight planes of movement
  3. begin mobility and ADL training concurrently, emphasizing independence in transfers and ambulation.

- *As the fracture stabilizes*
  1. progress WB on physician's order
  2. begin active exercises in standing posture
  3. begin to work on speed as well as power
  4. customize exercises to include the patient's interests
  5. discontinue THPs on physician's order
  6. begin aerobic conditioning
  7. emphasize gait maneuverability, functional gait speed and endurance, and negotiating uneven surfaces including stairs
  8. focus on normalizing ADL skills, weaning off unnecessary assistive devices.

- *As the fracture heals*
  1. progress to FWB on physician's order
  2. normalize gait pattern on all surfaces (with device)
  3. emphasize proprioceptive and balance retraining
  4. teach independence in all ADL activities with device
  5. encourage continued WB exercises for life.

- Do not prescribe unnecessary equipment or exercise.

OSTEOARTHRITIS

With increasing age, a common complaint at the hip is osteoarthritis (OA). For reasons not presently understood, the articular cartilage of WB joints undergoes progressive degeneration that apparently begins with a decrease in the concentration of proteoglycans. This results in a loss of strength and ability of the cartilage to absorb shock. The subchondral bone is then more susceptible to repetitive fatigue fractures.[45(pp608,609)] In response to these stresses, the subchondral bone remodels itself, eventually forming spurs and subarticular cysts, which contribute further to the degeneration of the articular cartilage.[46(p29)]

Interestingly, the two most widely accepted theories proposed to explain the causes of OA are opposite in nature, but not mutually exclusive: (1) habitual overuse (i.e., the wear-and-tear theory) and (2) habitual disuse with loss of cartilage nutrition. Both are suspected of somehow causing abnormal mechanical stresses within the hip joint that trigger the destruction of the articular cartilage. Other factors that possibly predispose a person to developing OA of the hip are:

- genetics
- hip joint infection
- hip flexion contracture
- femoral or acetabular fractures with malunion
- avascular necrosis of the femoral head
- slipped capital femoral epiphysis
- developmental dislocation of the hip
- Legg-Calvé-Perthes disease[47(p6)]

Clinically, the patient complains about some or all of the following symptoms:

- gradual progression of a dull hip pain in the inguinal area that can also refer to the medial knee joint
- pain that increases with activity and decreases with rest
- morning stiffness
- pain and difficulty in walking
- loss of functional mobility

On evaluation, the therapist may also find the following signs:

- antalgic gait (pain on WB side)
- gluteus medius limp
- capsular pattern (ROM limited in extension, IR, and abduction)
- possible flexion, adduction, and/or external rotation (ER) contractures
- decreased strength
- disuse atrophy

Roentgenograms of the hip joint may show joint-space narrowing, subchondral bony sclerosis, bone cysts, or osteophyte formations[20(p8)]; however, radiographs cannot reveal the severity of the patient's symptoms.[45(pp608,609)]

Conservative Treatment of the Osteoarthritic Hip

The conservative approach to the treatment of OA is to unload the affected hip as much as possible to prevent further cartilage destruction. The doctor may also prescribe nonsteroidal anti-inflammatory drugs and order physical therapy to increase ROM and strength.

Exercise Program

The exercise program is initiated to attain two important goals: (1) restoration of normal ROM and (2) improvement in hip strength. The losses of motion and strength can result from disuse as well as from the disease process itself. Therefore, a complete reconditioning program needs to be designed for the LEs, including an aerobic component.

The application of heat modalities (hydrocollator pack or ultrasound) to the hip region prior to exercising reduces muscle spasm and pain. PNF is an excellent method of rehabilitating the LE of the patient with hip OA. The PNF LE skill pattern Diagonal 1 (D1) in supine position is an efficient form of exer-

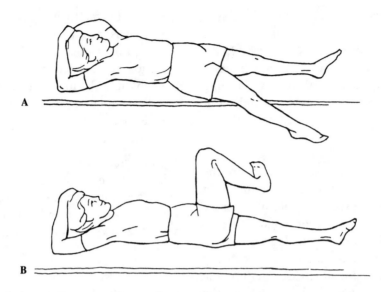

Figure 4–10 Proprioceptive neuromuscular facilitation D1 pattern. (A) Start with hip in extension, abduction, and internal rotation; knee in extension; and foot in plantarflexion and eversion. (B) Bring hip into flexion, adduction, and external rotation; knee into flexion; and foot into dorsiflexion and inversion. Reverse to starting position.

cise for patients with OA (Figure 4–10). The D1 flexor component encompasses hip flexion, adduction, and ER. The D1 extensor component encompasses hip extension, abduction, and IR—the three motions most often lost because of OA of the hip. The exercises can be assisted or resisted, and the therapist can adjust the timing of the exercise as needed. The D1 exercise restores strength and ROM simultaneously, and reconditions the entire LE. In addition, exercises specifically directed at strengthening the hip abductors can be beneficial.[48(p3)] As the patient progresses, an aerobic activity such as bicycle riding should be added to the program. Impact aerobics and jogging activities should be discouraged.

The therapist must also evaluate the patient's entire lower quarter for muscle imbalances and posture. By maintaining proper skeletal alignment, the impact loading on the hip may be reduced.[47(p10)] The reader is referred to the muscle imbalance section later in this chapter.

Passive ROM activities, such as gentle stretching at the end of available range and joint mobilization (inferior glide and lateral distraction) to the hip capsule, are also indicated for the osteoarthritic hip. However, excessive stretching can exacerbate hip arthritis. The myofascial release leg pull technique may be helpful, but caution should be taken if the hip joint is acutely inflamed.

If a therapeutic pool is available, the upright exercises in Figure 4–13 can be performed in the water. In addition, different leg movements such as the "flutter" and "frog" kicks are excellent for improving strength and coordination in the LEs. The flutter kick can be practiced in both supine and prone po-

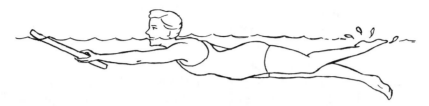

Figure 4–11 Prone flutter kicking with a kickboard. Knees should be kept in relative extension and the ankles should be relaxed. The use of a kickboard increases the intensity of the exercise.

sitions. For a more strenuous workout, kickboards can be used (Figure 4–11). The therapeutic pool is a perfect modality for the patient with OA. The heated environment soothes the musculature, and the buoyant quality of the water prevents excessive hip joint pressure during WB activities.

Mobility Program

The affected hip must be protected from unnecessary stresses while the patient undergoes the mobility retraining program. Sidelying on the painful hip for prolonged periods should be avoided. However, the patient should be encouraged to lie prone for at least 15 minutes daily to prevent loss of hip extension.

Standing up from a sitting position should be achieved with help from the upper extremities to unload the hip. Armrests on chairs and grab bars in the bathroom therefore are recommended.

The therapist should bring the patient through the entire developmental sequence. Sitting and quadruped exercises with a physioball can increase strength and proprioception in unstable postures. These functional exercises will improve the patient's balance, coordination, and confidence in all positions. Finally, the therapist should instruct the patient on how to get on and off the floor.

Ambulation Program

One of the most beneficial ways to unload the hip is to hold a cane or crutch in the opposite hand. A slower ambulation velocity also reduces the hip joint reaction force. If the patient is already exercising in the water, ambulation activities should be performed there as well. The patient needs to be able to maneuver on all surfaces and in all directions safely and with confidence. Ambulation on uneven surfaces, such as grass or gravel, provides necessary proprioceptive training. Balance activities in bilateral standing without device should be included in the program. The patient must learn to monitor pain and fatigue and to rest appropriately to prevent further articular damage. If a patient deteriorates to the point of needing bilateral support in order to ambulate, surgical intervention (osteotomy or THA) usually is indicated.

Activities of Daily Living Program

Most ADL elements can be taught safely in bilateral standing, although the patient should be encouraged to sit and rest as needed. Lifestyle modifications to unload the hip initially involve minor changes such as carrying smaller loads of laundry or lighter bags of groceries, or installing railings on stairways. Modifications of activities should also include stressing the importance of weight reduction in overweight or obese patients. Loss of weight can significantly improve function (and general health) and reduce hip symptoms.[48(p4)] In addition, the patient should be encouraged to participate in nonimpact sport activities, such as swimming, "mall walking," and golf.

Summary of the Conservative Treatment of the Osteoarthritic Hip

- Unload the affected hip as much as possible.
- Strengthen the entire LE, especially hip abduction.
- Restore joint ROM, especially hip extension, abduction, and IR.
- Optimize skeletal alignment and muscle balance of the entire lower quarter.
- Use a cane in the opposite hand during WB activities to minimize the joint reaction forces.
- Encourage nonimpact aerobic activities.
- Modify activities (including ADL) to reduce joint reaction forces.

Surgical Treatment of the Osteoarthritic Hip

If conservative management is unsuccessful, the orthopaedic surgeon has two options for helping the elderly patient with severe OA of the hip: proximal femoral osteotomy and THA. (Hip arthrodesis is usually reserved for younger patients or heavy laborers.)[48(p5)] THA is discussed in greater detail later in this chapter.

Proximal Femoral Osteotomy

The pain resulting from OA of the hip can be relieved by an osteotomy, which redistributes some of the WB stresses by changing the skeletal alignment of the femur. By removing a wedge of bone from the medial side of the femur (Figure 4–12), all muscle tension is reduced and healthy cartilage is rotated into a WB position.[49(pp148,149)] Osteotomy is most suited for the young elderly patient with a stable hip joint and with limited articular damage.[48(p4)]

In general, the conservative treatment for the OA patient outlined above can be used for rehabilitating the patient with osteotomy

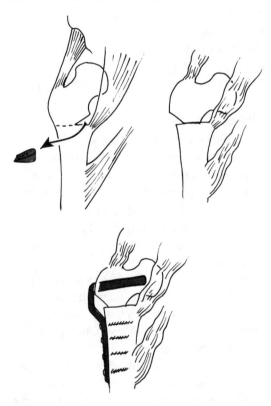

Figure 4–12 Proximal femoral osteotomy. *Source:* Reprinted with permission from G.A. Shankman, Orthopaedic Management of the Hip and Pelvis, *Fundamental Orthopaedic Management for the Physical Therapist Assistant*, p. 197, © 1997, Mosby-Year Book, Inc.

with the exception of WB status and activities. Because the femur has been surgically fractured, protected WB is ordered until complete healing occurs. Ambulation and ADL skills are taught with a walker or crutches. After full WB orders are received, the therapist slowly progresses the patient through a pain-free functional exercise program including mini step-ups, one-quarter wall squats, and treadmill training.[50(p197)] Total body conditioning with nonimpact aerobic activities has also been found to be useful.

RHEUMATOID ARTHRITIS OF THE HIP

Unlike OA, rheumatoid arthritis (RA) is a systemic inflammatory disease that primarily affects synovial tissues. It is common worldwide, affecting more than 3.6 million persons (mostly women) in the United States.[51(pp130–131)] The etiology remains unknown, but is suspected to involve genetics[52(p25)] or infectious agents.[53(p40)] A person is diagnosed with RA if at least four of the seven criteria listed below have been present for at least 6 weeks:

1. morning stiffness of at least 1 hour in and around joints
2. arthritis of three or more areas
3. arthritis of hand joints
4. symmetric arthritis
5. rheumatoid nodules
6. serum rheumatoid factor
7. roentgenographic changes[52(p24)]

When RA affects the hip joint, severe arthrosis, deformity, pain, and disability ensue. In the early stages of the disease, the patient complains of decreased ambulation endurance and difficulty with prolonged standing, squatting, and negotiating stairs. As the disease progresses, the patient displays increasing muscle weakness, especially in the gluteal muscles and hip flexors.[47(p9)] Protrusio acetabuli (the intrapelvic protrusion of the acetabulum) is the end stage of hip RA and is caused by the WB pressure eroding the joint surface. The femoral head often flattens, causing an antalgic or waddling-type gait as abductor muscle leverage is compromised; this results in the abductor muscles exerting more effort to control hip motion.[54(p25)]

Treatment of Rheumatoid Arthritis of the Hip

The treatment approach for the person with RA of the hip involves unloading the WB forces to prevent the progression of cartilage and bony destruction.

Modalities for Pain Relief

Heat and cold can be used successfully to decrease muscle guarding and pain in patients with RA. Superficial heat (e.g., hydrocollator packs, Fluidotherapy, paraffin baths) is thought, paradoxically, to cool inflamed joints,[55] while deep heating (e.g., ultrasound) raises joint temperature.[56(p1)] Cold therapy (e.g., ice packs, ice massage, vapocoolant spray) applied for less than 6 minutes increases joint temperature; however, prolonged cold application (more than 10 minutes) has been found to decrease joint temperature. Many of the studies on the effects of thermal therapy reach conflicting conclusions. No consensus on the best treatment is yet possible. There are even some indications that placing deep heat over inflamed joints is harmful. In general, there appears to be no major differences between heat and cold in clinical outcome or patient preference, but both modalities have had a positive effect on patient symptoms.[54(p87)]

Exercise Program

During acute exacerbations, isometric exercise appears to be the treatment of choice for maintaining strength with little joint motion. Isometrics should be performed at various hip joint angles because there is little transference of strength gains throughout range. Isometrics are also appropriate to use as stabilizing exercises for the trunk and pelvis. As the inflammation subsides, low resistance isotonic training is appropriate.

In general, if pain lasts longer than 2 hours after exercising, the intensity of the exercise program is too great and should be adjusted. Aquatic exercises, as shown in Figure 4–13, can also increase muscle strength while protecting the hip joint from excessive joint reaction forces. Light stretching is also important to maintain or increase flexibility. Stretches should be held for 10 to 30 seconds in sets of three to five repetitions.[54(p99)] In addition, aerobic exercise (such as walking, Tai Chi, and bicycle riding) has been beneficial, increasing aerobic capacity, walking time, and physical activity.[57(p1396)]

Mobility Program

The emphasis of the mobility program is to make the patient functional in bed, transfers, and ambulation while unloading the hip as much as possible. Since RA usually affects many joints, one joint cannot be protected at the expense of another. Patient education on joint protection and the need for rest periods is important.

Ambulation Program

The emphasis of this program is on *functional* ambulation. If assistive devices are needed, they must also protect the joints of the wrist and hand, which are commonly affected by RA. Platform walkers and crutches can unload the hip greatly without stressing the small hand joints, but they tend to be bulky and fatiguing to use. Preambulation exercises of mini wall squats, supported heel-offs, and mini step-ups may be helpful in restoring sufficient strength for gait; however, these activities may be too strenuous for patients with severe involvement of the feet and knees. Functional ambulation (the ability to walk to a destination in order to do something of importance) should be stressed over correcting gait deviations and progressing assistive devices. Stair climbing of even one step should be taught because many buildings and sidewalks require the ability to negotiate a 7-inch step.

Activities of Daily Living Program

Because of the multijoint involvement of RA, the ADL program needs to be individually tailored to the patient's many impairments and needs. Hip RA mainly compromises instrumental ADL because it affects the ability to ambulate for even short distances. The patient should be encouraged to perform and try out various approaches to problems that limit independence, while adhering to joint protection and energy conservation principles. Many adaptive devices are available and should be evaluated and prescribed by the occupational therapist. (For more information on adaptive devices, the reader is referred to the texts at the end of this chapter.)

Summary of Treatment of Rheumatoid Arthritis of the Hip

- Unload the affected hip (usually bilateral) as much as possible.

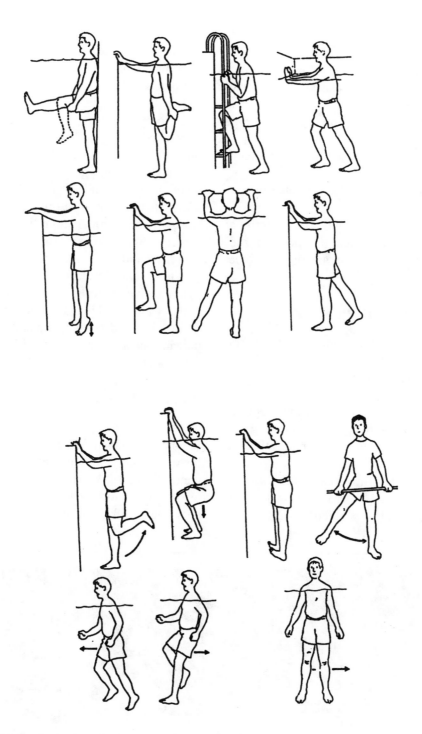

Figure 4–13 Pool exercises for lower extremity strengthening. *Source:* Reprinted from V.A. Brander, Rehabilitation Following Hip, Knee, and Shoulder Arthroplasty in *Rehabilitation of Persons with Rheumatoid Arthritis*, R.W. Chang, ed., p. 162, © 1996, Aspen Publishers, Inc.

- Use heat or cold modalities to decrease pain and muscle guarding.
- Use strength training of the LEs to prevent progressive weakness and maintain function.
- Stretch the affected joints gently to optimize flexibility.
- Stress functional mobility and ambulation.
- Teach joint protection and energy conservation principles.
- Prescribe ambulation and functional (adaptive) equipment that does not sacrifice the integrity of one joint to protect another.

TOTAL HIP ARTHOPLASTY

In 1938 Philip Wiles implanted the first THA. Many other pioneers (e.g., Moore, Bohlman, Judet, Charnley, and McKee) continued the work, each one refining the process. The evolution of total joint replacements continues today with ongoing experiments using different materials and designs.[23(pp3-4)]

Unlike hip fracture treatment, which is emergency surgery performed on frail elderly patients, THA is elective surgery performed on healthy elderly patients. The operation usually takes 2 to 3 hours and the patient may require up to three units of packed red blood cells.[58(p1)] Approximately 200,000 THAs are performed each year, achieving good to excellent results in nearly all cases. Advanced age is no longer a contraindication, with patients more than 80 years of age successfully undergoing the procedure to maintain quality in their lives. (Not surprisingly, in this oldest surgical group, there were more minor complications from surgery, slightly longer hospitalizations, and slower rehabilitation.)[59(pp131,132)]

The rehabilitation of the patient with a THA involves education, reconditioning, and gait retraining. The therapist needs to be aware of the different THAs and the special precautions associated with differing surgical approaches.

Prosthetic Hardware

A THA usually consists of a metallic femoral component and an ultrahigh molecular weight polyethylene acetabular component (Figure 4–14). This metal-to-plastic interface allows for a stable fixation with a low coefficient of friction. With concern growing

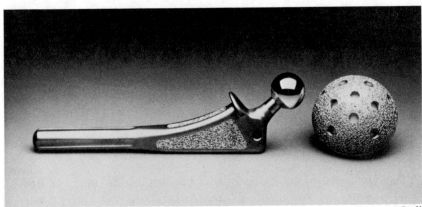

Figure 4–14 Total hip replacement (porous-coated). Courtesy of Zimmer Inc., Warsaw, Indiana.

over particulate matter causing lysis of bone in implants, other designs are being proposed, including ceramic-on-polyethylene components and the metal-on-metal interface that was discarded 20 years ago.[60(pS244)]

The components can either be cemented or uncemented. (See section on acrylic cement earlier in this chapter.) In general, the results from both have been similar, except that the uncemented prosthesis causes more thigh pain and tends to cost more. [48(p7),61(pp163,164),62(p105)] The best-of-both-worlds scenario created the hybrid arthroplasty, which uses a cemented femoral component with an uncemented acetabular component. The hybrid eliminates the increased thigh pain experienced with uncemented femurs, as well as the loosening of the acetabular component that occurred with cemented fixation.[63(pp2,8),64(p155)]

Over the past 30 years, THAs have evolved in response to failures caused initially by infection and component loosening.

As we enter the new millennium, the next hurdle to overcome in joint replacement is the loss of skeletal bone, which is augmented by the body's response to stress shielding and particulate debris (Figure 4–15). New prosthetic materials that will protect bone loss from occurring will have to be designed for joint replacement to be successful in the future.[65(p194)]

Prosthetic Dislocation

Dislocation of the femoral component from the acetabular component occurs in 1 to 8% (3% average) of primary THA operations. Dislocations are due primarily to patient factors and surgical factors. The patient factors include weak or imbalanced hip muscles,[66(p45)] preexisting femoral anteversion, marked genu valgus, a history of previous hip operations, and lack of compliance with postoperative hip precautions.[48(p9)] (See total

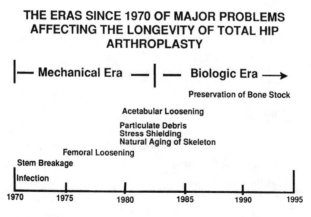

Figure 4–15 Early mechanical problems that limited the longevity of total hip replacement largely have been solved. The increased longevity of total hip replacement for periods from 10 to 15 years allows the manifestation of long-term biologic adaptation to these mechanical constructs. The effects of natural aging and bone resorption secondary to particulate debris or stress shielding pose threats to the preservation of sufficiently strong host bone. *Source:* Reprinted with permission from R. Poss, The Shape and Strength of the Human Femur, *Clinical Orthopaedics and Related Research*, Vol. 274, p. 200, © 1992, J.B. Lippincott Company.

hip precautions below.) The surgical factors include using a posterolateral surgical approach (rather than an anterolateral approach), malaligning the prosthesis, performing a trochanteric osteotomy,[67(p201)] and being a less experienced surgeon.[68(p206)] In addition, postoperative hip ROM that exceeds the ROM allowed by the THA can contribute to dislocation.

Total Hip Precautions

To insert the THA, the surgeon must open the hip capsule and dislocate the affected hip. The surgeon can choose one of three ways to gain access to the hip joint: (1) anterolateral approach, (2) lateral approach, or (3) posterolateral approach. The affected anatomical structures and the standard movement precautions associated with the different surgical approaches are described in Table 4–2. Some surgeons prefer more strict limitations on movement, especially with-

in the first 6 weeks postoperatively when most dislocations occur. For posterolateral approach, these severe THPs include no hip flexion beyond 90°, no hip IR, nor adduction past neutral. For anterior approach, these severe THPs include no hip extension past 0° (as would occur in normal walking), no hip ER, nor adduction past neutral. The movement precautions prescribed are solely determined by the orthopaedic surgeon and can vary considerably from hospital to hospital and doctor to doctor. The therapist must maintain good communication with the physician to know which THPs to use following surgery. In an unscientific polling of seven orthopaedic surgeons in the Boston area in 1997, four preferred standard THPs and three preferred severe THPs.

For anterolateral approach, the patient avoids activities that place the hip in extension, adduction, and ER, such as bed mobility and standing while turning away from the operative side.[48(p10)] For posterolateral ap-

Table 4–2 Standard Total Hip Precautions (THPs) for Different Surgical Approaches

Surgical Approach	Anatomical Structures Affected	Contraindicated Motions
Anterior	Tensor fasciae latae Gluteus medius	Simultaneous hip extension and external rotation
Lateral	Gluteus medius Greater trochanter (osteotomy)	Simultaneous hip flexion, adduction, and internal rotation
Posterolateral	Tensor fasciae latae Gluteus maximus External rotators	Simultaneous hip flexion, adduction, and internal rotation

Many orthopaedic surgeons order the simultaneous contraindicated motions shown in the table above; however, some order severe THPs limiting hip flexion to less than 90°, hip adduction to neutral, and hip internal rotation to neutral (for a posterolateral approach). Most surgeons discontinue the THPs after 3 months, but some prefer to maintain them indefinitely.

Data from *Common Disorders of the Hip*, M.C. Singleton and E.F. Branch, eds., © 1986, Haworth Press.

proach, the patient avoids the following types of activities:

- excessive trunk or hip flexion while putting on socks or shoes
- rolling in bed without a pillow between legs
- crossing legs, especially avoiding IR
- keeping legs together when sitting (Do not sit like a lady!)
- sitting in low chairs or soft chairs
- leaning forward in bed to pull up sheets or blankets

- lying on the operated side (unless approved by doctor)
- any contorted or torqued positions

THPs may be discontinued by the orthopaedic surgeon after 3 months.[58(p3)] By that time, a strong pseudo-capsule will have formed about the hip and the patient can resume normal activities (Table 4–3). Five of the 7 surgeons polled in 1997 discontinued THPs in 3 months. Some physicians, however, prefer to maintain THPs indefinitely for their patients.

Table 4–3 Approximate Time Frames to Resume Activities after Total Hip Arthroplasty (THA)

Activity	Approximate Time Frame in Postoperative (PO) Weeks
Drive a car*	3–6
Swim	6
Return to work part-time*	6
Resume sexual intercourse*	after discharge from hospital with THPs
Lie on operated side	8 weeks or sooner on physician approval
Ride a stationary bicycle	8
Sleep without pillow between legs	8
Use regular toilet	8
Cross nonoperative leg over operative leg	8–12
Put on own shoes and socks (without dressing aids)	8–12
Return to work full-time*	12
Play golf or bowl‡	12–16
Do low-impact aerobics‡	16–32
Play doubles tennis‡	24–32

Until the physician has discontinued total hip precautions (THPs), the patient must receive orders before initiating any of these activities.

Source: Data from Thomas RL, "Management of hip fracture in the geriatric patient: A team approach in the institutional setting," *Topics in Geriatric Rehabilitation*, 1996;12(1):66.

*Brander VA, Stulberg SD, Chang RW, "Life after total hip arthroplasty," *Bulletin on the Rheumatic Diseases*, 1993;42(3).

‡Holpit LA, "Preoperative and postoperative physical therapy for the total shoulder, hip, and knee replacement patient," *Orthopaedic Physical Therapy Clinics of North America*, 1993;2(1):113.

Treatment of the Patient with a Total Hip Arthroplasty

The therapist usually finds treatment of the patient with a THA a rewarding experience. Because the patient has opted for surgery, he or she usually is in good general health and is highly motivated to get better. Unlike the patient with a hip fracture, this patient has been in constant pain for years. Elective surgery provides immediate relief from years of pain and disability. Over the past decade, the average length of stay in the acute care hospital has been reduced from three weeks to less than one week. Patients now adhere to an accelerated exercise and mobility program while strictly maintaining THPs. Some patients require a longer rehabilitation course than described below.

Phase 0 (Preoperative Planning)

At this time, the therapist has the rare luxury of teaching the patient about the rehabilitation process before surgery. Because patients are now admitted to the hospital the night before surgery, this education process usually occurs in the form of a presurgical consult or group class. It is important to instruct the patient in diaphragmatic breathing and coughing to prevent any respiratory complications after surgery. The therapist can also teach THPs, transfer techniques to the unaffected side, and crutch walking. LE antiembolic exercises, such as isometric quadriceps and gluteal sets and ankle pumps,[69(p1198)] are also taught.

Phase I (PO Days 0 to 5)

Exercise Program. On the day of surgery, the patient is seen bedside for instruction in deep breathing, coughing, isometric gluteal sets and quadriceps sets, ankle pumps, and THPs. On PO Day 1, the patient begins therapy twice a day bedside for LE isometrics, ankle pumps, contralateral limb strengthening, UE strengthening, and review of THPs. On PO Day 2, the patient can add active-assisted straight-plane exercises (Figure 4–8) in the supine position. (Take care that the patient does not get tangled in the sheets.) The therapist should prevent hip flexion past 70 to 90°, and adduction and IR past neutral if a posterolateral surgical approach has been used. PNF skill patterns and passive stretching are contraindicated, as they may contribute to hip dislocation. By PO Days 3 to 5, the patient attends therapy in the physical therapy gym twice a day, adding sitting exercises, and progressing the mat program to active exercises.[70(p12),71(p162),72(pp87–88)]

Mobility Program. During Phase I, a trapeze can facilitate bed mobility while unloading the hip. The patient must be instructed in performing mobility functions while maintaining the appropriate THPs. Beginning on PO Day 1, the patient begins assisted bed-to-stand and bed-to-chair transfers to the unaffected side. Use of the upper extremities is encouraged to unload the hip. The therapist should be alert for any signs of orthostatic hypertension. If present, the therapist may need to use a tilt table to slowly get the patient to upright. On PO Day 3, the patient begins toilet transfers on a raised toilet seat. On PO Days 4 to 5, the patient learns to perform bed mobility and transfers with less assistance. The ability to transfer independently by PO Day 5 is one of the functional milestones necessary for discharge to home.[48(p10),70(p12),71(p164),72(pp87,88),73(p111)]

Ambulation Program. The patient with an uncemented THA is usually TDWB for the initial recovery phase. The patient with a cemented THA usually begins PWB on the affected side, although some doctors order unrestricted WB immediately. On PO Day 2 or 3, assisted ambulation begins on level surfaces in the parallel bars or with a walker.[70(p12)] If an anterolateral approach has been used, the patient avoids using a swing-through gait pattern to avoid hip hyperextension and the potential for dislocation of the THA. Independence in ambulation with a device (even for short distances) is one of the functional milestones necessary for discharge to home.[48(p10)] On PO Day 5, the patient begins to maneuver in all directions on level surfaces and begins climbing stairs with railings in the physical therapy gym.

Activities of Daily Living Program. Beginning PO Day 1, the patient attends occupational therapy twice a day for ADL training and upper extremity (UE) strengthening and endurance training.[74(pp24,25)] The patient must incorporate the THPs into all ADL tasks, such as grooming, dressing, and toileting activities. Putting on socks and shoes without excessively moving the hip into flexion and rotation becomes an enormous challenge. Long-handled shoehorns and dressing sticks are necessary at this time. The therapist should discourage the use of pantyhose and girdles, as they may constrict blood flow. If the patient has PWB orders, grooming can be performed in a bilateral standing position. If the patient is TDWB, ADL activities should be performed in sitting or supine position. If a patient is using a wheelchair, a piece of plywood should be placed between the sling seat and the wheelchair cushion to prevent excessive hip IR with flexion. The patient also may require a small abductor wedge to maintain proper hip alignment while in supine or sitting position.

The catheter is usually removed around PO Day 2. Patients who received a posterior surgical approach should cleanse the perineal area from an anterior direction, and those who received a lateral approach should cleanse the perineal area from a posterior direction to prevent excessive hip abduction from occurring.[74(p27)] For most patients with THAs, raised toilet seats with toilet frames or grab bars are a necessity. (Patients less than 5 feet tall can usually maintain THPs on a regular toilet.)

Most patients are unable to perform ADLs independently before discharge from the acute care hospital. To be discharged directly home, the patient will require a caregiver for meal preparation and other instrumental ADL, as well as light assistance in mobility, dressing, and bathing. See Table 4–4 for summary of Phase I treatment of THA.

Phase II (PO Weeks 1–3)

At this time, the patient has either been discharged to home with community care support (i.e., visiting nurse association) or has been transferred to a subacute rehabilitation facility for approximately 2 weeks. The patient's pain level drops dramatically, allowing easier performance of the ADL and exercise programs. Strict THPs remain in effect during this phase.

Exercise Program. The patient should continue supine and sitting exercises (Figure 4–8), with emphasis on concentric and eccentric muscle control. Light resistance (Theraband™ or 1 to 3 lb cuff weights) can be added as needed; but motor control, not strengthening, should be emphasized at this point. The exercises can also be performed faster to stimulate Type II muscle fibers. The therapist should ensure that

Table 4–4 Summary of Phase I (PO Days 0–5) Treatment of THA

PO Day	Exercise	Mobility	Ambulation	ADL
0 (bedside)	Deep breathing Coughing Quad & gluteal sets Ankle pumps	Use trapeze to unload hip THP instruction		
1 (bedside)	LE isometrics Ankle pumps UE strengthening Contralateral limb strengthening	Assisted bed-to-stand and bed-to-chair transfers THP instruction	WB orders per MD	
2 (bedside)	Continue as above Add active-assisted straight-plane exercises in supine	Continue bed mobility and transfers with trapeze THP instruction	Begin assisted ambulation with device on level surfaces	Begin washing and dressing with assistive devices
3–4	Continue as above Add sitting exercises Progress mat program to active exercise	Begin toilet transfers Decrease assistance in basic transfers THP instruction	Progress distance	Begin toilet transfers and toileting activities
5	Continue as above Progress repetitions Prescribe ambulation device for discharge	Independence in basic transfers THP instruction	Beginxz stairs Maneuver on level surfaces	Prescribe assistive devices for discharge

Sources: Topics in Geriatric Rehabilitation (1996;12(1):12), Copyright © 1996, Aspen Publishers, Inc, and *Clinical Orthopaedics and Related Research* (1995;316:87–88), Copyright © 1995, Lippincott-Raven Publishers.

hip flexion does not exceed 90° for patients with a posterolateral approach. Bridging and SLR are still unsafe due to the enormous joint reaction forces they generate at the hip (two to four times the body weight). The orthopaedic surgeon may restrict hip abduction exercises if a lateral approach was used. The patient with a cemented THA begins the standing exercise program (Figure 4–9) to rehabilitate the hip joint in its position of function. Patients with uncemented THAs should be introduced to the standing exercise program only after receiving PWB orders from the orthopaedic surgeon. External support must be provided. If available, therapeutic pool activities can add some variety to the program. UE strengthening continues and aerobic conditioning can be initiated.

Mobility Program. Strict THPs remain in effect during this entire rehabilitation phase. Bed mobility and transfers may continue to be difficult for the patient, but should be emphasized. If no cardiopulmonary contraindications are present, the patients should begin to lie prone for 15 minutes daily to prevent hip flexion contractures. The therapist should be insistent on this issue because muscle imbalances can cause unneeded complications, including dislocations, further along the rehabilitation road.

Ambulation Program. For the patient with a cemented THA, high-level gait training can be started. The therapist begins to "normalize" the patient's gait, slowly discontinuing the abducted or waddling gait pattern. For patients who had an anterolateral approach, a swing-thru gait is still contraindicated. Patients with uncemented prostheses must maintain protected WB (usually TDWB-to-PWB) as ordered by the doctor. All patients must learn to maneuver in varied directions and on all surfaces, including stairs, with the appropriate device. The therapist should measure ambulation velocity and endurance at this time to ensure that the patient's walking speed is safe and functional.

Activities of Daily Living Program. The patient with a cemented THA should be independent in most basic ADL tasks, including bathing and dressing with assistive devices. The patient can begin some light homemaking tasks or easy meal preparation while manipulating the walker or crutches. The patient with an uncemented THA should

continue to work on grooming and dressing activities in sitting and upright positions while maintaining THPs and WB precautions. Most instrumental ADL, including driving cars (or riding in them), continue to be contraindicated at this time.

Phase III (PO Weeks 3–6)

At this time, the patient has either been discharged home with community health services or has been discharged to a skilled nursing facility for longer term rehabilitation. A pseudo-capsule should be forming about the hip, and other soft tissues (whether split or retracted) should be healing. Strict THPs remain in effect. Around PO 6 weeks, the patient usually has a follow-up visit with the orthopaedic surgeon, who may order increased WB.

Exercise Program. Resistive exercise with light weights (under 5 lb) or Theraband™ continues to be used to restore normal strength and endurance. Hip abduction exercises may still be contraindicated in some patients. Most patients will be able to perform the standing exercise program shown in Figure 4–9 with varying amounts of support and resistance. The therapist should also instruct the patient in stretches for both the gastrocnemius and soleus muscles, lumbar stretches (with caution), and encourage the patient to continue prone-lying to stretch the hip flexors.

Mobility Program. Strict THPs remain in effect. At home, the patient should be encouraged to sit on a firm chair (preferably with armrests) and to avoid low or upholstered sofas and chairs (usually the patient's favorite). Most patients can safely transfer to either side. Car transfers need to be taught at this time in preparation for the patient's

6-week postoperative medical checkup. To maintain THPs during the car ride, the patient may need to sit on pillows and recline the backrest. The patient should avoid sitting "normally" in a car (with hips flexed over 90°) to avoid posterior dislocation in the event of a sudden stop.[75(p327)]

Ambulation Program. The patient with a cemented THA can progress to a cane when ready, but a walker should be kept at the bedside at night for safety purposes. A Trendelenburg gait (abductor lurch) is often still present due to abductor weakness. Patients who received a posterolateral approach can begin supervised sidestepping and backward walking using small steps for short distances. (Agility exercises, such as cross-overs, are obviously still contraindicated.) If possible, the therapist should encourage the patient to walk with a cane (and perhaps a companion) outdoors for progressive distance and speed. By PO Week 6, many patients can regularly walk 1 to 5 blocks.[58(p3)] Patients who are FWB can begin step-over-step stair climbing with railing and cane. The patient should try to use the powerful gluteus maximus, quadriceps, and gastrocnemius muscles to negotiate the stairs instead of compensating with excessive trunk undulations. Patients who are PWB continue to negotiate stairs one at a time to protect the prosthetic fixation.

Activities of Daily Living Program. The patient with a cemented THA should now be independent in light meal preparation. Dressing activities still require long-handled shoehorns and dressing sticks in order to maintain THPs. Heavier household tasks, such as vacuuming, making beds, or doing laundry, are still contraindicated. Patients with uncemented THAs have to maintain both WB and movement precautions, making even simple ADL activities tedious and physically draining. Assistance in meal preparation and other household tasks is still required, but at a lesser level.

Many patients resume sexual activity at this time. Although they have questions about safely resuming intercourse, they generally do not ask about it and health care professionals do not often offer unsolicited advice on this topic. Vanderbilt Medical Center has created a two-page handout on sexual activity after THA (one for each gender) that is routinely given to all patients before discharge. (See Exhibits 4–2 and 4–3.) The format is informative and nonthreatening, and opens the door to further communication between patient and health care provider.

Phase IV (PO Weeks 6–12)

Except for patients with severe complications, the majority of patients have returned home to complete the rehabilitation process. After the follow-up visit with the orthopaedic surgeon, most patients receive FWB as tolerated orders. (However, WB orders are still dependent on physician preference, and some patients continue with light WB only.) As the healing process continues, the THPs are now followed less strictly, with many patients being allowed to drive a car or return to work part-time. Patients can now be seen in an outpatient therapy department or private practice to advance their programs.

Exercise Program. The patient continues the resistive exercise program to restore strength and endurance, with emphasis on standing exercises. Resistance can be increased to the 5 to 10 lb range. Patients who have avoided abductor training can now initiate a strengthening program. Patients with an anterior approach should still avoid

Exhibit 4–2 Home Care Instructions. Total Hip Replacement: Sexual Activity—Female

HOME CARE INSTRUCTIONS
TOTAL HIP REPLACEMENT: SEXUAL ACTIVITY—FEMALE

INTRODUCTION:

Before your discharge, your physical therapist and occupational therapist will give you written instructions on your exercise program and the everyday activities you can safely perform at home.

This instruction sheet should be compatible with the instructions given to you by your therapist. The purpose of this instruction sheet is to provide you with information that will assist you to resume sexual activity.

PURPOSE:

Many patients have questions about resuming sexual activity after having a hip replacement, and often one is embarrassed to ask these questions. This sheet will offer several suggestions. It is up to you as an individual to select what is acceptable to you. Sex is, after all, a very personal and private matter.

Communication with your sexual partner is very important. You may want to share these instructions with your partner. It is especially important that you let your partner know what feels good to you as well as what causes you pain or discomfort.

INSTRUCTIONS:

It is important that you be in a comfortable position before you start sexual activity. Being in a comfortable position will make sudden movements less likely.

−OVER−

continues

Exhibit 4–2 continued

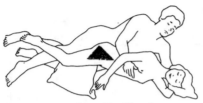

Woman lies on side with pillow between legs. The man enters from behind. The shaded triangle is the hip that had surgery.

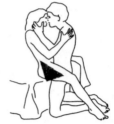

Woman sits on bed. Man kneels in front of woman. The shaded triangle is the hip that had surgery.

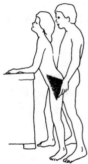

Both partners are standing. The man enters from behind. The woman uses a walker or table for support. The shaded triangle is the hip that had surgery.

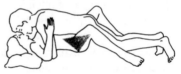

After 6 Weeks: Man above, woman below, face-to-face coital position. The shaded triangle is the hip that had surgery.

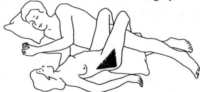

After 6 Weeks: The female lies on her back with knees flexed over male. The man enters from behind. The shaded triangle is the hip that had surgery.

CALL YOUR DOCTOR IF YOU HAVE:
    Any persistent pain
    Temperature above 100°
    Redness or drainage from incision
    Chest or calf pains, swelling, tenderness, or redness

IMPORTANT PHONE NUMBERS:
    Vanderbilt University Hospital—
    Physician—
    Home Health Agency—

Courtesy of Department of Nursing, Vanderbilt Medical Center, 1988, Nashville, Tennessee.

Exhibit 4–3 Home Care Instructions. Total Hip Replacement: Sexual Activity—Male

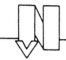

HOME CARE INSTRUCTIONS
TOTAL HIP REPLACEMENT: SEXUAL ACTIVITY—MALE

INTRODUCTION:
   Before your discharge, your physical therapist and occupational therapist will give you written instructions on your exercise program and the everyday activities you can safely perform at home.
   This instruction sheet should be compatible with the instructions given to you by your therapist. The purpose of this instruction sheet is to provide you with information that will assist you to resume sexual activity.

PURPOSE:
   Many patients have questions about resuming sexual activity after having a hip replacement, and often one is embarrassed to ask these questions. This sheet will offer several suggestions. It is up to you as an individual to select what is acceptable to you. Sex is, after all, a very personal and private matter.
   Communication with your sexual partner is very important. You may want to share these instructions with your partner. It is especially important that you let your partner know what feels good to you as well as what causes you pain or discomfort.

INSTRUCTIONS:
   It is important that you be in a comfortable position before you start sexual activity. Being in a comfortable position will make sudden movements less likely.

-OVER-

continues

Exhibit 4–3 continued

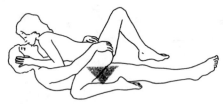

Woman above, man below, face-to-face coital position. The shaded triangle is the hip that had surgery.

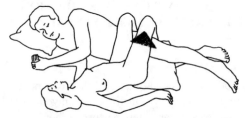

The woman lies on her back with knees flexed over male. The man enters from behind. The man keeps a pillow between his legs. The shaded triangle is the hip that had surgery.

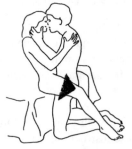

Woman sits on bed. The man kneels in front of woman. The shaded triangle is the hip that had surgery.

CALL YOUR DOCTOR IF YOU HAVE:
    Any persistent pain
    Temperature above 100°
    Redness or drainage from incision
    Chest or calf pains, swelling, tenderness, or redness

IMPORTANT PHONE NUMBERS:
    Vanderbilt University Hospital—
    Physician—
    Home Health Agency—

Courtesy of Department of Nursing, Vanderbilt Medical Center, 1988, Nashville, Tennessee.

bridging. Stretching of the ankle plantar flexors and hip flexors continues to be imperative.

As the patient begins to "feel better," the desire and motivation to continue daily exercising begin to wane. The therapist must educate the patient on the importance of continuing strengthening exercises on the functional outcome of the procedure. Multiple studies have shown that hip muscle weakness persists 2 years post-THA, jeopardizing the stability of the implant.[76(p73),77(pp118–120)] Another study has correlated muscle imbalance as the major factor contributing to prosthetic dislocation.[66(p45)] All investigators urge continued exercising to restore strength.

Mobility Program. For most patients, THPs can now be followed more loosely, because the risk of dislocation is markedly reduced after 6 weeks.[48(p9),73(p113)] However, some doctors maintain strict THPs through 3 months. Patients should still be encouraged to avoid soft or low upholstered chairs. The therapist should bring the patient through the development sequence as a precursor to learning how to get on and off the floor. With planning and supervision, the affected hip can be maintained in 90° or less of flexion throughout developmental sequence.

Ambulation Program. The patient with an uncemented THA is probably now at WB as tolerated status and can begin the high-level gait activities discussed previously. Patients at FWB can work on more advanced closed-chain activities: step-ups and step-downs, sidestepping with larger steps, backward walking, and forward walking for speed and endurance. Emphasis should be on restoring a normal gait pattern. Patients can

usually advance their ambulation endurance to 45 minutes daily. To ambulate safely in the community (e.g., cross streets, shop, bank), the patient should also be able to walk at a velocity of 150 to 208 ft/min (44.5 to 63.5 m/min)[37(pp1372,1373)] At PO Month 3, Brown et al[78(pp1260,1261)] found the average walking velocity of patients with THA to be 144 ft/min, which is just below the safe speed needed in a moderate sized community. Therefore, it is probably a good idea to train the patient to be able to ambulate quickly for a short distance (to cross a street or catch a bus), even if the patient's self-selected walking speed falls below safety minimums.

The ability to accelerate and quickly decelerate to avoid an oncoming pedestrian (or skateboarder) is also important and should be trained. This usually requires proprioceptive and advanced balance retraining, which can be initiated on a small balance board with the patient supported in a door frame and the therapist providing minimal assistance for safety purposes (Figure 4–16). Sidestepping with greater speed and around obstacles can also help teach the patient how to maneuver quickly and safely.

Activities of Daily Living Program. Patients should be completely independent in basic ADL and can now initiate many instrumental ADL safely. Patients are usually allowed to return to driving, but they should be cautioned that their LE reflexes will be slowed on the affected side, limiting their ability to "break" quickly in an emergency. Only light lifting is allowed at this time (under 10 lbs); therefore, groceries should be lightly bagged and heavy loads of laundry should be split. Yardwork, snow removal, washing floors, and other heavy household tasks are contraindicated.

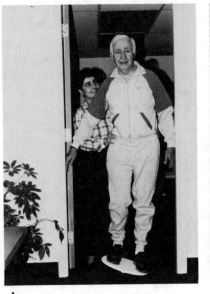
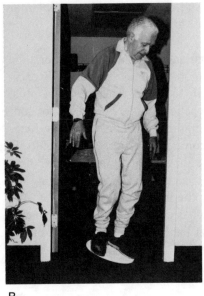

A   B

Figure 4–16 Advanced proprioception and balance retraining. During this difficult activity, the patient begins (A) while supported in a doorway; the therapist provides assistance as needed for safety. The patient progresses (B) to independent balance and proprioception work in all directions.

Phase V (PO Month 3 on)

Therapy has generally been discontinued by Phase V; however, the therapist needs to be able to answer the patient's questions regarding return to normalcy. Most physicians discontinue THPs in part or in total at this time. Patients can return to work full time if desired. Common sense dictates that extremes of hip ROM and torqued positions still should be avoided as much as possible.

What type of lifestyle can the patient expect in the future? Within 6 months of surgery, patients can return to golf, bowling, swimming, and doubles tennis; but high-impact sports have been very detrimental to the stability of the prosthesis and should be avoided.[73(p113),76(pp76,77),79(pp29–31)] By 1 year postoperatively, the patient is ambulating at 180 ft/min, or 69% of the normal velocity (262 ft/min) for elderly people. By 2 years postoperatively, the majority of patients with THAs can ambulate without device or with only a straight cane at a velocity of 218 ft/min, or 84% of normal.[78(pp1260,1261),80(p1385)]

Summary of Treatment of the Patient with a Total Hip Arthroplasty

- Know the type of THA (cemented or uncemented) and the WB order.

- Know the surgical approach and the appropriate THPs.

- Preoperatively, instruct the patient in respiratory exercises, isometric gluteal and quadriceps sets, ankle pumps, and THPs.

- *During the acute recovery phase (PO Days 0 to 5)*
  1. maintain strict THPs
  2. begin isometrics and straight-plane isotonic exercises
  3. begin reconditioning exercises to unaffected extremities
  4. begin transfers to the unaffected side
  5. begin assisted ambulation on level surfaces
  6. use appropriate dressing and toileting equipment.

- *From 1 to 2 weeks postoperatively*
  1. maintain strict THPs
  2. add light resistance to the exercise program
  3. begin working on speed as well as control
  4. begin isotonic exercise in standing posture if FWB
  5. begin prone-lying to stretch out hip flexors
  6. emphasize independence in bed mobility and transfers
  7. ambulate in all directions with appropriate device
  8. emphasize independence in basic ADL (with device).

- *From 3 to 6 weeks postoperatively*
  1. maintain strict THPs
  2. progress resistive exercise when appropriate
  3. customize the program to the patient's interests
  4. stretch out hip flexors and Achilles tendon
  5. teach car transfers
  6. advance patients with uncemented THAs to FWB on physician's orders
  7. ambulate for progressive distance and speed

  8. emphasize independence in basic ADL (with device).

- *From 6 to 12 weeks postoperatively*
  1. maintain THPs, but less strictly
  2. return to driving, sexual activity, part-time work
  3. continue progressive resistive exercise
  4. begin developmental sequence with THPs
  5. begin high-level gait activities
  6. begin proprioceptive and balance activities
  7. normalize gait pattern on all surfaces
  8. work on ambulation velocity and maneuvering ability
  9. begin instrumental ADL, wean off assistive devices.

BURSITIS

There are at least 13 bursae about the hip, 4 of which are seen clinically (Figure 3–2). Bursitis can be caused by direct trauma, friction from an underlying tendon, or from infection. Medically, the doctor may choose to aspirate the bursa, inject it with anesthetic or cortisone, surgically excise it, or prescribe conservative treatment.[81(p297)] The symptoms of bursitis respond well to standard therapeutic intervention: anti-inflammatory medication, ice, ultrasound, moist heat, massage, and exercise; however, simply treating the symptoms without regard to the cause is unjustified. The therapist must evaluate the patient and determine the reason for the bursitis in order to prevent its recurrence.

Iliopectineal Bursitis

The iliopectineal bursa is the largest bursa in the body, communicating with the hip joint in about 15% of adults. Bursitis is generally caused by friction from the iliopsoas tendon, which lies on top of it. It commonly is found in patients with OA of the hip. The patient complains of pain in the groin or the anterior portion of the hip joint that worsens on passive hip flexion, extension, or ER.[82(p61)] On evaluation, hip flexor tightness or a leg length discrepancy usually is discovered. In addition to the use of therapeutic modalities (e.g., ice, ultrasound) to decrease symptoms, the therapist must also gently stretch the hip flexors, strengthen the surrounding musculature, or prescribe corrective shoe orthotics as needed.

Trochanteric Bursitis

There are two bursae in the region of the trochanter: one between the greater trochanter and the gluteus maximus muscle and the other between the tendons of the gluteus maximus and the vastus lateralis muscles. The patient complains of tenderness and pain just lateral to the greater trochanter, which can radiate down the lateral thigh.[82(p62)] The pain can be provoked by hip rotation. Other symptoms may include pain while crossing legs, climbing stairs, playing golf, and lying on the affected side. The iliotibial band (ITB) may be tight. The cause of the bursitis can be direct trauma, as from a fall, or microtrauma as might occur from compensatory IR of the femur from excessive foot pronation.[81(p297)] The therapist needs to assess the postural alignment of the entire LE to determine the causal factors. Along with rest and modalities to reduce the symptoms, the therapist may need to prescribe corrective shoe orthotics, stretch out the ITB, and restore muscle balance to the hip.

Ischiogluteal Bursitis

This bursa is located between the ischial tuberosity and the gluteus maximus. The patient complains of local tenderness when sitting, which is immediately relieved upon standing. The patient may display an antalgic gait pattern and may have restricted hip flexion.[83(p502)] The cause of this bursitis is usually prolonged sitting on a hard surface. Sedentary people are at risk as well as avid bicyclists. Other common causes include men who keep thick wallets in their back pockets and people with muscle imbalances of the hamstrings and gluteus maximus. (See muscle imbalance section later in this chapter.) The treatment includes removal of the stimulus by padding hard sitting surfaces, removing the wallet from the back pocket, modalities for symptomatic relief, and exercises to restore muscle balance to the hip. (Anecdotally, patients report that "sitting on an ice pack" offers better relief than ultrasound.)

Summary of Treatment of Bursitis

- Determine the cause of injury.
- Reduce the patient's symptoms with the appropriate modalities.
- Treat the cause of the injury to prevent recurrence with stretching, strengthening exercises, and/or prescription orthotics.

MUSCLE IMBALANCES AT THE HIP

The body has many movement options available to it to achieve its functional objectives. Those options are based in part on the skeletal alignment of the joints. If the joints are optimally aligned, minimal strain is placed on the surrounding soft tissues and efficient motor function can occur.[84(p14)] When the joints come out of alignment because of postural habits, trauma, or alterations in muscle recruitment, the system becomes unbalanced, causing movement to become painful and jerky. (This is similar to a car needing its front end aligned for a smooth ride to occur.)

Sahrmann[84(p21)] has identified two muscle faults that can cause painful syndromes to occur: alterations in muscle length and alterations in muscle dominance. These can occur separately or in combination. She theorizes that these faults can alter the axis of rotation of the joint (the path of instantaneous center of rotation [PICR]), which can also set off pain in the area.

Postural Faults and Changes in Muscle Length

Posture is an expression of personality, as well as a complex reaction to a multitude of environmental influences.[85(p2)] For the elderly person, the effects of aging and disuse often combine to cause increased flexion in the body. The changes in muscle length and function that result from aging, trauma, and lifelong postural habits can cause painful conditions to arise in the hip or low back region, decreasing the ability to move fluidly and efficiently. Although many patients will be unable to correct some of the fixed deformities that can occur over time, even minor corrections may be enough to lessen the pain and increase function.

Many dysfunctions at the hip arise from alterations in optimal position of the lumbopelvic region. According to Kendall, McCreary, and Provance,[86(pp86,87)] a person with an anterior pelvic tilt usually has elongated and weak anterior abdominals and hamstrings, along with shortened and strong hip

flexor muscles (Figure 4–17A). A person with a posterior pelvic tilt has an elongated and weak iliopsoas, along with strong and tight hamstrings (Figure 4–17B). In addition, uneven iliac crest heights can cause the gluteus medius to be lengthened and weak on the high side, and tight and strong on the low side.[84(p21)]

Other dysfunctions arise from alterations in femoral alignment, with the internal and external rotators being out of balance. These can occur from postural habit (common in former dancers) or from poor alignment of the foot causing compensatory changes up through the entire lower quarter. (It also can occur from excessive femoral anteversion or retroversion.)

The ability to walk with a normal gait pattern is greatly affected by loss of full hip extension. This can cause compensatory forward trunk lean, increased lumbar lordosis, a flexed knee in mid stance (Figure 4–18), an increased anterior pelvic tilt, or loss of the trailing thigh in terminal stance. The loss of hip extension can be attributed to hip flexor tightness, ITB tightness, or a painful arthritic hip.[87(pp246–252)]

In general, many elderly patients adopt a flexed knee posture to compensate for loss of hip extension. This requires the quadriceps to fire to maintain upright position, increasing the energy cost of standing and walking.

Treatment of Muscle Length Dysfunction

The treatment of muscle length dysfunction is straightforward and logical. Shortened muscles must be stretched, lengthened muscles must be kept out of overstretched positions, and motor relearning needs to occur to integrate the changes into functional gains. Before stretching, heat modalities may be used to prepare the soft tissues. In addition,

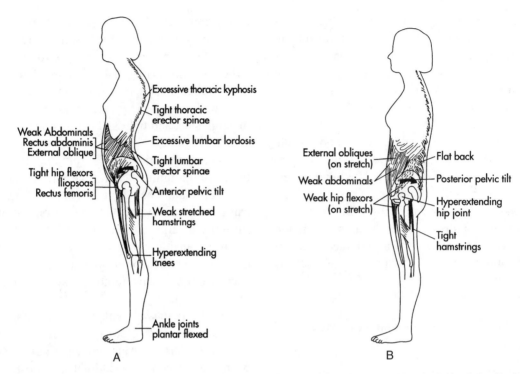

Figure 4–17 Alterations in muscle lengths with anterior pelvic tilt (A) and posterior pelvic tilt (B). *Source:* Reprinted with permission from A. Hartley, Hip and Pelvis Assessment, *Practical Joint Assessment: Lower Quadrant*, 2 ed., p. 114, © 1995, Mosby-Year Book, Inc.

the stretch should be prolonged in the geriatric population (minimum of 30 seconds) to be effective. It is imperative that the patient maintain control over lumbopelvic alignment while stretching tight hip musculature. This is most easily accomplished by having the patient stretch from a supine position when possible (Figures 4–19 and 4–20). However, stretches can also be performed in sitting and standing (Figures 4–21 and 4–22).

Muscles that are "too long" and are displaying "stretch weakness" also need to be restored to optimal length. The therapist needs to teach the patient how to contract these muscles in their shortened position.[84(p12)] Avoiding postures that place stretches on these muscles is obviously important.

To integrate the new range of motion into walking or other activities, the patient needs to perform high-level gait and agility exercises. Depending on the patient's balance and functional level, these exercises can include:

- balance work on a foam mat
- balance work on the wobble board (Figure 4–16)
- forward walking with large strides
- forward walking for speed
- forward walking with elastic tubing resistance (Figure 4–23)
- backward (retro) walking
- sidestepping
- cross-over (carioca) stepping
- maneuvering around obstacle courses

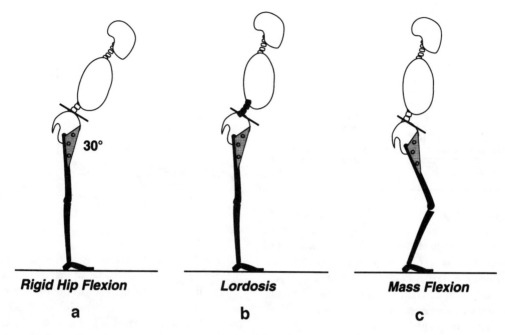

Figure 4–18 Inadequate hip extension in midstance. (a) Without compensation, the pelvis and trunk are tilted forward. Bolted plate indicates a rigid contracture. (b) Lumbar lordosis can restore an erect trunk. (c) Knee flexion equal to the fixed hip flexion can right both the pelvis and trunk. *Source:* Reprinted with permission from J. Perry, Hip Gait Deviations, *Gait Analysis*, p. 247, © 1992, Slack Incorporated.

- floor-to-stand transfers
- stair climbing

Alteration in Muscle Dominance

Movement imbalance can also arise from problems in recruitment of muscles. This is essentially a "coordination problem" and can change the pattern of muscle dominance.[84(p3)] In general, the two-joint muscles, which are normally secondary movers, take over initiation of movement from the one joint prime movers. These longer muscles cannot stabilize the joint properly, causing a deviation in the PICR. Sahrmann lists three common faults involving accessory muscles dominating the prime movers at the hip:[84(p21)]

1. tensor fascia lata and ITB over gluteus medius
2. hamstrings over gluteus maximus
3. tensor fascia lata and rectus femoris over iliopsoas

Treatment of Alterations in Muscle Dominance

Correcting problems in muscle recruitment requires motor retraining, not strengthening per se. The therapist must not allow substitution of muscles to occur during exercise. Biofeedback can be helpful to ensure the correct muscle is firing (or sometimes to make sure that the undesired muscle is not firing). To recruit the gluteus medius, hip abduction is performed without allowing hip flexion or IR to occur. To restore gluteus

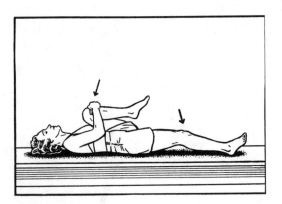

Figure 4–19 Iliopsoas stretch in supine. Flex one hip and knee and hold firmly against chest with hand clasp. Extend opposite leg, and attempt to flatten the back of the knee against table to lengthen hip flexors. *Source:* Reprinted with permission from L. Daniels and C. Worthingham, *Therapeutic Exercise,* 2 ed., p. 60, © 1977, W.B. Saunders Company.

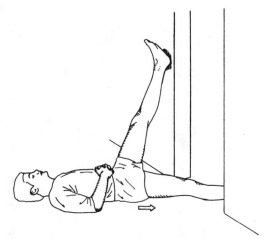

Figure 4–20 Self-stretching of the hamstring muscles in supine. Additional stretch can occur if person moves buttock closer to the door frame. *Source:* Reprinted with permission of C. Kisner and L.A. Colby, *Therapeutic Exercise: Foundations and Techniques,* 3 ed., p. 407, © 1996, F.A. Davis Company.

maximus as prime mover, the patient can lie prone with knee bent and extend the hip. The patient then progresses to lifting the leg with the knee extended. To restore iliopsoas as prime mover, the patient can begin in long sitting and do a "Sit-Back" (Figure 4–24), ending up supine on the mat. As with all motor relearning, it is necessary to incorporate the new pattern into a functional activity. This can be accomplished by having the patient tighten the gluteals while walking, or performing one-legged balance without tilting the pelvis. Although the exercises are not strenuous, they are specific, and the patient sees results within 1 to 7 days of initiating the program.

Summary of Treatment of Muscle Imbalance

- Determine the physical impairments (postural faults, short muscles, weak muscles, incoordination, etc.) that are contributing to the painful condition.
- Correct the muscle imbalances through stretching tight muscles, strengthening lengthened muscles in their shortened ranges, and motor retraining.
- Do not allow muscle substitution to occur.
- Emphasize corrected movement patterns through high-level gait and activities.

Sitting/Hamstring/Calf Stretching

Purpose: stretch hamstrings and calf muscle; training to keep pelvis immobile while moving legs.

Sit with your back straight, pelvis erect, and arms resting at your sides.

___ Sit with back against wall.

Slowly straighten your knee, being sure not to let your pelvis rock backward. (Don't slump and let your low back round out.)

After your knee is as straight as possible, move your ankle so that your foot points upward toward your knee (stretches your calf).

___ Move at ankle.

___ Lead with big toe side of foot. Do not lead with toes.

Relax and lower your leg to the starting position.

Repeat the sequence with the other leg.

Repeat _____ times with each leg.

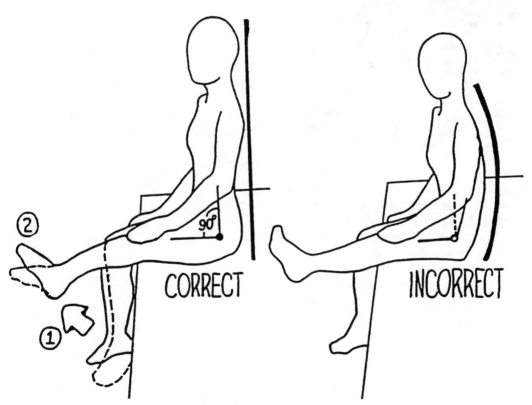

Figure 4–21 Sitting hamstring stretch. *Source:* Reprinted with permission from S. Sahrmann from "Exercises for Correction of Muscle Imbalances," St. Louis, Missouri, Copyright © 1990.

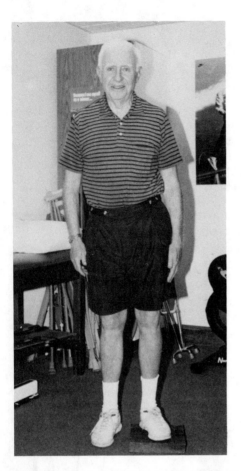

Figure 4–22 Tensor fascia lata (TFL) and iliotibial band (ITB) stretch in standing. According to Kendall, McCreary, and Provance, to stretch a tight left TFL/ITB, place a board under the left foot and keep equal weight on both feet. Keep good hip alignment, allowing no internal hip rotation. Perform a posterior pelvic tilt to add hip extension to the stretch. Hold 1–2 minutes.[84(p60)]

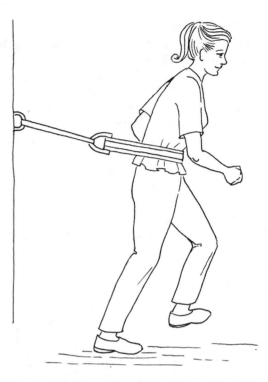

Figure 4–23 Forward walking with resistive tubing to integrate new range into gait pattern. *Source:* Reprinted from T. Goldstein, Functional Exercises for the Lower Extremities, *Functional Rehabilitation in Orthopaedics*, p. 78, © 1995, Aspen Publishers, Inc.

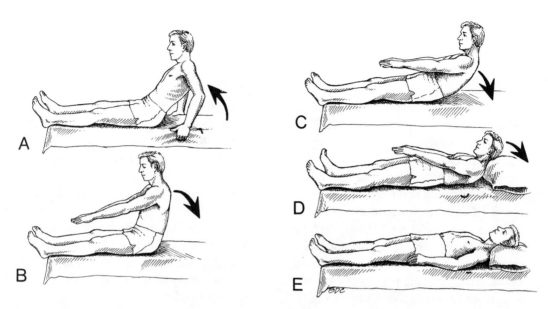

Figure 4–24 Slow sit-back exercise to improve strength and coordination of the abdominal and hip flexor muscles as the spine "rolls down" on the table. This exercise requires a less demanding lengthening contraction, rather than the shortening contraction of a sit-up. (A) pushing the torso up (arrow) with the arms from the supine to the seated position. This avoids loading the flexor muscles of the trunk and hips. (B) beginning of the slow sit-back, lumbar spine flexed. (C) rolling the back down onto the table, maintaining spinal flexion so that each spinal sement reaches the table in succession. (D) completion of slow sit-back. (E) period of full relaxation with abdominal (diaphragmatic) breathing. Three cycles of this slow sit-back exercise should be performed daily to provide full benefit. *Source:* Reprinted with permission from J.G. Travell and D.G. Simons, *Myofascial Pain and Dysfunction: The Trigger Point Manual*, Vol. 2, p. 107, © 1983, Lippincott Williams & Wilkins.

DOCUMENTATION TIPS

Referrals

Due to shorter hospital stays, patients are quickly being transferred from one health care provider to another. A person with a hip fracture can be discharged from the acute care hospital in 5 days, the subacute rehabilitation unit (or hospital) after 2 more weeks, the skilled nursing facility after 4 more weeks, and finally to home (if lucky) to be seen by yet another therapist. In a perfect world, the medical record would arrive with the patient at each level of care and provide the therapist with all pertinent data needed to treat the patient effectively. This is not a perfect world; therefore, it is incumbent upon the therapist at each level to pass along a referral to the therapist at the next level of care. This often consists of the therapist's discharge summary, which, by the time it is dictated and sent to the next level, is useless.

Communicating needed patient information through the health care system is a challenge. A referral must be sent with the patient. It can be very brief, but should include the following information in detail regarding patients with hip dysfunction:

- specific diagnosis (i.e., right subcapital hip fracture on December 21, 2001)

- surgical intervention: type of fixation hardware, surgical approach, cemented or uncemented, ROM available in operating room, complications, etc
- WB orders and any movement precautions
- mobility status: bed, transfers, ambulation, stairs, amount of assistance, etc
- premorbid status: general health, ADL, community or institution living, etc
- cognition

In addition, but only if the therapist has time, strength, ROM, and balance status can be sent along. This information is relatively unimportant compared to the necessity of knowing what type of fracture, fixation, and precautions are in place.

Referrals need to be written as though Murphy's Law rules the day. The acute care therapist cannot assume that the subacute therapist will get even the most basic information, the subacute therapist cannot assume that the nursing home therapist will ever get any information either, and so on and so on. Although no one in any profession enjoys "doing paperwork," providing important information in the referral is imperative for quality patient care.

REFERENCES

1. Kennedy EM. Hip fracture outcomes in people 50 and over—Background paper. U.S. Congress, Office of Technology Assessment. OTA-BP-H-120, U.S. Government Printing Office, Washington, DC, 1994.

2. Martin AD, Silverthorn KG, Houston CS, Bernhardson S, Wajda A, Roos, LL. The incidence of fracture of the proximal femur in two million Canadians from 1972–1984. *Clin Orthop.* 1991;266: 111–118.

3. Ebert FR, Jacobsen SJ, Smith GS. Relative rates of fracture of the hip in the United States—Geographic, sex, and age variations. *J Bone Joint Surg.* 1995;77-A(5):695–702.

4. Bean N, Bennett KM, Lehmann AB. Habitus and hip fracture revisited—skeletal size, strength and cognition rather than thinness. *Age and Aging* 1995; 24(6):481–484.

5. Madhok R, Melton LJ, Atkinson EJ, O'Fallon WM, Lewallen DG. Urban vs rural increase in hip fracture incidence—age and sex of 901 cases in 1980–89 in Olmsted County, USA. *Acta Orthop Scand.* 1993; 64(5):543–548.

6. Cooper C, Coupland C, Mitchell M. Rheumatoid arthritis, corticosteroid therapy and hip fracture. *Annals Rheum Dis.* 1995;54(1):49–52.

7. Hemenway D, Feshkanich D, Colditz GA. Body height and hip fracture—A cohort study of 90,000 women. *Internat J Epidem.* 1995;24(4):783–786.

8. Michelson JD, Myers A, Jinnah R, Cox Q, Van Natta M. Epidemiology of hip fractures among the elderly. *Clin Orthop.* 1995;311:129–135.

9. Parker MJ, Twemlow TR. Spontaneous hip fractures—44/872 in a prospective study. *Acta Orthop Scand.* 1997;68(4):325–326.

10. Chua D, Jagial SB, Schatzker J. An orthopedic surgeon survey on the treatment of displaced femoral neck fracture—opposing views. *Canadian J Surg.* 1997;40(4):271.

11. Koval KJ, Zuckerman JD, eds. *Fractures in the Elderly.* Philadelphia:Lippincott-Raven Publishers; 1998.

12. Shih CH, Wang KC. Femoral neck fractures:121 cases treated by Knowles pinning. *Clin Orthop.* 1991; 271:195–200.

13. McAndrew M. The treatment of geriatric hip fractures. *Top Geriatr Rehabil.* 1996;12(1):32–37.

14. Boguch ER, Ouellette G, Hastings DE. Intertrochanteric fractures of the femur in rheumatoid arthritis patients. *Clin Orthop.* 1993;294:181–186.

15. Thomas RL. Management of hip fracture in the geriatric patient: A team approach in the institutional setting. *Top Geriatr Rehabil.* 1996;12(1):59–69.

16. *Zimmer Product Encyclopedia.* Warsaw, IN: Zimmer USA; December 1981.

17. Chiu FY, Lo WH. Undisplaced femoral-neck fracture in the elderly. *Arch Orthop Trauma Surg.* 1996;115(2):90–93.

18. Waddell JP. The treatment of unstable intertrochanteric hip fractures. *Techniques Orthop.* 1989;4(2): 41–47.

19. Corzatt R, Bosch A. Internal fixation by the Ender method. *JAMA.* September 1978;240.

20. Kozinn SC, Wilson PD Jr. Adult hip disease and total hip replacement. *Clin Symp.* 1987;39(5):2–32.

21. Bauer TW, Geesink RT, Zimmerman R, McMahon JT. Hydroxyapatite-coated femoral stems. *J Bone Joint Surg.* 1991;73-A(10):1439–1452.

22. Lo WH, Chen WM, Huang CK, Chen TH, Chiu FY, Chen CM. Bateman bipolar hemiarthroplasty for displaced intracapsular femoral neck fractures—uncemented vs cemented. *Clin Orthop.* 1994;302:75–82.

23. Morscher E, ed. *The Cementless Fixation of Hip Endoprostheses.* Berlin, West Germany: Springer-Verlag; 1984.

24. Sauffer RN. Ten-year follow-up study of total hip replacement. *J Bone Joint Surg.* 1982;64-A:983.

25. Harris WH. Total hip replacement: "cement versus cementless" resolution. *Bull Rheum Dis.* 1994; 43(5):1–4.

26. Koval KJ, Friend KD, Aharonoff GB, Zuckerman JD. Weight-bearing after hip fracture—a prospective series of 596 geriatric hip fracture patients. *J Orthop Trauma.* 1996;10(8):526–530.

27. Lauritzen JB, Petersen MM, Lund B. Effect of external hip protectors on hip fractures. *The Lancet* 1993;341:11–13.

28. Cameron ID, Quine S. External hip protectors: likely non-compliance among high risk elderly people living in the community. *Arch Gerontol Geriatr.* 1994; 19:273–281.

29. Cummings SR, Nevitt MC, Browner WS, Stone K, et al. Risk factors for hip fracture in white women. *New Engl J Med.* 1995;332:767–773.

30. Young Y, Brant L, German P, Kenzora J, Magaziner J. A longitudinal examination of functional recovery among older people with subcapital hip fractures. *JAGS*. 1997;45(3):288–294.

31. Van der Sluijs JA, Walenkamp GHIM. How predictable is rehabilitation after hip fracture? A prospective study of 134 patients. *Acta Orthop Scand*. 1991; 62(6):567–572.

32. Frankel VH, Nordin M. *Basic Biomechanics of the Skeletal System*. 2nd ed. Philadelphia: Lea & Febiger; 1989.

33. Gould JA III, Davies GJ, eds. *Orthopaedics and Sports Physical Therapy*. St. Louis: CV Mosby Co; 1985.

34. Guccione AA, Fagerson TL, Anderson JJ. Regaining functional independence in the acute care setting following hip fracture. *Phys Ther*. 1996;76: 818–826.

35. Harrison R, Balstrode S. Percent weight bearing during partial immersion in the hydrotherapy pool. *Physiotherapy Practice*. 1987;3:60–63.

36. Woolfenden JT. Aquatic physical therapy approaches for the extremities. *Orthop Phys Ther Clinics N Amer*. 1994;3(2):209–230.

37. Robinett CS, Vondran MA. Functional ambulation velocity and distance requirements in rural and urban communities. *Phys Ther*. September 1988;68: 1371–1373.

38. Jarnlo GB, Thorngren KG. Standing balance in hip fracture patients: 20 middle-aged patients compared with 20 healthy subjects. *Acta Orthop Scand*. 1991;62(5):422–426.

39. Scotece GG, Perry D, Thermann K. Pelvic dysfunction in geriatric patients acute status post hip surgery. Research presentation at Washington State American Physical Therapy Association Fall Meeting, October 1997.

40. Sherington C, Lord SR. Home exercise to improve strength and walking velocity after hip fracture; a randomized controlled trial. *Arch Phys Med Rehabil*. 1997;78:208–212.

41. Ceder L, Ekelund L, Inerot S, et al. Rehabilitation after hip fracture in the elderly. *Acta Orthop Scand*. 1979;50:681–688.

42. Koval KJ, Skovron ML, Aharanoff GB, Meadows SE, Zuckerman JD. Ambulatory ability after hip fracture—a prospective study in geriatric patients. *Clin Orthop*. 1995;310:150–159.

43. Folman Y, Gepstein R, Assaraf A, Liberty S. Functional recovery after operative treatment of femoral neck fractures in an institutionalized elderly population. *Arch Phys Med Rehabil*. 1994;75(4): 454–456.

44. Jette A, Harris B, Cleary P, et al. Functional recovery after hip fracture. *Arch Phys Med Rehabil*. 1987;68:735–740.

45. Cyriax J. *Textbook of Orthopaedic Medicine*. 7th ed. London, England: Bailliere Tindall; 1978.

46. Singleton MC, Branch EF, eds. *Common Disorders of the Hip*. New York: Haworth Press; 1986.

47. Beattie P. Degenerative diseases affecting the hip and sacroiliac joints. Course notes from The Hip and Sacroiliac Joint, Orthopaedic Section APTA, February 1997.

48. Evans BG. Operative and nonoperative management of hip pathology. Course notes from The Hip and Sacroiliac Joint, Orthopaedic Section APTA, April 1997.

49. Radin EL, Rose RM, Blaha JD, Litsky AS. *Practical Biomechanics for the Orthopedic Surgeon*. 2nd ed. New York: Churchill Livingstone Inc, 1992.

50. Shankman GA. *Fundamental Orthopedic Management for the Physical Therapist Assistant*. St. Louis: Mosby-Year Book; 1997.

51. Raney RB, Brashear HR. *Shands' Handbook of Orthopaedic Surgery*. 8th ed. St. Louis: The Mosby Company; 1971.

52. Smith CA, Arnett FC. Epidemiologic aspects of rheumatoid arthritis. *Clin Orthop*. 1991;265:23–35.

53. Wilder RL, Crofford LJ. Do infectious agents cause rheumatoid arthritis? *Clin Orthop*. 1991;265: 36–41.

54. Chang RW, ed. *Rehabilitation of Persons with Rheumatoid Arthritis*. Gaithersburg, MD: Aspen Publishers, Inc; 1996.

55. Lehmann JF, Silverman DR, Baum BA, Kirk NL, Johnstone VC. Temperature distributions in the human thigh, produced by infrared, hot pack and microwave application. *Arch Phys Med Rehab*. 1966; 47:291.

56. Harris ED, McCroskery PA. The influence of temperature and fibril stability on degradation of cartilage collagen by rheumatoid synovial collagenase. *N Eng J Med*. 1974;290:1–6.

57. Minor MA, Hewett JE, Webel RR, Anderson SK, Kay DR. Efficacy of physical conditioning exer-

cise in patients with rheumatoid arthritis and osteo-arthritis. *Arthritis Rheum.* 1989;32:1396–1405.

58. Brander VA, Stulberg D, Chang RW. Life after total hip arthroplasty. *Bull Rheum Dis.* 1993;42(3):1–5.

59. Pettine KA, Aamlid BC, Cabanela ME. Elective total hip arthroplasty in patients older than 80 years of age. *Clin Orthop.* 1991;266:127–132.

60. Black J. Metal on metal bearings. A practical alternative to metal on polyethylene total joints? *Clin Orthop.* 1996;329S:S244–S255.

61. Rorabeck CH, Bourne RB, Laupacis A, et al. A double blind study of 250 cases comparing cemented with cementless total hip arthroplasty. *Clin Orthop.* 1994;298:156–164.

62. Healy WL. Economic considerations in total hip arthroplasty and implant standardization. *Clin Orthop.* 1995;311:102–108.

63. Total Hip Replacement. NIH Consensus Statement 1994;12(5):1–31.

64. Harris WH. Hybrid total hip replacement. *Clin Orthop.* 1996;333:155–164.

65. Fackler CD, Poss R. Dislocation in total hip arthroplasties. *Clin Orthop.* 1980;151:169–178.

66. Pierchon F, Pasquier G, Cotten A, Fontaine C, Clarisse J, Duquennoy A. Causes of dislocation of total hip arthroplasty—CT study of component alignment. *J Bone Joint Surg.* 1994;76B(1):45–48.

67. Turner RS. Postoperative total hip prosthetic femoral head dislocations. *Clin Orthop.* 1994;301: 196–204.

68. Hedlundh U, Ahnfelt L, Hybbinette CH, Weckstrom J, Fredin H. Surgical experience related to dislocations after total hip arthroplasty. *J Bone Joint Surg.* 1996;78B(2):206–209.

69. McNally MA, Cooke EA, Mollan RAB. The effect of active movement of the foot on venous-blood flow after total hip-replacement. *J Bone Joint Surg.* 1997;79-A(8):1198–1201.

70. Shelton S. Rehabilitation following total hip arthroplasty. *Top Geriatr Rehabil.* 1996;12(1): 9–22.

71. Scott CM, Gatti L. Physical therapy following total hip and total knee replacement. *Orthop Phys Therap Clin N Amer.* 1993;2(2):161–172.

72. Flanagan SR, Ragnarsson KT, Ross MK, Wong DK. Rehabilitation of the geriatric orthopaedic patient. *Clin Orthop.* 1995;316:80–92.

73. Holpit LA. Preoperative and postoperative physical therapy for the total shoulder, hip, and knee replacement patient. *Orthop Phys Therap Clin N Amer.* 1993;2(1):97–118.

74. Stinnett KA. Occupational therapy intervention for the geriatric client receiving acute and subacute services following total hip replacement and femoral fracture repair. *Top Geriatr Rehabil.* 1996;12(1):23–31.

75. Brotzman SB, Cameron HU, Boolos M. Rehabilitation after total joint arthroplasty. In: Brotzman SB, ed. *Handbook of Orthopaedic Rehabilitation.* St. Louis: Mosby-Year Book; 1996.

76. Long WT, Dorr LD, Healy B, Perry J. Functional recovery of noncemented hip arthroplasty. *Clin Orthop.* 1993;288:73–77.

77. Shih CH, Du YK, Lin YH, Wu CC. Muscular recovery around the hip joint after total hip arthroplasty. *Clin Orthop.* 1994;302:115–120.

78. Brown M, Hislop HJ, Waters RL, Porell D. Walking efficiency before and after total hip replacement. *Phys Ther.* October 1980;60:1259–1263.

79. Kilgus DJ, Dorey FJ, Finerman GAM, Amstutz HC. Patient activity, sports participation, and impact loading on the durability of cemented total hip replacements. *Clin Orthop.* 1991;269:25–31.

80. Hageman PA, Blanke DJ. Comparison of gait of young women and elderly women. *Phys Ther.* September 1986;66:1382–1387.

81. Roos HP. Hip pain in sport. *Sports Med Arthroscopy Review.* 1997;5(4):292–300.

82. Winkel D. *Diagnosis and Treatment of the Lower Extremities.* Gaithersburg, MD: Aspen Publishers, Inc; 1997.

83. Magee DJ. *Orthopedic Physical Assessment.* 3rd ed. Philadelphia: WB Saunders Co; 1997.

84. Sahrmann S. Diagnosis and treatment of muscle imbalances associated with regional pain syndromes. Course Notes, 1990. Presented at the Massachusetts Chapter of the American Physical Therapy Association Annual Meeting, Danvers, MA; 1992.

85. Klein-Vogelbach S. *Therapeutic Exercises in Functional Kinetics.* Berlin, Germany: Springer-Verlag; 1991.

86. Kendall FP, McCreary EL, Provance PG. *Muscles: Testing and Function.* 4th ed. Baltimore: Williams & Wilkins; 1993.

87. Perry J. *Gait Analysis.* Thorofare, NJ: Slack Inc; 1992.

ADDITIONAL INFORMATION

For additional information on HipSaver hip external protectors, please contact:

The HipSaver Company, Inc.
566 Washington Street #673
Canton, MA 02021
(800) 358-HIPS

For additional information on adaptive devices for ADL:

Functional Rehabilitation in Orthopaedics, Goldstein TS, Chapter 14, Functional Exercise Equipment. Gaithersburg, MD: Aspen Publishers, Inc, © 1995.

Rehabilitation of Persons with Rheumatoid Arthritis, Chang RW, Chapter 15, Adaptive Equipment and Assistive Devices. Gaithersburg, MD: Aspen Publishers, Inc, © 1996.

5

The Knee Joint

The knee joint is considered to be one of the most complex joints in the human body. Over a lifetime, the knee is subjected to an accumulation of bumps, bruises, twists, and falls. In addition, articular diseases commonly affect this weight-bearing joint. When inflamed, the knee hinders the most basic locomotive abilities and functional activities. Prolonged stresses can cause progressive deformity and relentless pain.

ANATOMY OF THE KNEE JOINT

The knee "joint" actually consists of two distinct joints: the tibiofemoral and the patellofemoral joints. These joints act together to provide the stability required to support the body during weight bearing, as well as the mobility required for ambulation and activity.

The tibiofemoral joint consists of the two inferior femoral condyles and the two articulating surfaces of the tibial plateau. The medial femoral condyle is longer than the lateral condyle.[1(p1)] In addition, a lateral view of the distal femur reveals a flat surface for extension (i.e., for weight bearing) and a rounder surface for flexion.[2(p32)] The tibial plateau slopes posteriorly at a 10° angle. The medial tibial articulating surface is more oval and concave than its lateral tibial counterpart and faces inward.[1(p2)] The two tibial surfaces are separated by the tibial spines (also called the eminentiae intercondylaris). Thick hyaline cartilage (3 to 4 mm thick) protects the articulating surfaces of the knee. The fibrocartilaginous menisci lie between these two largest bones in the human body and help to distribute pressure and assist in joint lubrication. (See Figure 5–1.) The medial meniscus is C-shaped and firmly attaches to the joint capsule and medial collateral ligament (MCL). The lateral meniscus appears more like a closed ring and is loosely connected to the joint capsule.[1(p10)] Although the anterior and posterior horns of the menisci are anchored centrally, they can move forward and backward across the plateau.[2(p56)]

The patellofemoral joint is composed of the posterior surface of the patella and the trochlear groove on the anterior surface of the distal femur. The lateral femoral wall is higher than the medial wall and helps to hold the patella on track. The patellar surface has a large lateral facet, a smaller medial facet, and an "odd" facet (located medially to the medial facet). In addition, the posterior surface of the patella is protected by the thickest articular cartilage (5 to 6 mm thick) in the body.[2(p36)]

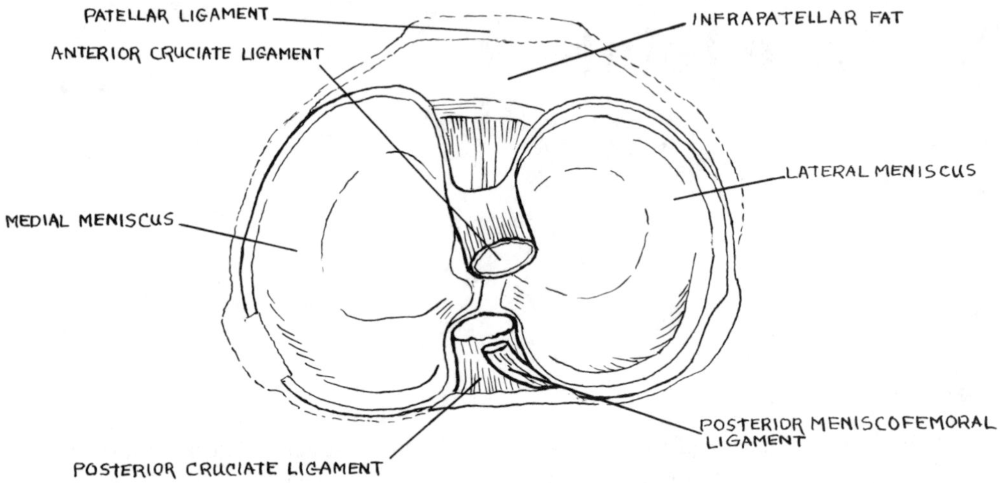

Figure 5–1 The tibial surface of the knee joint. The medial surface is the primary weight-bearing surface. The medial meniscus is C-shaped and firmly attaches to the joint capsule and medial collateral ligament. The lateral surface is less concave and is covered by the ring-shaped lateral meniscus. The tibial attachments of the anterior cruciate ligament and posterior cruciate ligament are also shown.

The superior tibiofibular joint is an arthrodial plane joint composed of the fibular head articulating with the tibial facet on the rim of the tibial condyle. Occasionally, the tibiofibular joint communicates with the tibiofemoral joint.[3(p249)] Although it is not considered part of the knee joint, it figures prominently in the mechanics and pathomechanics of the knee.

Ligaments

The knee is encompassed by an extensive joint capsule, including ligamentous structures that help to control the movements of the joint. Because the osseous components of the knee provide little (if any) stability, the soft tissue structures are important in maintaining joint integrity. Figures 5–1 and 5–2 show some of the ligamentous and bony structures of the knee.

The Cruciates

The anterior cruciate ligament (ACL) arises from the medial aspect of the tibia and traverses posteriorly, laterally, and upward to attach to the supracondylar notch of the lateral condyle of the femur. It is a strong, spiraled ligament that becomes increasingly taut from 60° of flexion toward full knee extension. It consists of two distinct bands of fibers, with the posterolateral band being larger. The ACL resists forward movement of the tibia on the femur, internal rotation of the tibia, and valgus/varus forces. With aging, the ACL weakens considerably and can tear easily.[2(pp108–114)] In the presence of arthritic disease, the ACL is often destroyed.[4(p54)]

The posterior cruciate ligament (PCL) originates at the posterior edge of the tibia and travels anteriorly and upward, to attach to the medial femoral condyle. It is vertically oriented and resists posterior displacement of the

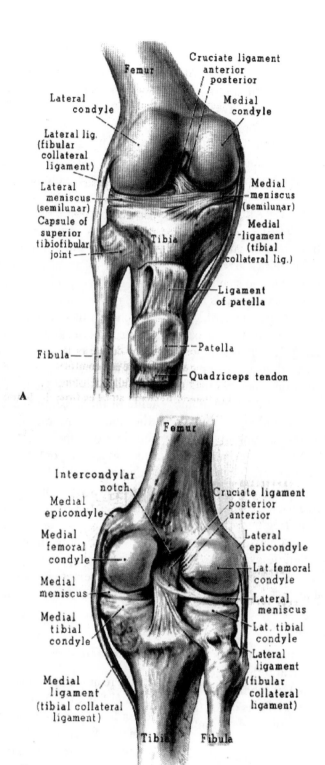

Figure 5–2 Anterior (A) and posterior (B) aspects of the knee depicting ligamentous and capsular structures. *Source:* Reprinted with permission from S.W. Jacob and C.A. Francone, *Structure and Function in Man,* 5 ed., pp. 125 and 127, © 1982, W.B. Saunders Company.

tibia on the femur and internal tibial rotation. Like the ACL, the PCL consists of two major bands of fibers, with the anterior fibers comprising the bulk of the ligament. The posterior fibers are most taut in full flexion, and the anterior fibers are most taut in full extension.[5(p24)] The entire ligament is least tense in midflexion (45° to 75°).[2(pp116–118),6(p71)] Although it has twice the strength of the ACL,[5(p28)] it also weakens greatly with increasing age and can be destroyed by articular disease.[7(p726)]

The cruciates work together to stabilize the knee mechanically with varying bands being taut and relaxed at different ranges of knee motion. Both cruciates wrap around each other and tighten during flexion and internal tibial rotation and unwind during extension and external tibial rotation. They contribute significantly to the successful "screw home mechanism" of the knee in full extension.[5(p25)]

The cruciates also have an important sensory contribution to normal knee function. Four distinct mechanoreceptors have been identified in both cruciate ligaments: Ruffini endings, Pacinian corpuscles, Golgi tendon organlike endings, and free nerve endings. These mechanoreceptors cause changes in the gamma muscle spindle system around the knee, directly affecting both position sense and functional joint stability.[8(pp173–175)]

The Capsular Ligaments

In general, the capsular ligaments maintain some degree of tension throughout the range of motion (ROM) of the knee as they guide and control the movements of the tibia, femur, and patella. They are mostly taut in full extension.

Superficially, the MCL attaches from the femoral medial epicondyle to the tibia. The lateral collateral ligament is extracapsular and connects the femoral lateral epicondyle to the fibular head.[1(pp22,25)] The collateral ligaments resist any varus or valgus stress to the knee. The patellar retinaculum is a continuous sheet of collagenous material between the patella, quadriceps, and femur. It ensures transverse stability of the patella and helps to keep the patella within the trochlear groove.[2(p85)] On the lateral side, the retinaculum is reinforced with fibers from the iliopatellar band and iliotibial tract.[9(p141)]

Deep to the collateral ligaments are the capsular ligaments. Medially, the deeper portion of the capsule can be divided into anterior, middle, and posterior ligaments. Each attaches to the medial meniscus and helps to control external rotation of the tibia.[2(p122)] The posterior ligament also blends with the semimembranosus muscle and is often called the posterior oblique ligament. On the lateral side of the knee, the capsule thickens from the lateral femoral condyle to the fibular head to form the arcuate ligament, which encompasses the popliteus muscle.[1(p25)] In most people, the fabellofibular ligament arises from the styloid process of the fibular head and inserts in the lateral femoral condyle under the gastrocnemius muscle.[10(pp9,10)] Along with the tendons in the area, these capsular ligaments help control varus/valgus stresses and tibial external rotation and secondarily control tibial anterior and posterior translations.[9(p141)]

Bursae and Synovial Tissues

There are approximately 12 bursae located around the knee. Most of them separate tendons from each other or from bony prominences. Anteriorly, four bursae are located around the patella (Figure 5–3):

1. suprapatellar bursa
2. prepatellar bursa
3. deep infrapatellar bursa
4. superficial infrapatellar bursa

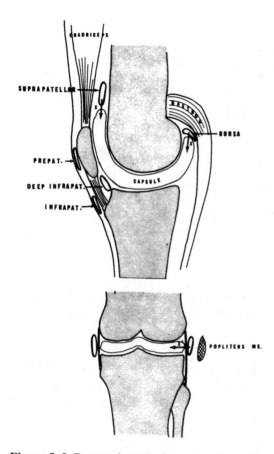

Figure 5–3 Bursae about the knee. Bursae noted: suprapatella, also termed the quadriceps femoral bursa, may communicate with the knee capsule; prepatellar, between the skin and patella; infrapatella (superficial), between the skin and infrapatellar ligament; deep infrapatellar, between infrapatellar ligament and tibia; and bursae between the lateral head of the gastrocnemius and joint capsule, the fibular collateral ligament and biceps or popliteal tendon, and the popliteal tendon and the lateral femoral condyle. X indicates possible communication with the joint capsule. *Source:* Reprinted with permission from R. Cailliet, *Knee Pain and Disability,* 3 ed., p. 12, © 1992, F.A. Davis Company.

Medially, there are bursae at the pes anserinus insertion, around the MCL, at the semimembranosus tendon, and at the medial gas-

trocnemius insertion. Laterally, there are bursae separating the lateral collateral ligament from the popliteus as well as the biceps femoris. There are also bursae located at the insertions of the lateral gastrocnemius and the popliteus. At least three of the above bursae (the suprapatellar, the popliteal, and the medial gastrocnemius) communicate with the knee joint.[1(p47)]

The synovial membranes that comprise the bursae also line the joint capsule and provide lubrication and nutrition to the articular surfaces. The plicae, which are the inward folds of the synovium, are normally soft, pliant, and highly elastic. The plicae follow a medial course (in a C shape) from the lateral patellar tendon to the medial wall of the knee joint to the infrapatellar fat pad to the ACL[11(pp171–173)] (Figure 5–4). Usually the synovium, plicae, and bursae contribute quietly to normal joint function; but when injured by trauma or disease, each of these soft tissue structures can cause high levels of pain and dysfunction.

Muscles and Motion

The tibiofemoral joint has a ROM of 0° to 135° from extension to full flexion. There is no appreciable loss of knee ROM with normal aging. When the joint is fully extended, no passive rotation, abduction, or adduction is possible. When the joint flexes to 30°, up to 10° of passive abduction and adduction becomes possible. When the joint flexes to approximately 90°, 45° of external tibial rotation and 30° of internal rotation can be obtained. Beyond 90°, the range of internal and external rotation decreases due to soft tissue restrictions.[12(p116)]

For these motions to occur, the articular surfaces of the femur must slide and roll upon the tibial plateau. Conjunct rotation occurs during the terminal phase of knee exten-

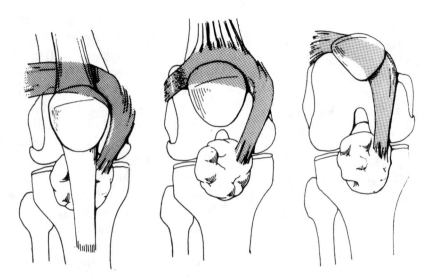

Figure 5–4 Plica from the anterior to posterior view on a right knee. *Source:* Reprinted from T.A. Blackburn et al., An Introduction to the Plica, *The Journal of Orthopaedic and Sports Physical Therapy,* Vol. 3, No. 4, p. 172, © 1982, Williams & Wilkins.

sion as well as the initial phase of knee flex-ion because of three factors:

1. the architecture of the joint (the longer medial femoral condyle)
2. the offset location of the two fixed axes of rotation of the knee[13(pp266–267)]
3. the controlling ligaments

When the foot is fixed and the knee is ex-tending, the femur rotates internally on the tibia. (The tibia rotates externally on the fe-mur in a foot-free position.) This is the "screw-home" mechanism of the knee, which brings the joint into its close-packed position—full extension. During the initial phase of flexion, the femur rotates externally on the tibia when the foot is fixed, unlocking the joint.[1(p50)] If rotation fails to occur, the ar-ticulating surfaces of the tibia and femur are forced to withstand abnormal forces that can damage the joint.

During flexion and extension, the patella also glides along the femur. As the knee

flexes, the patella glides caudally approxi-mately 7 cm, while the articulating surface of the patella actually moves proximally. (Figure 5–5) At full extension, the patella is proximal to the trochlea. At approximately 20°, the patella contacts the femur with both medial and lateral facets, with more pressure on the lateral surface. Around 30° to 45°, the patella centralizes and becomes "seated" in the femoral sulcus. Between 30° and 70°, the patella becomes very prominent. From 90° to 135°, the patella rotates, sinking into the intercondylar groove, and engages the "odd facet."[12(p122),14(pp536,537),15(pp132,133),16(p287)] Because many people fail to bring their knees into full flexion often enough, the "odd facet" is often a site of degenerative changes and pain due to disuse.[2(p38)]

The amount of knee motion necessary to perform most activities of daily living (ADL) for the elderly population is 0° to 105°. Lack of adequate knee motion usually does not prevent most people from performing ADL,

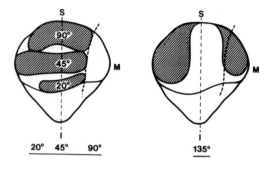

Figure 5–5 Patellar contact points during range of motion. *Source:* Reprinted from W. Woodall and J. Welsh, A Biomechanical Basis for Rehabilitation Programs Involving the Patellofemoral Joint, *The Journal of Orthopaedic and Sports Physical Therapy,* Vol. 11, No. 11, p. 536, © 1990, Williams & Wilkins.

because the surrounding joints compensate for the loss. Table 5–1 shows the ROM necessary to perform some common ADL.

The quadriceps femoris and the hamstrings are the two major muscle groups of the knee joint. They act together with the ankle dorsiflexors and plantarflexors in a consistent coordinated pattern of firing for differing functional activities.[17(p645)] Isolating each individual muscle for strength training must be followed by integrated activities in order to be functional. It is beyond the scope of this text to go into specific muscle actions, and the reader is referred to Table 5–2 for a recap of the basic muscle actions and innervations. Additional muscle actions are discussed in Chapter 6 under knee disorders. For example, the vastus medialis oblique acts to keep the patella on track throughout range[18(p11),10(p12)] and is often weak in patients with anterior knee pain. It is discussed extensively under patellofemoral pain disorders.

Innervation

The knee receives its nerve supply chiefly from the femoral and sciatic (tibial and common peroneal branches) nerves. Specific muscle innervations are described in Table 5–2. Because the front of the knee is derived largely from the second and third lumbar segments, diffuse pain can be referred from the hip region. Pain can also be referred to the back of the knee from an L-5 disc lesion, as this area is developed from the first and second sacral segments.[19(pp622,623)]

The sensory distribution to the knee comes from the L-3, L-4, and L-5 nerve roots, which supply the superior, medial, and lateral aspects of the knee, respectively. The S-2 dermatome covers a longitudinal band on the posterior aspect of the thigh and knee.[20(pp190,191)] As mentioned previously, the receptor afferents provide proprioceptive information from the joint capsule, cruciate ligaments, and muscle tendons. A study by Petrella et al[17(p235)] found that knee joint proprioception diminished in the elderly (age range 60–86 years), but that regular activity attenuated the decline.

Blood Supply

The knee joint has an intricate and complex blood supply. The popliteal artery gives off five genicular branches. The two superior genicular branches supply the distal femur. The middle genicular supplies the cruciate ligaments and the synovium of the joint. The two inferior genicular branches supply the menisci and the tibial plateau (Figure 5–6). These genicular arteries also anastomose with each other and with the descending branch of the lateral circumflex femoral, the circumflex fibular, and the anterior and posterior tibial recurrent arteries to form deep

Table 5–1 Mean Tibiofemoral Motions Necessary for Activities of Daily Living

Activity of Daily Living	Extension-Flexion (0° to 135°)
Walking*	
Stance phase	15°–40°
Swing phase	15°–70°
Stair climbing	
Step over step (up and down)	0°–83°
One step at a time	
Up	
First leg	0°–73°
Second leg	0°–62°
Down	
First leg	0°–43°
Second leg	0°–76°
Standing up from a chair	0°–93°
from a toilet[†]	0°–105°
Stooping to lift an object	0°–117°
Tying a shoe	0°–106°

Note: At least 10° of tibial rotation and abduction/adduction also must be available.

Sources: Physical Therapy (1972;52[1]:34–42), Copyright © 1984, American Physical Therapy Association.

The Knee Joint (p 24) by P Evans, Churchill Livingston, © 1986.

[†]*Clinical Management in Physical Therapy* (1987;7[1]:6), Copyright © 1987, American Physical Therapy Association.

and superficial networks to supply the entire knee joint.[21(pp680,681)]

KINETICS OF THE KNEE JOINT

To prescribe an appropriate rehabilitation program, the therapist must understand how forces are transmitted or absorbed about the tibiofemoral, patellofemoral, and superior tibiofibular joints.

The Tibiofemoral Joint

In determining the joint reaction force on the tibial plateau during dynamic activities, five forces must be considered:

1. the ground reaction force (or body weight)
2. the patellar tendon force
3. the point of application (the patella tendon insertion on tibial tuberosity)
4. the acceleration of the tibia
5. the mass moment of inertia (the torque needed to accelerate the tibia)[12(p126)]

If a therapist desires to minimize the tibiofemoral joint reaction force, the following adjustments to the program could be made:

• Reduce weight-bearing status to partial weight bearing or non-weight bearing.

Table 5–2 Knee Motions, Muscles, and Innervations

Motion	Primary Muscles	Secondary Muscles	Innervation
Flexion 0°–135°	Semimembranosus		Tibial: L-5, S-1, S-2
	Semitendinosus		Tibial: L-5, S-1, S-2
	Biceps femoris		
	Long head		Tibial: L-5, S-1, S-2
	Short head		Peroneal: L-5, S-1, S-2
		Gastrocnemius	Tibial: S-1, S-2
		Popliteus	Tibial: L-4, L-5, S-1
		Sartorius	Femoral: L-2, L-3
Extension 0°	Quadriceps femoris		Femoral: L2-4
	Rectus femoris		
	Vastus medialis		
	Vastus lateralis		
	Vastus Intermedius		
	Tensor fasciae latae		Superior gluteal: L-4, L-5
External tibial rotation 0°–15°	Biceps femoris		
	Long head		Tibial: L-5, S-1, S-2
	Short head		Peroneal: L-5, S-1, S-2
	Tensor fasciae latae		Superior gluteal: L-4, L-5
Internal tibial rotation 0°–15°	Semimembranosus		Tibial: L-5, S-1, S-2
	Semitendinosus		Tibial: L-5, S-1, S-2
	Popliteus		Tibial: L-4, L-5, S-1
		Gracilis	Obturator: L-2, L-3
		Sartorius	Femoral: L-2, L-3

Sources: Gray's Anatomy, ed 35 (pp 562–564, 570, 574–576) by R Warwick and PL Williams (eds), Churchill Livingstone Inc, © 1973. *Knee Pain and Disability* (pp 16–29, 39) by R Cailliet, FA Davis Co, © 1973.

- Perform submaximal quadriceps exercise.
- Perform exercises slowly (decrease tibial acceleration).
- Perform exercises without weights (decrease the mass moment of inertia).

The tibiofemoral joint reaction force is also affected by the condition of the menisci, articular cartilage, and soft tissue structures. Removing the menisci decreases the contact surface area and can increase the joint reaction force by three times that of a knee with the menisci intact. As they do on the hip joint, ADL place stresses on the knee joint well in excess of the body weight. During normal gait, the tibiofemoral joint reaction force is two to four times the body weight and is greater than four times the body weight during stair climbing.[12(pp127,128)]

Shearing forces also occur at the tibiofemoral joint. Unlike compressive joint reaction forces (which are applied perpendicular to the tibial plateau), shear forces are applied parallel to the tibial plateau. In a study on knee exercises,[22(p518)] a difference in

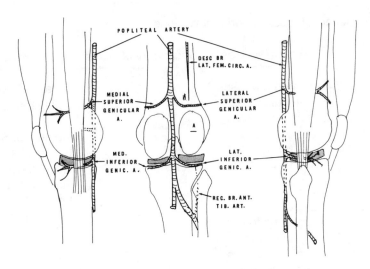

Figure 5–6 Blood supply of the knee joint. The popliteal artery has five branches in the area of the knee joint. *Source:* Reprinted with permission from R. Cailliet, *Knee Pain and Disability,* 3 ed., p. 12, © 1992, F.A. Davis Company.

the direction of the shear force at the tibiofemoral joint was found to be dependent on whether the exercises were performed in the open or closed kinetic chain. The open chain exercises produced significantly less posterior shear force (or PCL stress) than the closed chain exercises, but open chain terminal extension (40° to 0°) produced an anterior shear force (or ACL stress), while closed chain exercises did not. The therapist can therefore design an exercise program to protect the cruciate ligaments from potentially damaging shear forces.

The Patellofemoral Joint

The patella acts as a single axis pulley that deflects the quadriceps tendon, increasing its angle of pull on the tibia and thereby giving a mechanical advantage to the quadriceps muscle group.[23(p301)] At around 45° of extension, it lengthens the quadriceps lever arm by 30%.[12(p128)]

The patellofemoral joint reaction force is influenced by body weight and quadriceps muscle force. Both the quadriceps muscle force and the patellofemoral joint reaction force increase with increased knee flexion.[12(p139)] With increasing flexion from 30° to 60°, the contact surface of the patella increases from 2.6 cm^2 to 3.6 cm^2, helping to distribute the load over a greater area.[24(p37)] With normal patella alignment, the knee can easily withstand the demands of everyday living. If the patella is tilted or displaced, the contact area is altered and the joint reaction force may act on a smaller area, causing damage. In general, to minimize the patellofemoral joint reaction force, exercising in the 20° to 50° range should be limited as the compressive force significantly increases in this range. Table 5–3 shows the approximate patellofemoral joint reaction forces associated with different activities.

The Superior Tibiofibular Joint

The superior tibiofibular joint has great ability to withstand high tensile forces and provides compensatory motion to accommo-

Table 5–3 Approximate Patellofemoral Joint Reaction Forces during Therapeutic Activities

Therapeutic Activity	Patellofemoral Joint Reaction Force (in Units of Body Weight)
Sitting (knee flexed 90°)	0
Walking	½
Stair climbing (7½-inch rise, up or down)	3½
Deep knee bends	7½
Resisted exercise (20 lb)	
0° (straight leg raising)	½
0°–15° (short arc quad)	¾
20°–50°	1½
60°–75°	⅔
80°–90°	½

Source: Data from *Acta Orthopaedica Scandinavica* (pp 131–137), © 1972, Monksgaard International Publishers, Ltd.

date the movement of the tibia during weight bearing. It also accepts one-sixth of the static weight-bearing load of the knee. Although it is not part of the knee joint, injury to the superior tibiofibular joint can directly affect the mechanics of the knee, causing a nagging pain at the lateral aspect.[25(pp129,131)] Dysfunction of the superior tibiofibular joint can occur indirectly from an injury to the inferior tibiofibular joint or nearby ankle structures.

SUMMARY

- The knee joint consists of the tibiofemoral joint and the patellofemoral joint.
- The joint capsule, ligaments, menisci, and musculature maintain the knee's structural integrity.
- The knee is innervated by the femoral nerve and by the tibial and common peroneal branches of the sciatic nerve.

- Afferent mechanoreceptors provide important proprioceptive input influencing functional knee stability.
- Five genicular arteries supply the knee joint.
- The functional ROM of the tibiofemoral joint is 0° to 105°. With the knee flexed, 10° of rotation, abduction, and adduction are also necessary for normal joint function.
- During terminal knee extension, conjunct tibial external rotation occurs in the foot-free position because of the longer medial femoral articulating surface, the offset location of the two axes of rotation, taut ligaments, and muscular action.
- During knee flexion, the patella slides distally, while the articular surface moves proximally.
- The patella acts as a pulley, increasing the lever arm of the quadriceps mechanism by 30%.

- The tibiofemoral joint reaction force greatly exceeds the body weight during most ADLs.
- The patellofemoral joint reaction force is minimal during walking, but increases dramatically during stair climbing and squatting activities.
- The superior tibiofibular joint accepts one-sixth of the weight-bearing load of the knee joint.

REFERENCES

1. Cailliet R. *Knee Pain and Disability*. 3rd ed. Philadelphia: FA Davis Co; 1992.

2. Evans P. *The Knee Joint*. Edinburgh, Scotland: Churchill Livingstone; 1986.

3. Semonian RH, Denlinger PM, Duggan RJ. Proximal tibiofibular subluxation relationship to lateral knee pain: A review of proximal tibiofibular joint pathologies. *J Orthop Sports Phys Ther*. 1995;21(5):248–257.

4. Rand JA, Dorr LD, eds. *Total Arthroplasty of the Knee*. Rockville, Md: Aspen Publishers, Inc; 1987.

5. Van Dommelen BA, Fowler PJ. Anatomy of the posterior cruciate ligament: A review. *The Am J Sports Med*. 1989;17(1):24–29.

6. Bach BR, Daluga DJ, Mikosz R, Andriacchi TP, Seidl R. Force displacement characteristics of the posterior cruciate ligament. *The Am J Sports Med*. 1992;20(1):67–72.

7. Kleinbart FA, Bryk E, Evangelista J, Scott WN, Vigorita VJ. Histologic comparison of posterior cruciate ligaments from arthritic and age-matched knee specimens. *J Arthrop*. 1996;11(6):726–731.

8. Johansson H, Sjolander P, Sojka P. A sensory role for the cruciate ligaments. *Clin Orthop*. 1991;268:161–178.

9. Greenleaf JE. The anatomy and biomechanics of the lateral aspect of the knee. *Oper Techn Sports Med*. 1996;4(3):141–147.

10. Engle RP. *Knee Ligament Rehabilitation*. New York: Churchill Livingstone, 1991.

11. Blackburn TA, Eiland WG, Brandy WD. An introduction to the plica. *J Orthop Sports Phys Ther*. 1982;3(4):171–177.

12. Frankel VH, Nordin M. *Basic Biomechanics of the Skeletal System*. 2nd ed. Philadelphia: Lea & Febiger; 1989.

13. Hollister AM, Jatana S, Singh AK, Sullivan WW, Lupichuk AG. The axes of rotation of the knee. *Clin Orthop*. 1993;290:259–268.

14. Woodall W, Welsh J. A biomechanical basis for rehabilitation programs involving the patellofemoral joint. *J Orthop Sports Phys Ther*. 1990;11(11):535–542.

15. Laforgia R, Renna A, Mocci A, Specchiulli F. Biomechanical aspects of the patellofemoral joint. *J Sport Traumatol*. 1994;16(3):131–146.

16. Goodfellow J, Hungerford DS, Zindel M. Patellofemoral joint mechanics and pathology: Functional anatomy of the patellofemoral joint. *J Bone Joint Surg*. 1976;B-58(3):287–290.

17. Petrella RJ, Lattanzio PJ, Nelson MG. Effect of age and activity on knee-joint proprioception. *Amer J Phys Med Rehabil*. 1997;76(3):235–241.

18. McConnell J. Patellofemoral Course Notes; 1988.

19. Cyriax J. *Textbook of Orthopaedic Medicine*. London, England: Bailliere Tindall; 1978.

20. Hoppenfeld S. *Physical Examination of the Spine and Extremities*. New York: Appleton-Century-Crofts; 1976.

21. Warwick R, Williams PL, eds. *Gray's Anatomy*. 35th ed. Edinburgh, Scotland: Churchill Livingstone; 1973.

22. Wilk KE, Escamilla RF, Fleisig GS, et al. A comparison of tibiofemoral joint forces and electromyographic activity during open and closed kinetic chain exercises. *Am J Sports Med*. 1996;24(4):518–527.

23. Kramer P. Patella malalignment syndrome: rationale to reduce excessive lateral pressure. *J Orthop Sports Phys Ther*. 1986;8(6):301–309.

24. Marder RA, Swanson TV, Sharkey NA, Duwelius PJ. Effects of partial patellectomy and reattachment of the patellar tendon on patellofemoral contact areas and pressures. *J Bone Joint Surg*. 1993;75-A(1):35–45.

25. Radakovich M, Malone T. The superior tibiofibular joint: the forgotten joint. *J Orthop Sports Phys Ther*. 1982;3(3):129–132.

SUGGESTED READING

Grelsamer RP, McConnel J. *The Patella—A Team Approach*. Gaithersburg, MD: Aspen Publishers, Inc; 1998.

6

Treatment of Common Problems of the Knee Joint

By the time a knee enters its sixth decade, it is often the site of multiple complaints. Physical therapy and occupational therapy are usually reserved for patients who have severe pain or dysfunction that limits their independence in daily care.

KNEE FRACTURES

Fractures about the knee can involve the distal end of the femur (generally classified as supracondylar, intercondylar, or condylar), as well as tibial plateau fractures (see Figure 6–1). In addition, the patella is com-

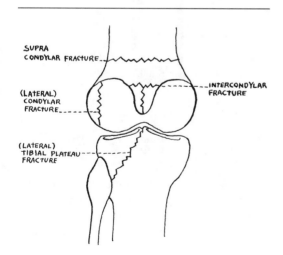

Figure 6–1 Fractures about the knee

monly fractured in the elderly. The therapist needs a firm understanding of the types of fractures and the surgical intervention required to stabilize the segments in order to provide appropriate treatment for patients with knee fractures.

Distal Femoral Fracture

Fracture of the distal femur is occurring with greater frequency, especially in nursing home residents. Complication rates in the frail elderly are high, with 9% of patients later requiring above-knee amputation for fracture displacement or infection. In addition, a high 1-year mortality rate (22%) and a significant decrease in function of the survivors occurs with this fracture.[1(pp22,24)]

In the elderly population, distal femur fractures usually result from a low-velocity injury, such as a simple fall. The fractures are generally classified into three major types (Figure 6–2):

1. Type A: extra-articular
2. Type B: partial articular or unicondylar
3. Type C: complete articular or bicondylar[2(p193)]

If the fracture is impacted or minimally displaced, the patient can wear a knee immo-

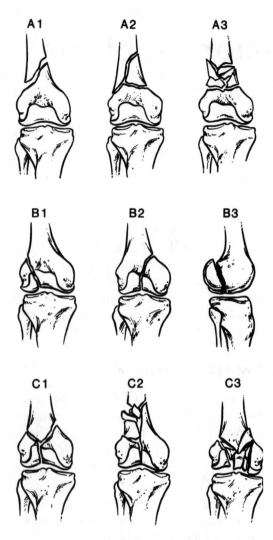

Figure 6–2 The Association for the Study of Internal Fixation (AO/ASIF) classification of distal femur fractures: type A, extra-articular; type B, unicondylar; type C, bicondylar. *Source:* Reprinted with permission from K.J. Koval and J.D. Zuckerman, *Fractures in the Elderly*, p. 194, © 1998, Lippincott-Raven Publishers.

bilizer and continue protected weight bearing until the fracture is healed. (The alternative treatment of skeletal traction and cast immobilization is not well tolerated by the elderly patient.) In most instances, the doc-

tor opts for surgical intervention for proper stabilization of the fragments. In the elderly, the surgeon often shortens the femur by impacting the proximal fragment into the distal fragment and then further stabilizes it with a blade plate (Figure 6–3).[3(pp39,43)] In addition to the blade plate, the following types of internal fixations are also commonly used:

- dynamic condylar screw (similar to hip compression screw)
- lag screws
- interlocked intramedullary nails
- flexible intramedullary nails (e.g., Zickel nails, Rush pins, Enders nails)
- total knee arthroplasty (TKA)[1(p22),2(pp197–198)]

The complication rate for surgical correction is high (22.4%) in the frail elderly and includes: respiratory infection, urinary tract infection, nonunion, loss of fixation, damage to the nerve or blood supply in the popliteal

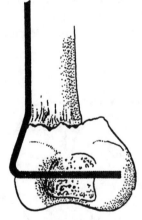

Figure 6–3 Blade plate fixation for distal femur fracture. In elderly patients or others with soft bone, it is best to shorten the femur and impact the proximal fragment into the distal fragment. *Source:* Reprinted from *Techniques in Orthopaedics* (1986;1[1]:43), Copyright © 1986, Aspen Publishers, Inc.

region, and loss of range of motion (ROM) and function.[1(p22),2(p200),4(p214)]

Tibial Plateau Fracture

Tibial plateau fractures (Figure 6–1) are common injuries, making up 8% of all fractures in the elderly.[5(p1455)] They are caused by either a compression force (as occurs in a jump or a simple fall) or a violent lateral force (as occurs in a car accident from the side). The lateral condyle is more frequently involved, resulting in split fractures (Schatzker Type 1) and a high incidence of soft tissue damage to the medial collateral ligament (MCL) (55%), the cruciates (69%), and the lateral meniscus (45%) in younger age groups.[4(p221),6(p389)] In the elderly, the subchondral bone is weaker, resulting in more split-depression (Type 2) and central depression (Type 3) fractures. The damaging force is dissipated by the collapsing bone, protecting the opposite collateral ligament[2(p203)] (Figure 6–4).

If the fracture fragments are stable (common in central depression fractures), the patient can be casted in 10° of flexion for two weeks. Some doctors opt to mobilize the knee first on a continuous passive motion (CPM) machine for a few days before casting. The patient is placed on protected weight bearing for 6 to 8 weeks.[7(p90)]

Surgery is the preferred treatment in unstable and displaced fractures.[8(p92)] Fractures of the medial plateau are difficult to stabilize. A medial parapatellar approach is generally used; the fracture is slightly over-reduced into valgus using lag screws; and fixation is with a buttress plate.[2(p213)] Fractures of the lateral plateau are somewhat easier to stabilize—depending on exact location, amount of comminution, and displacement. A lateral parapatellar incision or midline incision is used, any depressed articular

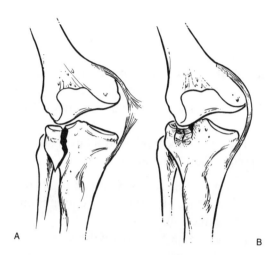

Figure 6–4 Differences in tibial plateau fracture with age. (A) Younger patients, whose strong subchondral bone resists depression, typically develop split fractures (Type 1); these patients are at the highest risk for collateral or cruciate ligament rupture. (B) In the elderly, the subchondral bone is less able to resist axial loading; these patients typically have depression (Type 3) or split-depression (not shown) fractures. As the bone compresses, the force is dissipated and protects the opposite collateral ligament from injury. *Source:* Adapted with permission from K.J. Koval and J.D. Zuckerman, *Fractures in the Elderly*, p. 194, © 1998, Lippincott-Raven Publishers.

fragments are elevated, bone is grafted to fill in defects, and fixation is with lag screws and buttress plate.[7(p93)7(pp209,210)] Any soft tissue injuries are also repaired.

Common complications following surgical repair of tibial plateau fractures include infection (8%), deep vein thrombosis (6%), and loss of knee flexion (42%).[7(pp97,98)]

Patellar Fractures

Because of the exposed nature of the patella, patellar fractures are common, comprising 1% of all skeletal injuries. Fractures are categorized as undisplaced or displaced; and further classified as transverse, vertical, or comminuted.[9(pp2111,2112)] Fractures in the elderly are caused by either direct trauma (from a fall or motor vehicle accident) or indirect trauma, such as from descending stairs or squatting.

There are three types of fracture that allow for conservative treatment:

1. vertical fractures with congruence of the articular surface and only minimal fragment dislocation
2. transverse fractures without joint involvement
3. transverse fractures involving the joint, but with only minimal fragment dislocation and incongruence of the articular surface[10(p198)]

Conservative treatment varies from surgeon to surgeon and may consist of initial joint aspiration, immobilization with a cast or splint for 2 to 6 weeks, and partial weight bearing (PWB) for 4 to 6 weeks. Surgical repair can involve the wiring of fragments together with Kirschner wire or an anterior tension band, screw fixation, partial patellectomy, or complete patellectomy.[9(p2112),10(pp198,199),11(pp177,178)]

A partial patellectomy has been shown to preserve some of the mechanical advantage of the extensor mechanism provided by the patella[12(p217)]; however, the smaller the patella fragment retained, the smaller the patellar contact area and the larger the joint reaction force occurring at the patellofemoral joint.[13(p44)]

Treatment of Knee Fractures

During the initial evaluation, the therapist should ascertain the following information in addition to the standard assessment presented in Chapter 2: the fracture site, the method of fracture reduction, any other known soft tissue injury (e.g., torn ligaments), and the weight-bearing orders. To evaluate function, the therapist may want to use the Iowa Knee Evaluation (Exhibit 6–1) or any other suitable functional scale.

Phase I (Postfracture Days 2 to 21)

During Phase 1, the knee usually is casted or splinted, although some doctors believe that immobilization is unnecessary and harmful. The joint is markedly swollen, hot, and painful. Weight bearing is limited on crutches or a walker. The therapist must protect the knee from unnecessary external and internal forces while returning the surrounding joints to previous function. The program is dependent on the location and severity of the fracture, amount of soft tissue involvement, and the attending physicians' view on mobility versus fracture stabilization.

Exercise Program. During the first week, the physician may order immediate CPM to prevent adhesions.[2(p201),10(p198)] Active ankle exercises and straight leg raising (SLR) in supine, side-lying, and prone positions (Figure 6–5) are initiated to prevent thrombosis[7(p95)] and begin strengthening the lower quarter muscles. (Depending on the fracture site and weight of the splint or cast, the patient may be unable to perform SLR at this time.) Except in the case of patellar fracture, the patient also performs "quad sets" and gluteal sets. Gentle ROM exercises usually begin after 1 or 2 weeks. If the patient suffered a distal femoral fracture, the therapist should not resist plantarflexion or passively stretch the Achilles tendon. The gastrocnemius attaches to the femoral condyles and could pull the fractured segments apart. Based on the initial evaluation results, the therapist should prescribe a reconditioning program as needed.

Exhibit 6–1 The Iowa Knee Evaluation

	No. of Points
Function (35 points)	
Instructions: Eleven activities of daily living are listed with a value. If the patient can perform the activity easily without restriction, give full value; if the patient cannot (or could not if he/she tried) perform the activity at all, give no points; if the patient can or could perform the activity but with difficulty, give an appropriate number of points between 0 and full value.	
Does most of housework or job, which requires moving about (5)	
Walks enough to be independent (5)	———
Dresses unaided (includes tying shoes and putting on socks) (5)	———
Sits without difficulty at table or toilet, including sitting down and getting up (reduce if additional aid is necessary) (4)	
Picks up objects from floor by squatting or kneeling (3)	———
Bathes without help (3)	———
Negotiates stairs foot over foot (3)	———
Negotiates stairs in any manner (2)	———
Carries objects, such as a suitcase (2)	———
Gets into an automobile or public conveyance unaided and rides comfortably (2)	———
Drives an automobile (1)	———
Total	———
Freedom from pain (maximum, 35 points; circle one only)	
Instructions: Circle the value that is overall most representative of the patient's pain, using the word descriptors. (Scoring should not be based simply on asking the patient the word descriptors in question form.)	35
No pain	
Mild pain with fatigue	30
Mild pain with weight-bearing	20
Moderate pain with weight-bearing	15
Severe pain with weight-bearing, mild or moderate at rest	10
Severe, continuous pain	0
Total	———
Gait (maximum, 10 points; circle one only)	
No limp, no support	10
Limp, no support	8
One cane or crutch	8
One long brace	8
One brace with crutch or cane	6
Two crutches with or without a brace	4
Cannot walk	0
Total	———
Absence of deformity or stability	
No fixed flexion of more than 10 degrees with weight-bearing	3
No fixed flexion of more than 20 degrees with weight-bearing	2
No fixed flexion of more than 30 degrees with weight-bearing	1
No varus or valgus deformity of more than 10 degrees with weight-bearing	3
No varus or valgus deformity of more than 20 degrees with weight-bearing	2
No varus or valgus deformity of more than 30 degrees with weight-bearing	1
No ligamentous instability	2
No locking, giving-way, or extension lag of more than 10 degrees	2
Total	———
Range of motion (10 points)	
Instructions: Total amount of flexion or extension, in degrees (normal, 150 degrees); assign 1 point for every 15 degrees.	
Total	
A normal knee receives 100 points; a score of 90 to 100 points is considered excellent function; 80 to 89 points is good function; 70 to 79 points is fair function.	———

Source: Adapted with permission from T.C. Merchant and F.R. Dietz, "Long-Term Follow-up after Fractures of the Tibial and Fibular Shafts," *The Journal of Bone and Joint Surgery*, Vol. 71-A, No. 4, p. 600, © 1989, Journal of Bone and Joint Surgery, Inc.

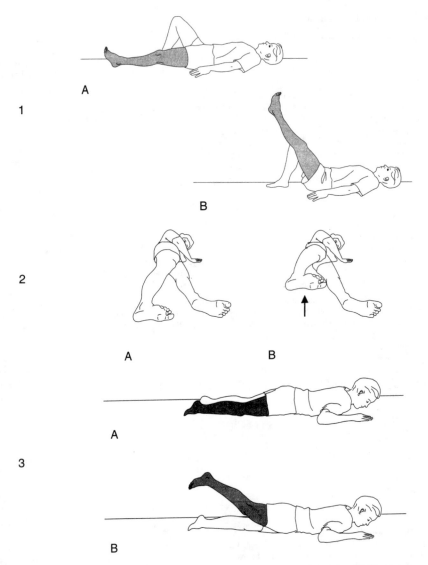

Figure 6–5 Straight-leg raising exercise in (1) supine, (2) side-lying, and (3) prone positions. A is starting position of exercise, B is ending position. These exercises can be done with a cast or splint on the knee to prevent movement of fracture fragments. Frail patients may have difficulty with these exercises. *Source:* Adapted from *Exercise Handouts for Rehabilitation*, C.B. Lewis, T. McNerny, pp. 63, 65, 67. Copyright © Aspen Publishers, Inc., 1993.

Mobility/Ambulation Program. A major portion of the therapist/patient program concerns returning the patient to independence in general mobility skills as soon as possible. The therapist instructs the patient in all aspects of bed mobility and transfers. The patient must ambulate slowly and unload the fractured lower extremity (LE) to minimize the tibiofemoral joint reaction force. Tibial plateau fractures are usually non-weight bearing (NWB) or touch-down weight bearing (TDWB) to prevent collapse of the fractured segment. If necessary, the patient can begin protected stair climbing with railings.

Activities of Daily Living Program. The therapist instructs the patient in the activities of daily living (ADL) tasks of grooming, toileting, and meal preparation from a seated position. Instrumental ADL—including driving—are contraindicated. If the patient wishes to resume sexual activity, he or she should lie supine with the involved extremity supported on a pillow. The pillow must be removed after intercourse to prevent muscle shortening.

Phase II (Postfracture Weeks 3 to 6)

During Phase II, sufficient soft tissue and bony healing should have occurred to allow for more aggressive therapy. Depending on the location and severity of the fracture, the orthopaedic surgeon may allow the splint to be removed for ROM and muscle-strengthening purposes. The therapist now can evaluate the exposed knee. The therapist should cautiously look for injury to the anterior cruciate ligament, meniscus, and collateral ligaments, as these structures are commonly damaged. (Standard ligamentous testing is contraindicated at this time as it can shear the fracture segments apart.) Weight-bearing orders are usually increased to PWB or weight bearing as tolerated with a splint and an ambulation device. Some patients may continue at NWB or TDWB.

Exercise Program. Prior to exercising, the therapist applies ice to the knee to help reduce pain and swelling. The patient with a tibial or a femoral fracture begins isotonic exercises within available ROM. If the patient cannot stop "splinting," biofeedback applied to the quadriceps or hamstrings can be beneficial to minimize cocontraction at the

joint. The patient progresses to lightly resisted isotonic or submaximal isokinetic exercise. The therapist may gently mobilize the patella to help regain ROM.

The patient with a patellar fracture continues SLR and begins quad sets and terminal knee extension exercises (0° to 20°) in supine and prone positions (Figure 6–6). Biofeedback can be used over the vastus medialis oblique (VMO) to help reeducate the muscle during terminal knee extension in the supine position. Resistive exercising in the midrange (20° to 50°) greatly increases the patellofemoral joint reaction force and should be avoided.

If a therapeutic pool is available (or a heated hotel pool), the patient with any type of knee fracture can begin the ROM and gentle strengthening exercises shown in Figure 4–13 in Chapter 4. Exercises should be done slowly and without buoyancy cuffs or swim fins.

Mobility/Ambulation Program. The patient now should be independent in all transfers. Gait training emphasizes maneuverability in all directions on even surfaces with a walker (or crutches) and a splint. If a therapeutic pool is available, the patient can begin to correct any gait deviations while in this protected environment. Stair climbing with appropriate ambulation device should be taught. The therapist must make sure that patients with tibial plateau fractures maintain proper weight bearing, especially during advanced ambulation activities such as stair climbing.

Activities of Daily Living Program. With PWB orders in effect, the patient continues to protect the fracture site by performing most ADL tasks in a sitting position. If the patient has good standing balance, grooming, dressing, and light homemaking can be worked on in upright positions holding onto

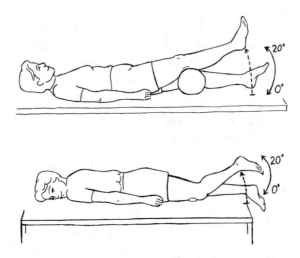

Figure 6–6 Terminal knee extension exercises in supine and prone positions. Supine exercising works the quadriceps group; prone exercising activates the hamstrings. A folded towel placed just proximal to the knee prevents patellar compression during prone lying.

furniture or countertops. Functional ambulation with an ambulation device and a splint should be approaching independence, except in the frail elderly who tend to need more time. Instrumental ADL, including driving, are still contraindicated at this time.

Phase III (Postfracture Weeks 6 to 12)

During Phase III, the fracture usually is healed and the orthopaedic surgeon orders full weight bearing (FWB). Almost all casts or splints are discontinued at this time, except for complex trauma patients or very frail patients. For many patients, Phase III marks the beginning of formal therapy. (Many doctors are reluctant to use up valuable therapy benefits while the patient is put in a cast and not ready for aggressive rehabilitation.) The therapist and patient goals are to return the joint (and the patient) to maximal function.

Exercise Program. The patient requires a minimal knee ROM of 0° to 105° for everyday function (see Chapter 5). Fractures about the knee tend to cause a loss of more flexion than extension. The therapist can use heat modalities or whirlpool therapy to prepare the soft tissues before using the following techniques to restore functional ROM:

- joint mobilization: especially inferior patella glide and posterior tibial glide
- passive stretch
- myofascial release (MFR): cross-hand technique (Figure 6–7)
- proprioceptive neuromuscular facilitation (PNF) techniques of "contract-relax" and "hold-relax"

As increased motion is achieved, the patient must exercise actively in this newly available ROM in order to maintain it. For patients with patella fracture, it is imperative to ensure the proper length of the hamstrings, iliotibial band (ITB), and gastrocnemius for proper patella tracking.

Along with sufficient ROM, the patient also needs adequate strength and control in the knee to walk, climb stairs, and perform skill activities. The patient can now tolerate

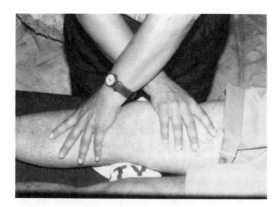

Figure 6–7 Cross-hand technique to fascia about the knee. This technique can also be used on the quadriceps muscle or the iliotibial band.

the full spectrum of exercise: isometrics, resisted isotonics, and isokinetics. The exercises must emphasize both concentric and eccentric work. As the knee is a weight-bearing joint, loaded exercises such as slight squats, leg presses, and step-ups and step-downs also should be performed. Resisted bicycle riding or use of a stair-climber increases both strength and ROM while providing an aerobic effect.

Patients with a healed patella fracture can now follow the intense strengthening and motor retraining program given to patients with patellofemoral dysfunction (shown later in this chapter.) The therapist may also discover that patients with a fracture of the distal femur or tibial plateau have developed secondary patellofemoral pain due to swelling, immobilization, or atrophy. They also need a patellofemoral program to complete the rehabilitation process.

Mobility/Ambulation Program. In the mobility/ambulation program, the patient now begins advanced balance and proprioception retraining. The patient strives for one-legged standing balance of 5 to 10 seconds with eyes open and works on the wobbleboard in standing position as shown in Figure 4–9 in Chapter 4. The patient also continues high-level gait training. In order to ambulate safely in the community (e.g., cross streets, shop, bank), the patient should be able to walk at a velocity of 150 to 208 ft/min (44.5 to 63.5 m/min) and be able to traverse a distance of about 1,000 feet.[14(pp1372,1373)] Although the ROM necessary for stair climbing step-over-step (0° to 83°) usually is present, the elderly patient commonly has difficulty or pain with the actual activity. Often, the problem lies at the ankle joint where the patient lacks sufficient dorsiflexor ROM or plantarflexor strength to achieve coordinated stair climbing. Task-specific exercise (e.g., progressive step-ups) may be required to achieve this goal.

Activities of Daily Living Program. The patient usually has sufficient ROM and strength to perform most self-care activities in the ADL program independently except for bathing in a bathtub. Unless the patient greatly desires a bath, a shower or tub seat is a safer alternative. The therapist now assesses the method the patient uses for advanced ADL tasks such as laundry, cooking, and shopping and makes recommendations for energy conservation, joint protection, and safety. If possible, the therapist also teaches the patient how to get on and off the floor. Although many patients will be unable to perform this skilled activity, it literally can be a lifesaver.

Summary of Treatment of Knee Fractures

- Know the type of fracture, the type of internal fixation, and the weight-bearing order.

- *During the first 3 weeks postfracture*
  1. protect the fracture site from unnecessary weight-bearing or rotational forces

2. begin CPM on physician order
3. begin isometric knee exercises and active hip and ankle exercises
4. do not stretch the Achilles tendon for patients with distal femur fracture
5. teach independence in all mobility skills, including ambulation with device
6. teach ADL tasks in sitting posture.

- *As the fracture stabilizes*
  1. begin active and active-assistive knee exercises within available ROM
  2. use biofeedback to enhance patient body awareness
  3. progress to lightly resisted isotonic and/or submaximal isokinetic exercise
  4. be aware of potential damage to ligaments, menisci, and other soft tissue structures
  5. continue gait training to improve maneuvering ability on level surfaces and stairs.

- *As the fracture heals*
  1. strive to attain knee ROM of 0° to 105° by using modalities, joint mobilization, MFR, PNF, and passive stretching
  2. maximize concentric and eccentric strength by using isometrics, isotonics, and isokinetics
  3. retrain the knee in a weight-bearing posture
  4. begin patellofemoral program for patients with patella fracture (and others as needed)
  5. retrain balance and proprioception with a small balance board
  6. train gait on all surfaces and stairs to eliminate gait deviations and improve ambulation velocity
  7. wean off ambulation devices
  8. teach energy conservation and joint protection during ADL.

OSTEOARTHRITIS

The most common form of arthritis in the knee is osteoarthritis (OA) involving the medial compartment of the tibiofemoral joint or the odd facet of the patella.[15(p48)] Although OA in the elderly is relatively nonprogressive, 39% of the "young" elderly complain of osteoarthritic symptoms at the knee, such as decreased ROM and function, joint swelling, and joint stiffness.[16(pp24,25)] Due to a decrease in the concentration of proteoglycans, the articular cartilage in weight-bearing joints begins to degenerate, with a resulting loss of strength and ability to absorb shock. In an effort to correct the problem, the subchondral bone remodels itself, eventually forming spurs and subarticular cysts[17(pp608,609)] (Figure 6–8).

Although the etiology of OA is presently unknown, there have been many theories advanced as to why cartilage begins to degenerate. Aside from genetics, factors that possibly predispose a person to developing OA of the knee are:

- increased age[18(p1446)]
- overuse[19(p244)]
- obesity[18(p1446),19(p244)]
- years of heavy labor[19(p243)]
- significant prior knee injury[19(p244)]
- increased bone mass[20(p21)]
- increased estrogen[21(p300)]

Medical intervention has revolved around symptomatic relief or replacement of the damaged joint surfaces with artifical components. As knowledge about this disease process grows, corrections and perhaps a cure become a possibility in the near future. Already isolated chondral defects have been repaired with autologous chondrocyte transplantation[22(p894)] and intra-articular injections of hyaluronate—a principal component of normal synovial fluid—have decreased pain

- joint tenderness
- joint crepitance
- capsular pattern: ROM limited mostly in flexion, slightly in extension
- moderately decreased strength (i.e., disuse atrophy)
- decreased ligamentous laxity (i.e., increased stiffness)[25(p189)]
- decreased proprioception[26(p53)]
- altered quadriceps coordination[27(p11)]
- decreased standing balance (with greater body sway)[28(p16)]
- marked loss of mobility skills, including basic transfers[29(p1435)]
- antalgic gait

Due to the major disability attributed to OA of the knee, the therapist should perform a functional assessment of the patient on the initial visit, using the Iowa Knee Evaluation (Exhibit 6–1) or any other suitable scale, such as the Arthritis Impact Measurement Scale.

The therapist must design a rehabilitation program that increases strength, ROM, balance, proprioception, coordination, mobility, and gait pattern, while protecting the osteoarthritic knee from unnecessary forces.

Exercise Program

ROM. Although the pathomechanics of the osteoarthritic knee may prevent it, the patient should attempt to regain 0° to 105° of ROM. After using a heat modality to prepare the soft tissues, the therapist can mobilize the joint to stretch the joint capsule, passively stretch tight musculature, or use MFR to release fascial restrictions (Figure 6–7). Stationary bicycle riding also provides an excellent way to gain ROM and is under direct patient control.

Strengthening. Short-term studies have indicated that exercising has increased physical capacity and decreased pain level in pa-

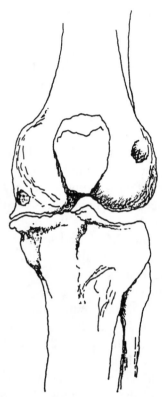

Figure 6–8 Osteoarthritis of the knee. Note the narrowing joint space and bony proliferation in the medial component, as well as the subchondral cysts. *Source:* Adapted with permission from C. Moncur, "The Older Person with Rheumatoid Arthritis and Osteoarthritis," *Orthopaedic Physical Therapy Clinics of North America*, Vol. 2, No. 3, p. 252, Copyright © 1993, W.B. Saunders Company.

and improved cartilage metabolism.[23(pp285,289)] There has also been some promising research into cartilage-modifying drugs, such as sulfated glycosaminoglycans, growth factors, and degradative enzyme inhibitors.[24(p851)]

Treatment of the Osteoarthritic Knee

On evaluation, the therapist may find some of the following signs and impairments in patients with moderate to severe OA:

tients with OA of the knee.[29(p1435),30(p68)] Additional studies have shown that increasing quadriceps strength is associated with maximal walking speed[31(p15),32(pM225)] and independence in both basic and instrumental ADL.[33(p1)] To improve strength and endurance in this population, a combination of isometric, isotonic, and isokinetic training has been highly successful.[34(p38)] The quadriceps can be trained eccentrically by performing a modified fencer's lunge (Figure 6–9). By widening the base of support, the exercise becomes progressively more difficult. Standing squats (0° to 25°) also help regain eccentric quadriceps control and strength. (Additional quadriceps strengthening exercises are discussed later in this chapter.) Many of the above exercises can be performed easily in a therapeutic pool. In addition, running, jumping, and, of course, swimming retrain the muscles while the buoyant quality of the water protects the arthritic joint.

Motor retraining. With both proprioception and coordination adversely affected in patients with OA of the knee, motor retraining needs to be done in addition to the simple strength and ROM exercises. Fisher and Pendergast designed the quantitative progressive exercise rehabilitation (QPER) program to improve motor unit activation in persons with OA of the knee. Their 2- to 4-month program (Exhibit 6–2) used a special table that easily allowed for exercising the quadriceps and hamstrings at differing muscle lengths. Exercise type included isometric, isotonic, ROM, and speed work. The hour program was conducted three times per week. The results showed significant increase in function, walking speed, cardiovascular function, pain reduction, and a 20% improvement in tibiofemoral joint space, suggesting that QPER may alter the degenerative process of OA.[35(pp47–49),36(p47)]

Although many clinicians will be unable to duplicate the conditions of Fisher and

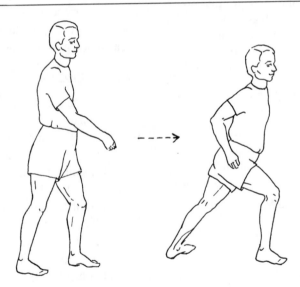

Figure 6–9 Modified fencer's lunge to promote eccentric contraction of the quadriceps. The patient aims the patella over the second toe while slowly lunging forward. If balance is impaired, furniture or an ambulation device can be used for support.

Exhibit 6–2 The 2-Month QPER Program

Week	Exercise
1	Isometric—5 × 5 s (2 days); 5 × 9 s (1 day) for quads (3 knee and 5 hip angles), hams (3 knee and 1 hip angle), each leg independently ROM—slow—5 × (all positions)
2	Isometric—5 × 9 s (all positions) Isotonic—5 ×—Resistance = 10% of max. strength measured for each position (all positions)
3	Isometric—5 × 9 s (all positions) Isotonic—5 × — Resistance = 20% of max. strength (all positions)
4	Isometric—5 × 9 s (all positions) Isotonic—5 × — Resistance — 30% of max. strength (all positions) Endurance—Hold resistance for a max. of 90 s or until fatigued. Repeat for quads and hams, each leg, only 1 position per day
5	Isometric—5 × 9 s (all positions) Isotonic—5 × — Resistance = 40% of max. strength (all positions) Endurance—90 s (1 position) Speed—5 × —Resistance = 20% of max. strength (all positions) Lift resistance as rapidly as possible through ROM
6	Isometric—5 × 9 s (all positions) Isotonic—5 × — Resistance = 50% of max. strength (all positions) Endurance—90 s (1 position) Speed—5 × —Resistance = 30% of max. strength (all positions)
7	Isometric—5 × 9 s (all positions) Isotonic—5 × — Resistance = 60% of max. strength (all positions) Endurance—90 s (1 position) Speed—5 × —Resistance = 40% of max. strength (all positions)
8	Isometric—5 × 9 s (all positions) Isotonic—5 × — Resistance = 70% of max. strength (all positions) Endurance—90 s (1 position) Speed—5 × —Resistance = 50% of max. strength (all positions)

The 3- and 4-month programs were similar with a less aggressive progression. The exercises were performed 3 times per week for up to 1 hour/day. *Abbreviation:* ROM = range of motion.

Source: Reprinted from *Journal of Back and Musculoskeletal Rehabilitation*, Vol. 5, No. 47, N.M. Fisher and D.R. Pendergast, "Application of Quantitative and Progressive Exercise Rehabilitation to Patients with Osteoarthritis of the Knee," p. 47, © 1995, with permission from Elsevier Science.

Pendergast's work, the important concepts of pain-free exercising, of recruiting muscles at varying lengths, and of ensuring that speed work is done (especially with elderly clients) can be incorporated into any rehabilitation program. Other types of proprioception and coordination work can be done on wobbleboards or foam rollers, or by using surface biofeedback while performing exercises and activities. Even rocking in a rocking chair has been shown to provide proprioceptive input to the ankle and knee.

Marching and kicking exercises while sitting on a physioball or air disc (e.g., Swisdisk™ or SitFit™) also work on motor retraining (Figure 6–10).

Mobility Program

It is crucial for the patient to be independent in sit-to-stand transfers, and most of the mobility program should address this issue. The patient with severe arthritis should use the upper extremities (UEs) to help unload the knees during this activity.

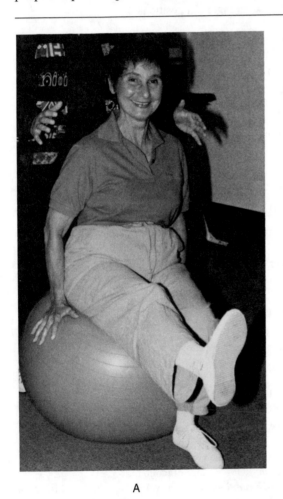

A

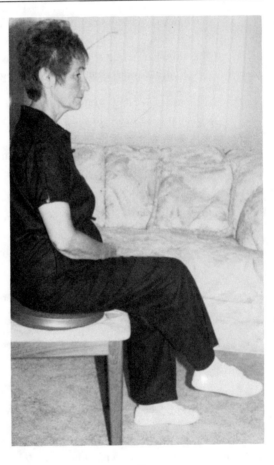

B

Figure 6–10 Motor retraining of lower quarter on a (A) physioball, for patients with good balance or modified on an (B) air disc for patients who are more frail or anxious. The air disc provides a degree of instability in a safer environment.

To teach the patient how to get on and off the floor, the therapist should bring the patient through the developmental sequence first. To prevent further damage to the arthritic knee(s), the patient should perform this activity each day on a padded but firm surface for a limited time only (5 minutes or less). Depending on the severity of the arthritis, some patients will be unable to tolerate this activity even with modifications.

Ambulation Program

The average arthritic patient ambulates at a greatly reduced velocity—125 ft/min[37(p1057)]—which is below the minimal velocity for safe ambulation in the community (150 to 208 ft/min),[14(pp1372,1373)] and about half the velocity of ambulation of healthy persons (262 ft/min).[37(p1057)] As mentioned previously, quadriceps strength is correlated with maximal ambulation velocity and must be worked on in the exercise program. In addition, Brinkmann and Perry[37(p1059)] found it necessary to focus attention on both the rate of motion and the ROM to improve ambulation velocity. Isokinetic exercise at high speeds is an excellent method for training rate of motion. If isokinetic equipment is unavailable, the patient can exercise isotonically with emphasis on speed and endurance. Fun activities such as kicking a ball (in sitting or supported standing position) also can improve rate of motion.

Patients with OA of the knee tend to display an abnormal gait pattern because of two physical impairments: genu varum and knee flexion contracture. The genu varum forces the patient to sway the trunk laterally during the stance phase to unload the medial compartment of the knee. Knee flexion contracture causes a more pervasive change in gait pattern. A 30° flexion contracture causes all phases of the gait cycle to be abnormal except for initial swing. Even a 15° flexion contracture results in a shorter step length and an increased demand on the quadriceps.[38(pp239–240,243)]

Although therapy may be unable to restore a completely normal gait pattern, the patient still should be able to ambulate functionally in the community. Ambulation devices, such as a cane or crutches, may be needed to decrease the tibiofemoral joint reaction force during the stance phase of gait. In addition, recent studies have shown that counterforce bracing for medial compartment OA can reduce pain and improve walking and stair climbing ability[39(p745),40(p251)] (Figure 6–11). The inability to get around in the community is one of the indications for a TKA.

Stair climbing is very stressful to both the tibiofemoral and patellofemoral joints. The therapist should teach the patient to negotiate stairs by unloading the LE until the surrounding musculature attains sufficient strength to protect the joint. Strength training should emphasize the gastrocnemius and

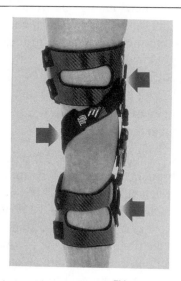

Figure 6–11 The Unloader™ Counterforce brace for the osteoarthritic knee with medial involvement. Courtesy of Generation II USA Inc., Bothell, Washington.

gluteus maximus muscles, which assist the quadriceps in stair climbing.

Activities of Daily Living Program

If knee flexion remains less than 90°, the ability to tie shoes, stoop to reach into low cupboards, and squat may be lost. The patient must compensate for this loss of knee motion by increasing available ROM at surrounding joints or through the use of assistive devices (e.g., dressing sticks, long-handled dusters). Pain also can be the limiting factor in achieving independence in functional activities. The therapist must educate the patient on body awareness, need for adequate rest, and joint protection.

In addition, gains made in strength, ROM, and balance may not easily transfer to functional activities. The patient may be locked into an old movement pattern (i.e., stuck in a rut) and be unable to change an old way of doing things (even if the old way hurts or is difficult). The therapist must encourage the patient to experiment with alternate methods, using the newfound gains from exercising. Through trial and error, the patient will learn to discard inefficient or painful movement strategies and replace them with efficient, less painful movement.

Summary of Treatment of the Osteoarthritic Knee

- Strive to regain 0° to 105° of knee ROM through joint mobilization, muscle stretching, and MFR.
- Maximize concentric and eccentric quadriceps strength by using a combination of isometrics, isotonics, and isokinetics.
- Work on motor retraining (coordination) by using functional exercises that recruit muscles at different lengths and that emphasize speed as well as stability.

- Attain independence in sit-to-stand and floor-to-stand transfers.
- Attain independent ambulation on all surfaces and stairs. Train ambulation velocity.
- Prescribe necessary ambulation and/or assistive devices, and braces.
- Teach body awareness, need for adequate rest, and joint protection.

RHEUMATOID ARTHRITIS OF THE KNEE

Rheumatoid arthritis (RA) generally affects larger joints such as the knee later in the progression of the disease. The course of RA may be less severe in patients more than 60 years of age, but the disease may have a more abrupt onset and is more likely to involve proximal rather than distal joints. The etiology remains unknown, but is suspected to involve genetics[41(p25)] or infectious agents.[42(p40)]

When RA affects the knee joint, quadriceps atrophy begins immediately. Loss of knee extension occurs early due to tightening of the joint capsule and hamstring muscles. Synovitis ensues, destroying the meniscus, cartilage, and cruciate ligaments. Joint destruction usually involves both the medial and lateral compartments of the knee (Figure 6–12A). The collateral ligaments stretch (especially the MCL) and contribute to the growing instability of the knee, as well as valgus or varus deformity.[43(pp120,121)] The patient usually complains of knee pain, swelling, and severe morning stiffness.[44(pp11,12)] On evaluation, the therapist also may find some of the following clinical signs:

- hot, edematous joint
- capsular pattern: ROM limited mostly in flexion, slightly in extension

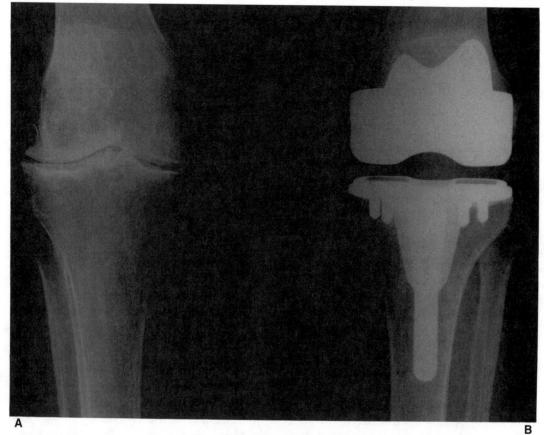

Figure 6–12 **A.** Rheumatoid arthritis destroys both the medial and lateral compartments of the knee. **B.** Uncemented, semi-constrained total knee arthroplasty. Courtesy of R. Wendell Pierce, MD.

- severe loss of strength (2 to 3/5)
- moderate loss of ROM
- loss of mobility skills, including basic transfers
- antalgic gait pattern
- systemic involvement: fatigue, subcutaneous nodules

Because the bulk of treatment is focused on restoring optimal function, the therapist should perform a functional assessment of the patient, using the Iowa Knee Evaluation (Exhibit 6–1) or any other suitable scale, such as the Arthritis Impact Measurement Scale (AIMS 2).

Treatment of Rheumatoid Arthritis of the Knee

The goals in treating RA of the knee are more modest than those for other knee problems. The progressive nature of the disease prevents restoration of normal knee function. During the chronic stages, the patient should strive for increased strength, endurance, ROM, and functional ability. In a study on the effects of detraining on patients with recent onset of RA, Hakkinen et al found that these patients required continuous physical exercise or else great strength losses occurred (especially in knee extension), which adversely affected functional capacity.[45(p1075)] During the acute stages, prevention of major losses in knee strength and ROM is a primary goal.

Pain Management

Pain is one of the major complaints of the patient with RA. Therapeutic modalities can be beneficial in pain management. Superficial heat (e.g., hydrocollator packs or warm, moist towels) may reduce muscle splinting and offer temporary pain relief. Deep heat (e.g., ultrasound) may be harmful to inflamed joints because it can cause further cartilage destruction,[46(pp275,276)] but can be used safely over muscles. Although ice packs or cold, wet towels offer anti-inflammatory as well as analgesic benefits, many patients resist using this modality. Transcutaneous electrical nerve stimulation (TENS) can be used effectively for localized pain relief, but the small control dials may be difficult for the patient with RA to manage. Gentle massage to tender muscles also relieves pain temporarily.

Patient education on work simplification, energy conservation, body mechanics, and joint protection may offer the best pain relief because the patient then may control everyday activities so that inflammation is prevented from occurring.

Exercise Program

During acute phases of RA involving the knee, the exercise program is designed to maintain as much strength as possible with the least damage to the inflamed joint. Therefore, the most appropriate form of exercise is isometrics, which is associated with low articular pressure.[46(p67)] The patient performs low-duration isometrics (one to three repetitions) frequently (five times) throughout the day. Resistive exercise is contraindicated at this time. Bed rest helps to reduce strain on the knee. To prevent flexion contractures while in bed, the therapist needs to educate the patient on the dangers of placing a pillow under the knee for comfort. However, forced stretching of tight hamstrings when large effusion is present can cause the joint capsule to rupture.[43(p121)]

During the more chronic phases of the disease, resistive exercise is indicated to maximize strength. A properly conditioned quadriceps muscle can protect an arthritic knee joint, since it acts as an energy absorber during gait and stair climbing.[46(p67)] The patient can exercise with free weights, Theraband™, or isokinetic machines within pain-free limits. PNF isometric techniques, such as "hold-relax" and "rhythmic stabilization," can be performed with maximal resistance in different parts of the range.[47(pp738,739)] The therapist should use cross-training principles when designing a rehabilitation program for patients with arthritis. By changing the pattern of joint loading on a daily basis, joint overload can be avoided.[48(p3)] In addition, the therapist must remember to schedule adequate rest breaks throughout the treatment session. Aerobic exercises—such as walking, bicycling, and swimming—can be very beneficial.[44(p19)] If available, the water environment provides generalized relaxation and reduces the compressive effects of gravity on weight-bearing joints, promoting more fluid, pain-free motion.[48(pp2,3)] The recommended pool temperature for patients with RA is 86° F.[49(p351)] (See Figure 4–13 in Chapter 4 for a sample of pool exercises.)

Many studies have documented the poor strength gains achieved by the population with RA, even with steady exercise. It is therefore important to reemphasize that the "strengthening" program plays its greatest role in maintaining strength, preventing contractures, and delaying the progression of increasing weakness.[50(p202)]

Mobility Program

The patient with RA benefits most from a rehabilitation program that emphasizes independence in basic mobility skills. The therapist should teach the fundamentals, such as rolling, bridging, and scooting in bed. Transfers, such as sit-to-supine and sit-to-stand, can range from difficult to impossible for this patient population, but they are necessary for patient independence. These transfers should be practiced on real beds (not just therapy mats) and on chairs of varying heights. The therapist should encourage the use of armrests whenever possible. The force of pushing down with the hands on the armrest creates a reaction force in the same direction as the quadriceps force. Combined with leaning forward, this greatly reduces the amount of quadriceps force (by more than one-third) needed to complete the task of rising to a standing postion[51(pp163,164)] (Figure 6–13).

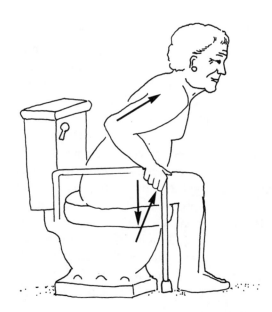

Figure 6–13 Pushing off on armrests significantly reduces the load on the quadriceps. *Source:* Reprinted with permission from S.L. Roberts and S.A. Falkenburg, *The Lower Extremity, Biomechanics: Problem Solving for Functional Activity*, p. 164, © 1992, Mosby Year-Book.

Ambulation Program

The average patient with RA ambulates at a velocity of only 88.5 ft/min,[37(p1057)] which is approximately half the minimal velocity necessary to ambulate safely in the community. Both rate of motion and ROM, therefore, should be trained in this population if the disease is in remission (i.e., chronic phase). At the very least, the patient should be able to ambulate at a faster speed for a short distance (45 ft) to cross a street safely. This can be accomplished with high-speed isokinetics, isotonics with emphasis on speed and endurance, and brisk walking.

Patients with RA of the knee often have knee flexion contractures that alter all phases of the gait cycle except for initial swing. They tend to take smaller steps because of loss of knee extension in terminal swing and because of pain. This places an additional burden on the quadriceps muscle, which is often weak to begin with. In addition, the knee tends to deform into valgus.[38(pp239,240,243)]

If a patient requires an ambulation device, the therapist must prescribe equipment that does not aggravate the joints of the wrist and hand. Extra padding on walker handles or platform attachments helps to protect the UEs from damaging forces.

Ambulating outdoors and climbing stairs are difficult for the patient with RA, but the ability to perform these activities can mean the difference between being socially active and being permanently homebound. The therapist and patient must work on these functional ambulation skills in order to achieve the patient's rehabilitation goals safely.

Activities of Daily Living Program

The most basic ADL tasks can be extremely difficult for the patient with RA because of the multijoint involvement of this disease. Raised toilet seats with toilet frames or grab bars and tub seats can make bathroom functions safer and easier. Some patients prefer to have their beds placed up on small blocks to make it easier to transfer. Otherwise, adaptive equipment should be kept to a minimum.

The therapist should watch the patient perform all normal activities—such as self-care, housework, and hobbies—to ensure that these tasks are being performed efficiently. To protect the knee from excessive strain, most activities should be adapted to the sitting position.[46(p238)]

Summary of Treatment of Rheumatoid Arthritis of the Knee

- During the acute stage of RA, prevent major losses of strength and ROM through short-duration isometrics (five times daily) and gentle stretching.
- During the chronic stage, maximize muscle strength, endurance, and aerobic capacity through full-spectrum exercising within pain tolerance.
- Design the exercise program with cross-training principles to prevent joint overload and schedule rest breaks during treatment sessions.
- Teach independence in bed mobility and all transfers.
- Improve ambulation velocity to at least 150 ft/min for approximately 45 ft to safely cross streets.
- Prescribe ambulation devices that do not strain the hand and wrist joints.
- Analyze all ADL tasks and recommend changes that protect the knee and conserve energy.

- Teach the patient about the concepts of work simplification, energy conservation, body mechanics, and joint protection. This will enable the patient to problem solve independently of the therapist.

TOTAL KNEE ARTHROPLASTY

In 1960, there were 831 reported cases of knee arthroplasty in the world.[52(p84)] In 1992, 167,000 TKAs were performed in the United States alone, and the rate of these operations continues to climb annually.[53(pM152)] Advanced age is no longer a contraindication, with patients 80 to 95 years of age having successful outcomes of markedly decreased pain and increased function from TKA surgery.[54(p48),55(pp79,80)] The primary reasons for replacing the knee joint are to eliminate severe pain and to restore ADL function in debilitated patients with OA and RA. The success rate for this operation is greater than 90%. Contraindications for this procedure are: active sepsis, prior knee infection, and absent quadriceps function. In the latter case, an arthrodesis is a better choice.[56(pp18,19)] The therapist needs to be aware of the different types of TKAs, as well as the different surgical approaches and closures, in order to treat this patient optimally.

Prosthetic Hardware

There are three basic types of TKA: totally constrained, semiconstrained, and totally unconstrained. The amount of constraint built into an artificial joint reflects the amount of stability that the hardware itself provides. As such, a totally constrained joint has the femoral portion physically attached to the tibial component and requires no ligamentous or soft tissue support. The semiconstrained TKA (Figure 6–12B) has two separate components that glide on each other, but the physical characteristics of the tibial component prevent excessive femoral glide. The totally unconstrained device relies completely on the body's own ligaments and soft tissues to maintain stability at the joint.

One of the first successful TKAs was the Waldius hinge. This totally constrained device allowed only 90° of flexion at the knee and no rotatory movement at all. The newer totally constrained TKAs (e.g., Spherocentric, Kinematic rotating hinge) employ triaxial hinge joints that allow for rotation. These TKAs are used primarily in grossly unstable knees that have been decimated by disease or cancer and account for less than 5% of devices used in total knee surgery.[57(pp121,122)]

Over the past 25 years, knee implants have been designed to reproduce the anatomical kinematics of the knee more closely and to allow for more normal ROM (Figure 6–14).[56(p36),58] Most semiconstrained knee implants (e.g., Total Condylar, Insall Burstein) require excision of the cruciate ligaments and rely on both prosthetic design and soft tissue balancing for stability. Totally unconstrained implants (e.g., Cloutier) usually maintain the posterior cruciate ligament and require good soft tissue balancing for stability. In general, the totally unconstrained implants afford the most normal ROM and gait;[58] however, both types of implants afford good stability and freedom from pain, which are the major reasons for performing the surgery.

The materials used in all total joint replacements need to display some unique properties to perform like a biological joint. The materials must be strong enough to withstand more than 1,000 lbs of pressure and have a coefficient of friction low enough to allow smooth gliding of the joint surfaces. This is quite difficult to achieve. Presently, the most common materials used in total joints are cobalt-chromium (CoCr) or titanium on ultrahigh molecular weight polyethylene (UHMWPE). In TKAs, CoCr is always used on the femoral weight-bearing surface due to its superior strength[59]; however, the coefficient of friction for the CoCr alloy on UHMWPE is 0.04, while the coefficient of friction for cartilage on cartilage (human joint) is considerably smaller at only 0.009. Work continues in the development of different alloys and materials (ceramics) for joint replacement.[56(pp29,30)]

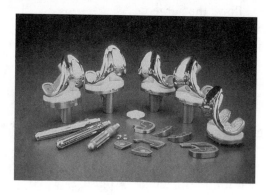

Figure 6–14 Total knee arthroplasty. Courtesy of Zimmer Inc., Warsaw, Indiana.

Total knee arthroplasties can be stabilized with or without cement. (See Chapter 4 for further information on acrylic cement.) Patient selection is important for uncemented TKAs. For example, patients with very soft bone will not have good results from a press fit prosthesis.[56(p181)] Hybrid TKAs (i.e., Miller-Galante) have uncemented femoral and patella components and cemented tibial components.[60(p78)] Results from cemented, uncemented, and hybrid TKAs have been similarly good, but the trend seems to be favoring a return to cemented prostheses.[59] Some surgeons delay weight bearing in patients with uncemented components, while others allow immediate weight bearing as tolerated.

Surgical Approach and Closure

There are three major surgical approaches for a standard TKA: the medial parapatellar retinacular approach, the midvastus split approach, and the subvastus (southern) approach. Because most surgeons use the standard anterior midline incision at the skin layer, a therapist looking at the suture line cannot know which deep surgical approach was used, except by reading the operative report.

The classic medial parapatellar retinacular approach (Figure 6–15) allows the surgeon excellent exposure of the knee, but splits the quadriceps tendon in its medial one-third. Due to involvement of the quadriceps, more postoperative patellofemoral complications occur with this type of approach.[61(pp58,61–62)]

The midvastus (or VMO splitting) approach also allows excellent exposure, while retaining the extensor mechanism (Figure 6–16). This allows excellent return of extensor function and less need for a retinacular release.[59,61(p56)]

The subvastus approach (Figure 6–17) preserves the integrity of the entire extensor

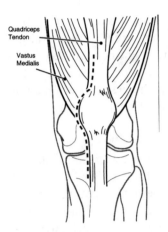

Figure 6–15 The classic medial parapatellar approach splits the quadriceps tendon in its medial 1/3. *Source:* Reprinted with permission from G.A. Engh, N.L. Parks, and D.J. Ammeen, "Influence of Surgical Approach on Lateral Retinacular Releases in Total Knee Arthroplasty," *Clinical Orthopaedics and Related Research*, Vol. 331, p. 58, © 1996, Lippincott-Raven Publishers.

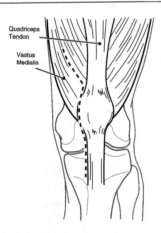

Figure 6–16 The midvastus (or VMO splitting) approach is shown going between the fibers of the vastus medialis and leaving the quadriceps tendon intact. *Source:* Reprinted with permission from G.A. Engh, N.L. Parks, and D.J. Ammeen, "Influence of Surgical Approach on Lateral Retinacular Releases in Total Knee Arthroplasty," *Clinical Orthopaedics and Related Research*, Vol. 331, p. 57, © 1996, Lippincott-Raven Publishers.

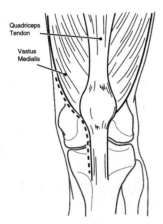

Quadriceps
Tendon

Vastus
Medialis

Figure 6–17 The subvastus approach maintains a fully intact vastus medialis obliquus. *Source:* Reprinted with permission from G.A. Engh, N.L. Parks, and D.J. Ammeen, "Influence of Surgical Approach on Lateral Retinacular Releases in Total Knee Arthroplasty," *Clinical Orthopaedics and Related Research*, Vol. 331, p. 57, © 1996, Lippincott-Raven Publishers.

mechanism, including the VMO. This decreases the likelihood of patellar subluxation and allows for rapid return of knee extension. This method does not expose the knee as well as the other approaches.[61(pp61,62),62(pp75–77)]

From a rehabilitation point of view, the surgical closure is of great interest. The classic closure technique is to suture the layers of the wound while the knee is extended. The knee is then flexed through range to make sure that no blockage to motion occurs. Some physicians advocate closing the wound with the knee in flexion to promote postoperative flexion; this method is technically more demanding. Many therapists and physicians anecdotally report that surgical closure in flexion helps restore motion in their patients. Several studies have been performed on this topic with mixed results. Reports range from no significant difference in ROM at all,[63(p86)] to improved flexion within the first week

postoperatively,[64(p65)] to significant improvement in flexion immediately postoperatively and up to 6 months later with patients requiring fewer home visits.[65(p74)] Research continues in this area.

Complications

Common complications following TKA include deep vein thrombosis, pulmonary embolus, infection, patellofemoral problems (including fracture, instability, patellar clunk syndrome, quadriceps rupture), peroneal nerve palsy, and supracondylar fracture.[9(pp270–278)]

Many patellofemoral problems seem to result from the design of the TKA itself[66(p197),67(p243)] and need to be addressed by the manufacturers. Due to the many patellofemoral problems seen, some physicians recommend not resurfacing the patella at all.[68(p156)] Some patellar complications arise 1 to 2 years after surgery. In tethered patella syndrome, a fibrous band forms, preventing the patella from seating properly in the femur. Patients complain of painful popping, catching, or jumping of the patella; this can be corrected by arthroscopic treatment.[69(p125)]

For patients 80 years and older, there is a slightly higher complication rate, with more infections and cardiovascular and neurologic problems.[70(p799)] Of particular concern is the much higher rate of decubitus ulcer development (11%) after TKA. All health care professionals should be cognizant of the potential for skin breakdown in the oldest old.[55(pp79,80)]

Unicompartmental Arthroplasty and Tibial Osteotomy

Other surgeries can be performed on patients with arthritis to relieve pain and promote function. Unicompartmental knee arthroplasty (UKA) replaces the joint surfaces on one side of the knee only (usually the medial compartment). UKAs provide better relief than tibial osteotomy and greater ROM (average 122°) than does a TKA,[71(p130)] as well as improved ambulation velocity and gait pattern.[72(p139)] With proper patient selection (i.e., patients with intact cruciate ligaments, no OA present in the other compartment), UKAs have had results equal to those of TKAs for much less cost. However, without proper patient selection, there tends to be a high failure rate for this procedure (12%), requiring revision surgery.[71(p135),73(pp209,212)]

Osteotomies have been performed for 40 years. The principle of tibial osteotomy is to realign the weight-bearing surface of the tibia to allow for better joint loading. By removing a wedge-shaped piece of bone, angular deformities about the knee can be corrected. The procedure is best performed on younger patients with OA, delaying the need for TKA for about 10 years.[56(pp21,22)]

Special Considerations for Patients with Rheumatoid Arthritis

TKAs have been successfully implanted in patients with RA, but the surgeon has greater difficulties to overcome when performing this operation. In general, the patient has a systemic, chronic disease that weakens both muscles and bone throughout the body.[74(p129)] Approximately 60% of these patients have cervical spine instability, which can cause serious problems with general anesthesia (including fatality by medullary compression).[75(p129)] Special equipment may be necessary in the operating room to accommodate patients with multiple joint contractures. In addition, extreme care needs to be taken to ensure sterility, as these patients have a higher risk of infection.[56(p255)] Despite these and other problems (i.e., blood transfusion, bone grafts, slower healing), the patient usu-

ally has good results from a cemented TKA, although not as good as patients with OA.[76(p330),77(p141)]

Treatment of the Patient with a Total Knee Arthroplasty

Prosthesis type, surgical technique, and prior knee deformity have a great impact on the outcome of TKA surgery. The rehabilitation program also plays a major role in returning the patient to functional independence.

Phase 0 (Preoperative Day 1)

As in all elective surgery, the therapist has the luxury of instructing the patient about the rehabilitation program before surgical insult. This generally occurs in a presurgical visit or class. The therapist teaches the patient deep breathing and coughing, transfer techniques, and walking with crutches. The therapist also introduces a short exercise program of isometric quadriceps and gluteal sets, SLR, hip abduction, and ankle circles and familiarizes the patient with the CPM machine, knee splint, and wheelchair.

Although it seems logical to medical professionals that patients would benefit from a preoperative exercise program before undergoing TKA surgery, current research does not support this hypothesis. In a recent study, patients who underwent a 6-week strengthening or cardiovascular program prior to TKA had the same postoperative results as the control group that did not exercise at all.[78(pp176,177)]

Phase I (Postoperative [PO] Days 1 to 6)

The hospital length of stay has dropped dramatically for this operation, with most patients being discharged to a rehabilitation facility or to home in 5 to 7 days after surgery.[79(p170)] Patients with RA may require longer hospitalization due to poorer healing. During the initial recovery phase, the TKA must be protected from external and internal forces to allow proper healing to occur. The joint is hot, edematous, and painful. Knee strength is Poor (2/5) and knee ROM is severely limited.

Exercise Program. During Phase I, the therapist applies ice to the patient's knee to reduce pain and swelling before and after treatment. Care should be taken using this modality to avoid a risk of transient peroneal palsy.[80(p86)] On PO Day 1, the patient begins an exercise program bedside consisting of isometrics (quadriceps and gluteal sets), ankle pumps and circles, and diaphragmatic breathing.[79(p169)] These exercises are performed independently by the patient every hour. On PO Day 2, the program progresses to short arc quads (terminal knee extension) and SLR with the knee splint on.[80(p88)] The therapist must make sure that the hamstrings are not cocontracting. On PO Day 3, the patient begins active heels slides while supine in bed (hamstrings) and sitting full arc motions of flexion and extension.[79(p169)] Some therapists advocate beginning passive knee flexion and extension at this time.[81(p8)] Starting on PO Day 4 until discharge, the patient begins exercising in the physical therapy department continuing the same exercises, but with greater intensity. Patients are also taught to self-stretch the knee into flexion while sitting (Figure 6–18). Based on the evaluation, the therapist also should initiate a conditioning program.

ROM. To increase ROM, the patient usually begins to use a CPM machine by PO Day 2 for 3 to 5 hours daily, but this may be delayed in patients with RA to promote healing.[82(p31)] Flexion is increased approximately 7° each day according to the patient's tolerance, although there is no clear consensus as to the best CPM protocol to use.[83(p360),84(p126)] Many studies support the short-term use of CPM in the acute care hospital[85(p208),86(p7),87(p421)]; however, CPM is not recommended beyond discharge, as it apparently has no long-term effects on knee ROM.[88(p228)]

An alternative method of using CPM was tried by Jordan et al,[89(pp231–232)] where he set the CPM machine in 70° to 100° of flexion in the recovery room and advanced extension over the next 2 days to 0°. He reported a decreased hospital stay and an increased ROM (average 120°) up to 1 year postoperatively.

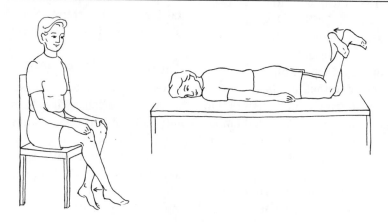

Figure 6–18 Self-stretching into flexion in sitting and prone positions

Two alternatives to using CPM consist of the "drop and dangle technique" and flexion/extension splinting. During the "drop and dangle technique," the patient sits bedside on PO Day 1 and slowly and gently allows the knee to "fall" into flexion.[90(p94)] The therapist supports the limb during this activity and monitors quadriceps firing. As soon as the quadriceps contracts, the therapist stops any further motion until the patient relaxes the muscle again.[59] The splinting method has been mostly used in Asia and consists of casting the knee into flexion and then extension on alternate days for 5 days.[91(pp178–179)] Both studies report good short-term results, with improved ROM over conventional CPM rehabilitation. Long-term studies still need to be performed.

Ideally, a ROM of 5° to 80° to 90° should be achieved after 1 week,[80(p88),81(p8)] but this is dependent on many factors, especially preoperative ROM. To work toward this short-term goal, the therapist can use any of the ROM protocols mentioned, although none have been proven to be better than another.

Mobility/Ambulation Program. The therapist/patient program emphasizes independence in bed mobility, transfers, and gait. For patients with RA, a trapeze should be used for the first few days. On PO Day 1, the patient begins bed-to-chair transfers with the knee splint on. Care should be taken not to pivot on the operated leg. A pillow may be placed on the chair so that less knee motion is necessary for independent transfers. On PO Day 2, the patient begins assisted ambulation in the room, weight bearing as tolerated with a walker (or crutches) and a knee splint. (Some doctors still prefer an initial period of protected weight bearing, especially for patients with an uncemented TKA.)

The splint can be removed (usually by Day 4) when the patient can perform active SLR without assistance. By PO Day 4, the patient begins ambulating in the physical therapy gym with a walker or axillary crutches. Emphasis is on heel-toe gait pattern and endurance. By PO Day 5, the patient is encouraged to walk on the nursing floor, if appropriate. Before discharge, the patient should be instructed in stair climbing using a railing and a cane or crutch for a limited amount of steps.[80(pp88,89),81(p8)]

Activities of Daily Living Program. At this acute stage, the patient uses a raised toilet seat with a toilet frame and performs most daily grooming and dressing activities while sitting. Adaptive equipment needs, such as reachers and long-handled shoehorns and sponges, should be assessed by the occupational therapist and provided by PO Day 2. The therapist begins teaching the patient about joint protection and energy conservation concepts so that the patient will be better able to solve problems independently.

The patient will be unable to perform most ADL, except the very basics of toileting and grooming, by discharge from the acute care hospital. If assistance is unavailable at home, the patient must go to a rehabilitation hospital for further therapy. (See Table 6–1 for a summary of Phase I treatment of TKA.)

Phase II (PO Weeks 1 to 3)

During this subacute phase, the patient has either been discharged to home with community care support (i.e., visiting nurse association) or has been transferred to a rehabilitation facility for about 2 weeks. The knee is still edematous and painful. The sutures usually have been removed by PO Day 10, but some patients with RA may be experiencing

Table 6–1 Summary of Phase I (PO Days 0–6) Treatment of TKA To Be Performed in Conjunction with Modalities of Ice, Elevation, and Compression To Control Edema

PO Day	Exercise	Mobility	Ambulation	ADL
0	Deep breathing Coughing Quad & glut sets SLR* Hip abduction Ankle pumps	Sit-to-chair transfer Education on CPM* machine		
1 (bedside)	Deep breathing LE isometrics Ankle pumps & circles ROM* program: CPM or "drop & dangle" method	Bed mobility Bed-to-chair transfers with splint		Assess adaptive equipment: reachers, long-handled sponges, and shoehorns
2 (bedside)	Continue as above Short arc quads SLR with splint UE* strengthening ROM program	Continue bed mobility and transfers Begin toilet transfers	Assisted ambulation in room WB* as tolerated with splint	Raised toilet seat Grooming and dressing while seated
3 (bedside)	Continue as above Heel slides in supine Sitting full arc motion: flexion and extension Passive flexion and extension ROM program	Decrease assistance in basic transfers	Independent ambulation with walker or crutches in room WB as tolerated with splint	Independent toileting and grooming Education on joint protection and energy conservation
4	Continue as above with increased intensity Add quadriceps and hamstring self-stretch	Independent in basic transfers	Gait training to improve pattern and endurance Discontinue splint (if able to SLR actively)	Continue as above

continues

Table 6–1 continued

PO Day	Exercise	Mobility	Ambulation	ADL
5–6	Continue as above Discontinue CPM machine		Independent ambulation on nursing floor Begin stairs with railing and cane	Independent dressing

*SLR = straight leg raise, CPM = continuous passive motion, UE = upper extremity, WB = weight bearing, ROM = range of motion

Sources: Journal of Orthopaedic and Sports Physical Therapy (1996;23[1]:8), Copyright © 1996 the Orthopaedic and Sports Physical Therapy Sections of the American Physical Therapy Association; *Sports Medicine and Arthroscopy Review* (1996;4[1]:88–89), Copyright © 1996 Lippincott-Raven Publishers; *Orthopaedic Physical Therapy Clinics of North America* (1993;2[3]:168–170), Copyright © 1993 WB Saunders Company.

healing problems. Knee strength generally is in the low Fair range (3−/5), and passive knee ROM is approximately 10° to 90°. The patient is ambulatory with a device but is still very limited in functional activities.

Exercise Program. The therapist continues to apply ice to the knee before and after the treatment session. Along with the isometric program, the patient progresses to active and lightly resistive isotonic exercises. To minimize the compression forces associated with isotonic exercise, resistance can be achieved safely and effectively through the use of rubber tubing. This is especially important for uncemented TKAs.[92(p9)] Light cuff weights (1 to 3 lbs) can be used with cemented TKAs. To reeducate the muscle properly, the patient also should work the quadriceps with a loaded exercise, such as a lunge (see Figure 6–9) or a modified leg press (simultaneous hip and knee extension as shown in Figures 6–19 and 6–20). Deep squats are contraindicated.

The therapist should realize that the introduction of an artificial joint to the knee increases the compression force of the tibiofemoral joint from the biological joint. During a mini squat (20° flexion), the joint reaction force is 3.5 times the body weight. This increases to 8 times the body weight at 40° flexion and then decreases to 6 times the body weight at 60° flexion[93(p109)]; therefore, over time, almost all exercises and functional activities will cause damage to the TKA.

The therapist must continue progressing ROM by using PNF, MFR, passive stretch, and patellar mobilization (especially inferior glide). Stationary bicycle riding is an excellent ROM exercise, but many of the "old" elderly have difficulty getting on the bicycle. The patient should be encouraged to self-stretch into flexion both in prone-lying and sitting positions (Figure 6–18). In most instances, the patient should attain 90° of flexion by PO Day 14. Otherwise, the orthopaedic surgeon will consider manipulating the joint to regain motion. Approximately 20% of all TKAs require manipulation, but whether manipulation really helps or causes more damage is still controversial.[94]

If a pool is available, a therapeutic pool program can be initiated. (See Figure 4–14.)

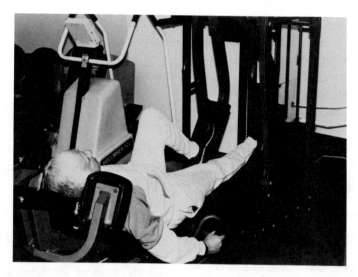

Figure 6–19 Modified leg press, shown on Nautilus. Both the hip and the knee extend together in a closed kinetic chain.

Problems with strength, ROM, proprioception, balance, and gait can be successfully addressed in the aquatic environment.

Mobility/Ambulation Program. The patient should be independent in all transfers at this time and also should be able to rise from most types of chairs, except low seats. Patients with RA may experience greater difficulty in mobility activities because of multiple joint involvement.

When the patient can perform SLR with less than a 5° extension lag, the knee immobilizer should be discontinued. (This generally occurs by PO Day 4, but frail patients may need more time.) The patient continues gait training, FWB with a device, on all surfaces including stairs. The patient performs stair climbing one step at a time with the good leg ascending first and the operated leg descending first. ("The good go to heaven, the bad go to hell.") This requires the least

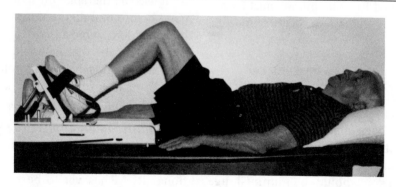

Figure 6–20 Modified leg press using the Shuttle® MiniClinic (Contemporary Design Company, Glacier, WA) to regain knee stability and strength

amount of ROM and strength. If the patient is having difficulty in retraining the quadriceps mechanism during stair climbing, biofeedback can be used. Generally, the patient needs to perform 4-inch step-ups and step-downs as a precursor exercise to integrate the entire lower quarter into the activity. The biofeedback device indicates when good quadriceps contraction is occurring during the eccentric phase (descending the step). Then the therapist must make sure that the patient is using the gastrocnemius and gluteus maximus muscles in conjunction with the quadriceps during stair climbing. These two powerful muscles help launch the patient up the stairs, requiring less quadriceps strength to perform the activity. (Sufficient ankle ROM and balance must also exist for the gastrocnemius to assist.)

Activities of Daily Living Program. The patient should be independent in all grooming, toileting, and dressing activities. Continued use of a raised toilet seat with grab bars is recommended. Light housekeeping, such as dusting, drying dishes, etc., can be performed if desired, but more intensive activities are still difficult. Driving is still contraindicated at this time. If the patient wishes to resume sexual activity, he or she should use a supine position and place a pillow under the involved LE. The pillow must be removed after intercourse to prevent muscle shortening.

Phase III (PO Weeks 3 to 6)

At this time, the patient has either been discharged home with community health services or has been discharged to a skilled nursing facility for continued rehabilitation. The soft tissues should be healing and the pain and edema should be diminishing. During Phase III, the therapist can aggressively address any remaining problems in strength, ROM, mobility, gait, and ADL. Knee strength is in the high Fair range (3+/5), with the hamstrings and quadriceps about equal in strength. Passive ROM is 5° to 100°.[95(pp26,27)] The doctor usually schedules a follow-up visit with the patient during this period.

Exercise Program. The patient should be independent in full-spectrum strengthening and ROM exercises. The therapist/patient program now emphasizes quadriceps strengthening in order to restore muscle balance to the hamstrings and quadriceps. (The hamstrings normally have less than two-thirds the strength of the quadriceps—or a 0.61 hamstring-quadriceps ratio.) This may prove difficult. A study by Huang et al found that a high hamstring-quadriceps ratio (0.86) exists up to 13 years following TKA surgery.[96(pp151–153)] In addition, the hip joint musculature, especially hip extension, has been found to weaken following knee surgery.[97] Resistive hip exercises need to be performed to restore proximal strength.

To restore functional ROM (0° to 105°) to the knee, the therapist continues to mobilize the patella, perform MFR, and passively stretch the muscles. Joint mobilization to the tibiofemoral joint is contraindicated in all uncemented prostheses and in many implant designs. The therapist must contact the surgeon before mobilizing this newly replaced joint. Stationary bicycle riding can be beneficial. The patient also should be instructed in more aggressive self-stretching techniques, such as stretching the knee with the affected leg on a stool or chair (Figure 6–21).

Mobility/Ambulation Program. Rising from a low seat or toilet still presents difficulties for the patient with a TKA, as functional ROM has yet to be restored to the joint. Gait training consists of weaning off ambulation devices, training ambulation ve-

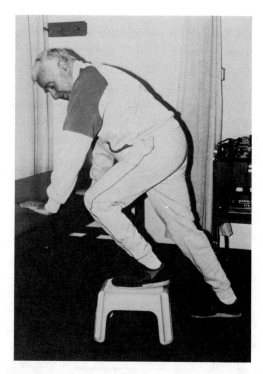

Figure 6–21 Quadriceps stretching on a stool. To further stretch the quadriceps, a chair can be used in place of the stool. A side benefit of this stretch is a simultaneous soleus stretch, which is often needed.

locity, and retraining one-legged standing balance and proprioception. Proprioception has been found to improve in patients after TKA, although the exact mechanism is not known.[98(p185)] The patient should be able to ambulate in all directions and on all surfaces for at least 500 feet. Pivoting on the surgical leg should still be avoided.[99(p117)] Although sufficient ROM usually exists to enable successful negotiation of stairs (0° to 83°), most patients continue to have difficulty in climbing stairs and need to practice step-ups. Patients with unconstrained TKAs usually have fewer problems with stair climbing than do patients with constrained arthroplasties. Excessive pelvic or trunk excursions during gait or stair climbing usually indicate insufficient ROM or strength of the involved knee.[94,95(p29)]

Activities of Daily Living Program. The patient should be independent in all basic ADL tasks, including light meal preparation. (Some patients with RA may be unable to perform some tasks because of inflammation or deformity of other joints.) Since most patients will be unable to squat or stoop, long-handled reachers may be necessary to obtain things off the floor. Instrumental ADL can still be problematical at this time. Although patients are physically able to drive, the ability of patients with total joint replacements to step on the break pedal quickly does not reach preoperative levels until 8 weeks following surgery.[100(p202)] Therapists should caution patients with right TKAs on this potentially dangerous situation.

Phase IV (PO Weeks 6 to 12)

It is perhaps important to point out that there is a percentage of patients that do not fit into the newer, leaner, faster rehabilitation system (some might say frenzy) that has gripped the United States over the past decade. Psychologically, they are simply not ready for "rehab in the fast lane." Many become depressed after surgery when they find themselves still in pain and with major losses of function with which to contend. If they have not progressed "fast enough," they may be sent to a nursing home (which some consider a fate worse than death.) Depression and anxiety can worsen as they wonder if they will ever go home again. In a study by Sinacore et al, functional outcome at 3 months post-TKA was most significantly predicted by psychosocial variables and not by physical or medical variables.[101(pM152)] These patients continue to need physical therapy and could definitely benefit from psychological intervention as well. For these patients, the rehabilitation process starts now. The pain has diminished significantly and the patients are finally ready, physically and mentally, to expend some serious energy into getting better. They enter Phase II or III at a less intensive level (two to three sessions/week) than previously described.

Except for the patients mentioned above and others with surgical complications, most patients have returned home to complete the rehabilitation process. Some patients have even been formally discharged from physical therapy at this time. These patients need to continue the rehabilitation process independent of formal therapy, which requires great mental discipline. Most patients continue to be seen one to two times per week in an outpatient setting, where their progress can be monitored and their program advanced.

Exercise Program. Emphasis on quadriceps strengthening and proximal hip muscle strengthening continues. The quadriceps weakness observed after TKA places the patellofemoral joint at great risk for dysfunction. As mentioned previously, some of the surgical techniques themselves contribute to patellar problems. With the swelling now decreased at the knee, the patellofemoral joint should be reassessed for tracking and muscle imbalance problems. A patellofemoral program (discussed later in this chapter) should be instituted when appropriate.

ROM should be approaching 0° to 115°, although the exact amount reached is usually dictated by presurgical ROM[102(p87)] and the constraint built into the prosthetic implant. The therapist should continue with soft tissue work and encourage the patient to maintain a vigorous stretching schedule to the entire lower quarter.

Mobility/Ambulation Program. Most transfers, including car transfers and rising from low chairs, should be independent. This goal may still be impossible to reach for patients with RA or other serious comorbidities. Standard floor-to-stand transfers should not be taught yet, as kneeling on the surgical knee and deep squatting are still contraindicated. The therapist should instruct the patient in an alternative method (Figure 6–22) of rising from the floor by using a chair, if sufficient UE strength is present. Frailer patients may be unable to accomplish this task, even though they are at a higher risk of falling.

The therapist should emphasize balance and proprioception activities in order to improve gait pattern and velocity. Skinner reports that gait pattern is altered in patients with TKA, probably due to problems in proprioception, balance, and muscle strength.[103(p78)] The patient should begin (or

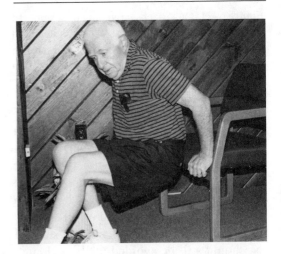

Figure 6–22 Floor-to-chair transfer. The patient with a TKA should not kneel on the operated knee or perform deep squats until approved by the physician. An alternate method of getting off the floor is to back up to a chair or stool and, by using the upper extremities, hoist oneself up onto the chair or stool. This obviously requires good upper extremity strength and may not be appropriate for all patients.

continue with) a more functional exercise program including some of the following activities:

- bilateral standing on a wobbleboard (Figure 4–9)
- one-legged balance
- ambulation on a foam mat
- toe-walking and heel-walking
- sidestepping
- backward walking
- stool walking (Figure 6–23)
- light jogging or skipping
- resisted ambulation with rubber tubing
- step-ups and step-downs
- fast walking

Any of these activities can be modified to assist the frailer patient or challenge the advanced patient. For example, sidestepping

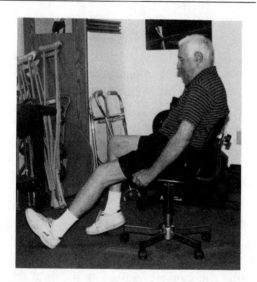

Figure 6–23 Stool walking. Sitting on an office chair, wheelchair, or clinic stool with casters, the patient plants the heels into the floor and propels the chair forward (using hamstrings and anterior tibialis) or pushes off with the toes to go backward. This activity strengthens and stabilizes both lower extremities. Altering the floor surface changes the difficulty of the exercise.

can be performed holding on to a railing in a nursing home corridor for a patient with balance problems, or can be performed on tiptoes without support. Distances for ambulation activities such as toe-walking or light jogging should be limited to around 20 feet initially, so as not to overload the joint.

To ambulate safely in the community, the patient should be able to walk at a velocity of 150 to 208 ft/min (44.5 to 63.5 m/min).[14(pp1372,1373)] Most patients with TKA achieve this velocity 1 to 3 years after surgery.[103(p83)] On the average, osteoarthritic patients with a TKA are able to walk significantly faster than rheumatoid arthritic patients with a TKA, but both populations still walk only 70% as fast as unaffected subjects. With more emphasis on gait speed, this population might be able to return to more normal walking speeds in a shorter time frame.

Negotiating stairs and descending ramps are still difficult for the patient, even 3 months after surgery. The patient should be assured that this is common and requires more time and strengthening of the quadriceps, especially eccentrically.

Activities of Daily Living Program. The patient should be able to perform all ADL, except for carrying heavy loads (more than 25 lbs), deep squatting, and sports or recreational activities. Sports activities, even golf and other low-impact sports, are contraindicated until 4 to 6 months postsurgery and then on physician approval only. In general, when the patient can return to high-level skill activity, common sense should rule the day. Repetitive loading can lead to fatigue failure of the prosthetic parts or bone/implant interface.[104(pp301,304)]

Although patients can successfully perform most ADL with TKA in Western society, Eastern cultures require greater knee ROM to fulfill societal roles. In addition, many religions require kneeling on benches or on the ground. For these patients, knee ROM of 105° is not functional. Full ROM is possible with certain designs of TKA, but the long-term effects of placing the artificial joint in such extreme range have not yet been determined.[91(p185)]

Summary of Treatment of the Patient with a Total Knee Arthroplasty

- Preoperatively, instruct the patient in respiratory exercises, isometric knee exercises, transfers, and crutch-walking.

- Know the type of TKA (constrained, cemented) and the weight-bearing order.

- *During the acute recovery phase (PO Days 1 to 6)*
  1. check wound for drainage and check skin for areas of breakdown
  2. apply ice, compression, and elevation to the knee before and after treatment
  3. begin isometric knee exercise
  4. begin active-assistive SLR with splint and terminal knee extension
  5. use CPM 5 hours daily, progressing motion 5° to 10° per day or use "drop and dangle" technique to regain knee flexion
  6. begin total body reconditioning
  7. begin bed-to-chair transfers and toilet transfers with a raised toilet seat
  8. begin gait training with an ambulation device and a splint.

- *During the semiacute phase (PO Weeks 1 to 3)*
  1. check skin integrity
  2. continue anti-inflammatory modalities
  3. progress exercise to resistive with tubing or light weights
  4. emphasize quadriceps exercises
  5. improve knee ROM by using PNF, MFR, patella mobilization, passive stretch, and bicycle riding
  6. teach independence in all transfers
  7. continue gait training without a splint
  8. begin stair climbing with railing
  9. train independence in basic ADLs.

- *From PO Weeks 3 to 6*
  1. emphasize quadriceps strengthening
  2. increase knee motion (5° to 105°)
  3. train one-legged standing balance (5 to 10 seconds)
  4. begin proprioception training
  5. gait-train on all surfaces, including stairs
  6. train independence in basic ADL.

- *From PO Weeks 6 to 12*
  1. emphasize quadriceps strengthening
  2. reassess patellofemoral joint
  3. increase knee motion to functional (0° to 105° or greater)
  4. train balance and proprioception with functional exercise
  5. wean off ambulation devices
  6. maximize ambulation velocity
  7. train independence in instrumental ADL.

OVERUSE INJURIES

The elderly patient is not immune to the many overuse syndromes that can affect the human knee joint, such as bursitis, tendinitis, or muscular strain. The therapist must determine the cause of injury (e.g., tight hamstrings, excessive kneeling) by evaluating the knee, hip, and ankle. For example, a patient with long-standing RA begins complaining about knee pain. The easiest assumption to make is that the disease has simply progressed to the knee; however, the patient's foot deformity could have worsened, causing abnormal stresses on the knee. Instead of knee exercises, the patient might require foot orthotics.

Bursitis

Prepatellar Bursitis

The prepatellar bursa lies superficial to the patella and is commonly injured from direct trauma, such as a fall or excessive kneeling.[4(p209)] When inflamed, it is commonly called "housemaid's knee" or "water on the knee." It is difficult to misdiagnose this condition, as the patient presents with a giant fluid sac on top of the patella, which is painful to touch.

Infrapatellar Bursitis

The deep infrapatella bursa usually becomes aggravated from overactivity, such as excessive squatting. It occurs commonly with infrapatella tendinitis. Active knee extension or any antigravity activities, such as getting up from a chair or stair climbing, exacerbate the bursitis.

Baker's Cyst

Any swelling on the posterior aspect of the knee can be called a Baker's cyst. It usually results from trauma or intra-articular effusion from one of many sources, including a tumor or a torn meniscus.[105(p670)] Because of this, a physician should determine the cause of this bursitis before the therapist begins treatment.

Treatment of Bursitis of the Knee

Bursitis responds extremely well to anti-inflammatory medication, "active" rest, therapeutic modalities, and exercise. The therapist should assess patella tracking and VMO activation, as any swelling at the knee can cause latent patellofemoral dysfunction. The activity that led to the overuse injury should be identi-

fied and modified to prevent recurrence. Occasionally, the physician has to aspirate or excise the bursa if swelling persists.[4(p209)]

Tendinitis

Patellar Tendinitis

Patellar tendinitis is usually an athletic problem developed from excessive quadriceps use and is often called "jumper's knee." In the elderly population, this syndrome can occur from mundane, everyday activities, if the optimal skeletal alignment of the knee has been altered by arthritis. In addition, tendinitis can occur from the patient beginning a new activity or even buying a new pair of shoes. The patient complains of pain at the anterior knee on stair climbing, kneeling, walking quickly, and jogging. Palpation of the tendon reveals thickening and point tenderness.

Hamstrings Tendinitis

Tendinitis at the hamstring insertion is most commonly caused by unwanted co-activation of the hamstrings during extension activities. After any knee injury or surgery, a muscle imbalance can occur whereby the hamstrings fire when they should be relaxed. This constant muscle action produces an overuse of the hamstrings and can set off posterior knee pain. Palpation or surface biofeedback over the hamstring muscle during knee extension reveals a contraction, when relaxation should be occurring. Simply asking the patient to "shut off" the noise from the biofeedback is the first step in treating this problem.

Treatment of Tendinitis at the Knee

As with any overuse injury, the cause of the dysfunction must be identified and corrected. Skeletal alignment should be checked, as it can often cause muscle imbalance. Tendinitis responds extremely well to ultrasound. The therapist can also perform MFR and cross-friction massage to the tendon. The patient should ice the affected tendon twice daily for 1 to 2 weeks. The physician may prescribe anti-inflammatory medication. The therapist prescribes pain-free open- and closed-chain exercises, which strengthen but do not aggravate the tendon. Biofeedback is helpful in retraining proper motor control. As the pain subsides, the therapist adds high-level balance, proprioception, and gait activities. ADL and sports function should be evaluated before the patient is discharged.

Summary of Treatment of Overuse Injuries

- Evaluate the knee, hip, and ankle or foot.
- Identify the cause of injury.
- Use modalities (e.g., ultrasound and ice) to treat the soft tissue.
- Prescribe pain-free therapeutic exercise to restore strength.
- Use biofeedback to retrain proper motor control.
- Treat the cause of injury to prevent recurrence.

MENISCAL TEARS

Tears to the menisci are common in the elderly population. Unlike in younger persons, a small rotatory force is often enough to cause a tear that can occur from a sudden turn or misstep. There has also been an increase in meniscal tears from sports-related injuries in the elderly population. The menisci are believed to have multiple functions at the knee joint:

- They make the tibiofemoral joint more congruent.
- They help distribute synovial fluid throughout the joint.
- They provide stability in all planes of motion.
- They provide increased contact area (2.5 times the area).
- They absorb energy or weight-bearing forces.[106(pp1130,1131)]

An injury or tear to the meniscus alters the biomechanical functioning of the tibiofemoral joint. The most common type of meniscal tear is the longitudinal tear, but transverse tears are more common in the aging population. The older patient may complain of a mild catching or clicking, swelling, pain on squatting, or a sensation of giving way. The most important diagnostic indicator of meniscal tear is localized tenderness at the medial or lateral joint line.[106(pp1136,1137)]

An acute, stable tear can heal with conservative treatment if it occurs in the outer one-third (vascularized zone) of the meniscus and if the cruciate ligaments are stable.[107(p154),108(p185),109(p811)] Tears in the central or inner thirds usually require surgical intervention (Figure 6–24). Since a total meniscectomy increases joint contact forces by more than 300%, most surgeons opt to perform a partial meniscectomy or a repair of the meniscus.

In general, arthroscopic surgery has replaced open surgery for meniscal injuries. Although good to excellent results occur in younger populations, this is not always the case in the older patient. Complications from medial meniscus surgery in patients over 50 years of age include osteonecrosis of the knee[110(p273)] and reflex sympathetic dystrophy.[111(p655)] Both these conditions can cause devastating loss of function in elderly patients.

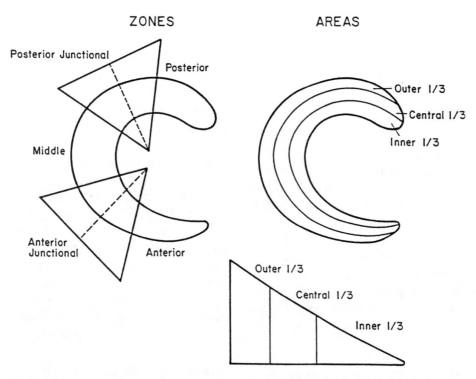

Figure 6–24 The zones and areas of the meniscus. Each zone represents one-fifth of the length of the meniscus and each area represents one-third of the width of the meniscus. The outer one-third is known to be vascularized, the central one-third is partially vascularized, and the inner one-third is avascular. *Source:* Adapted with permission from C.B. Weiss et al., "Non-Operative Treatment of Meniscal Tears," *The Journal of Bone and Joint Surgery,* Vol. 71-A, No. 6, p. 814, © 1989 by The Journal of Bone and Joint Surgery, Inc.

Treatment of Meniscal Injuries

Often times the orthopaedic surgeon does not order physical therapy for patients following arthroscopic meniscal surgery. Many patients are taught to use crutches and ice, and are given a home exercise program of isometrics and SLR on the day of surgery. As a whole, they do quite well and are able to return to their normal routine within about 6 weeks. Many patients, however, have residual motor control and weakness deficits, with problems in stair climbing and other high-level tasks.[112(p415)] These patients can benefit from a supervised rehabilitation program.

Exercise Program

PO Week 1. The patient begins isometric quadriceps sets, ankle pumps, and SLR, as well as self-assisted knee ROM exercises to tolerance. The therapist should use modalities, such as ice or compressive bandages, to minimize joint effusion.[112(p417),113(p972),114(p605)]

PO Week 2 to 4. If articular cartilage damage is present (which happens often in the elderly), aggressive isotonic and isokinetic exercise is delayed for 2 to 4 weeks.[113(p972),115(p168)] For most patients the following exercises can be added as tolerated:

- isometric quadriceps exercise at varying angles
- isometric hamstring exercise
- terminal knee extension
- stationary bicycle riding (1 to 5 min)
- hip isotonics[112(p417),113(p972),114(p605),115(p168)]

Major emphasis of the strengthening program is on the quadriceps group, which often remains weak after arthroscopic meniscectomy.[116(p18)] The patient continues to work for full knee ROM using self-stretching techniques (Figure 6–18) and wall glides.

Sometimes the therapist needs to perform MFR or light massage to the knee to prevent adhesions from forming, especially at the portal sites. The patient should be instructed in self-massage techniques at the portal sites.

PO Week 4 to 8. Patients with articular cartilage damage can begin the PO Week 2 to 4 program shown above. Other patients can move quickly to resisted isotonics and isokinetics, swimming, as well as closed-chain exercises. These can include

- mini squats
- step-ups
- modified leg presses (Figures 6–19 and 6–20)
- stool walking (Figure 6–23)
- sitting, wobbleboard

Patellar tracking should be assessed during these closed-chain exercises, and any patellofemoral dysfunction found should obviously be corrected before the patient is discharged. Bike riding is very beneficial for functional lower limb recovery[112(p425)] and should be gradually increased from 5 to 30 minutes. Full knee ROM should be achieved by 6 to 10 weeks postoperatively.[114(p606)]

Mobility/Ambulation Program

Aside from squatting, the patient is usually able to perform most transfers without assistance. Although some physicians restrict weight bearing, most patients are immediately weight bearing as tolerated with ambulation device or a knee immobilizer.[113(p972),114(p605)] As quadriceps strength improves, the patient is weaned off assistive devices and begins gait training. The patient needs to maneuver in all directions under control. By PO Week 6, most patients are ready for intensive balance and proprioceptive work, including standing wobbleboard, one-legged standing, or walking on a foam mat. Stair climbing progresses from 4-in step-up exercises to "normal" step-over-step pattern. Light jogging can begin after 3 months with physician approval.[114(p604)]

Activities of Daily Living Program

It usually takes the elderly patient a longer time to perform basic ADL after meniscal surgery. Depending on quadriceps strength, grab bars at the toilet may be necessary for a couple of weeks for safety. Instrumental ADL can be compromised, as the patient has difficulty carrying loads of laundry or groceries. Driving a car may be a problem if the right knee meniscus has been repaired. The patient should expect to require assistance in some form for at least 3 months following surgery. Return to prior function can take up to 6 months.[114(p606)]

Summary of Treatment of Arthroscopic Meniscal Surgery

- *PO Week 1*
  1. Minimize joint effusion with ice, TENS, and electrical stimulation.
  2. Begin knee isometrics, SLR, ankle pumps, and ROM exercises.

3. Ambulate weight bearing as tolerated with assistive device or splint.
4. Ensure all transfers and bed mobility are independent.
5. Train basic ADL.

- *PO Weeks 2 to 4*
  1. Minimize joint effusion.
  2. Continue PO Week 1 program for patients with articular cartilage damage.
  3. Progress other patients to: hamstring isometrics, terminal knee extension, hip isotonics, and light stationary bike riding. Emphasize quadriceps strengthening.
  4. Continue ROM stretching and self-stretching.
  5. Massage arthroscopic portal sites to prevent adhesions.
  6. Begin gait training without ambulation device for maneuverability.
  7. Train independence in all basic ADL without ambulation device.

- *PO Weeks 4 to 8*
  1. Begin more quadriceps intensive exercise for patients with articular cartilage damage.
  2. Progress other patients to resisted isotonics, isokinetics, and closed-chain exercise.
  3. Train balance and proprioception.
  4. Progress stair climbing to step-over-step.
  5. Begin low-level instrumental ADL.
  6. Return to full knee ROM in 6 to 10 weeks.
  7. Return to full function in 3 to 6 months.

PATELLOFEMORAL DYSFUNCTION

There are many disorders of the patellofemoral joint that can cause anterior knee pain. Some of these include: fracture, dislocation, tendinitis, bursitis, OA, and postural malalignment.[117(p334)] In addition, many of the same conditions have been given different names by various researchers, clinicians, and authors. This section will focus on the rehabilitation of anterior knee pain caused by muscle imbalance or skeletal malalignment.

The patient usually complains of sharp pain at the anterior knee on antigravity activities, such as getting out of a bathtub, rising from a chair, climbing or descending stairs, or getting out of a car. Walking on level surfaces at slow speeds causes little, if any pain. The therapist may find some of the following signs on evaluation:

- quadriceps weakness
- hamstring tightness
- gastrocnemius-soleus tightness
- ITB tightness
- tensor fascia lata (TFL) tightness
- lateral retinaculum tightness
- patella alta
- patella tilt (commonly inferior or lateral)
- patella glide (commonly lateral)
- patella rotation
- internal rotation of the hip
- crepitus
- large Q angle
- foot pronation
- rearfoot varus[117(p333),118(pp1424,1425),119(p265), 120(p235),121(p147),122(p155),123(pp18–23),124(p169)]

How the physical impairments listed above actually affect patellar alignment has been deduced and theorized, but not proven by research. In brief, the VMO portion of the quadriceps muscle actively pulls the patella in a medial direction and therefore helps keep the patella centered in the trochlear groove. Weakness of this muscle could lead to the patella tracking laterally, grinding the lateral facet into the femoral condyle.[120(p242)] Hamstring and gastrocnemius tightness causes increased flexion in the knee, thereby increasing the patellofemoral joint reaction force.[117(p334)] A tight ITB or lateral retinaculum has been shown to decrease the medial glide of the patella and increase tibial external rotation, altering patellar tracking.[121(p147),125(pp20,21)] Excessive patella glide, tilt, or rotation (Figures 6–25 and 6–26) changes the tracking of the patella in the femoral groove, which alters the contact sur-

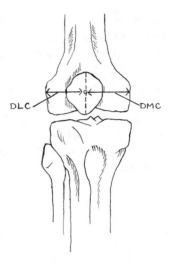

Figure 6–26 The patella glide measurement refers to the distance from the center of the patella to the medial femoral condyle (DMC) versus the lateral femoral condyle (DLC). Although the measurement itself has not been shown to be very reliable, most therapists assess this relationship in patients with patellofemoral syndrome. Many patients with anterior knee pain have a lateral glide of the patella (i.e., DMC > DLC).

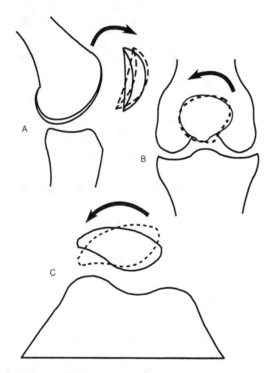

Figure 6–25 A, Sagittal plane rotation of the patella (flexion/extension). B, Frontal plane rotation of the patella (medial/lateral rotation). C, Transverse plane rotation of the patella (medial/lateral tilt). *Source:* Reprinted with permission from C.D. Ingersoll, "Rehabilitation of Patellofemoral Problems," *Orthopaedic Physical Therapy Clinics of North America*, Vol. 3, No. 3, p. 329, © 1994, W.B. Saunders Company.

faces and/or increases the torque in the knee.[117(p332)] A large Q angle, caused by femoral or tibial torsion may contribute to patellofemoral problems by increasing the lateral vector at the knee, pulling the patella laterally. Results from studies regarding the importance of Q angle in patellofemoral dysfunction are mixed.[126(p537)] Foot pronation and rearfoot varus have been found to correlate with increased patellofemoral pain,[122(pp155,156)] perhaps due to alterations in tibial rotation.

Patellofemoral dysfunction is most often associated with young women, yet anyone at any age is vulnerable. The elderly patient often develops patellofemoral dysfunction from one or more of the following problems:

- any swelling that occurs at the knee (due to bursitis, tibial plateau fracture, arthritis, etc.)

- extensor mechanism dysfunction from TKA surgery
- postural disorders: the tendency toward increased flexion in the elderly (e.g., tight hip and knee flexors) or the development of pronated feet

Treatment of Patellofemoral Dysfunction

Conservative treatment over the past decade has improved dramatically, decreasing the need for surgery. The major goal of therapy is to correct the impairments that alter patella alignment, thereby allowing it to track properly in the femoral groove.

Phase I (Days 1 to 14)

In this acute, initial phase, the patient reports sharp pain that is limiting everyday function. The therapy goals are to decrease or eliminate the pain, increase quadriceps strength in a pain-free range, increase flexibility of tight soft-tissue structures, and align the patella in the femoral groove.

Modalities. Modalities are extremely beneficial in the treatment of patellofemoral dysfunction. Ice and/or ultrasound around the periphery of the patella decreases pain and inflammation. Ultrasound at the TFL/ITB, hamstrings, patella tendon, and retinaculum can increase tissue distensibility. (Ultrasound is contraindicated over a TKA, but can still be used over muscle bellies.) Electrical stimulation can be used to decrease swelling or to help promote quadriceps firing. Biofeedback may help the patient recruit the VMO during the exercise program. (Research is mixed as to the efficacy of isolating the VMO or altering the timing of VMO firing.) Manual therapies, including massage, MFR, and patella mobilization, are necessary to increase the flexibility of the soft tissue structures.

Exercise Program. The patient must strengthen the quadriceps (including the VMO) in a ROM that causes minimal patellofemoral joint reaction forces and pain. Initially, the safest ROM is at 0° (quad sets and SLR) or terminal knee extension (0° to 20°). Although quadriceps activation is high with these types of exercise, the patella is not "seated" in the trochlear groove.[127(p386)] There is controversy as to whether terminal knee extension is best performed in the open- (Figure 6–6) or closed-kinetic chain. During closed-chain (or weight-bearing) exercise, the quadriceps works as a decelerator of knee flexion and an anterior stabilizer of the knee. Closed-chain terminal knee extension causes increased congruence of the patellofemoral joint[128(p110)] and a decreased patellofemoral joint reaction force.[129(p441)] Therefore mini squats, wall glides, knee extension in standing (Figure 6–27), and a modified leg press (Figures 6–19 and 6–20) appear to be a superior type of quadriceps exercise during this acute phase.

None of the above exercises has been proven to facilitate the VMO portion of the quadriceps more than the entire muscle as a whole.[130(pp39,40)] Theoretically, a cocontraction of the hip adductor muscles with the quadriceps should preferentially activate the VMO, due to the VMO's origin on the adductor magnus and longus muscles; however, clinical research has been conflicting on this subject.[127(pp389,390),131(p681)] Many clinicians continue to use the hip adductors in conjunction with knee exercises, such as quad sets, terminal knee extension, and wall squats with the hope that some facilitation is occurring. These exercises can be done with surface biofeedback over the VMO to ensure muscle recruitment (Figure 6–28).

The patient must also begin to stretch out tight muscles or fascial tissues in order to

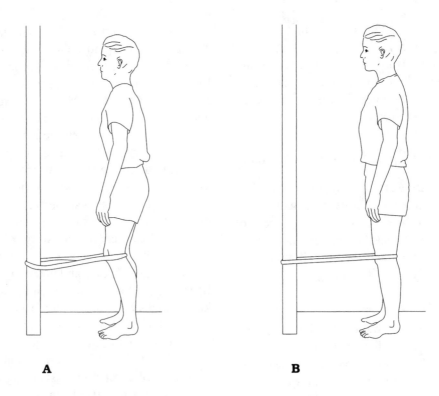

A   **B**

Patient Name: _____   **Date:** _____

Starting position: Standing with one end of an elastic tubing around your slightly bent involved knee and the other secured to a stationary object.

Exercise: Slowly pull your knee backward until it becomes straight.

Repeat _____ times.

Do _____ sessions per day.

Figure 6–27 Knee extension in the closed-chain with resistance. Terminal knee extension performed in weight-bearing posture has been found to be less irritating to the patellofemoral joint and can be initiated in the acute phase of treatment. *Source:* Adapted from *Exercise Handouts for Rehabilitation*, C.B. Lewis, T. McNerny, p. 85, Copyright © Aspen Publishers, Inc., 1993.

---

promote central tracking of the patella. The flexibility program should emphasize stretches to:

- the lateral retinaculum
- the ITB/TFL
- the hamstrings
- the rectus femoris
- the Achilles tendon

The patient should stretch each structure for a minimum of 30 seconds on a daily basis.

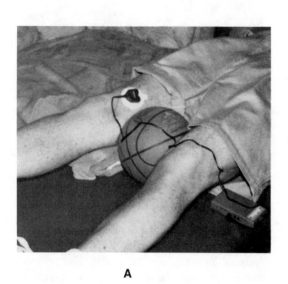

A

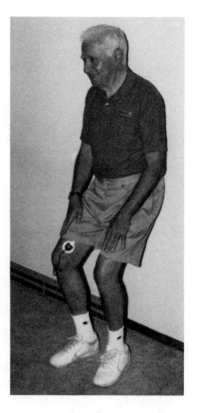

B

Figure 6–28 Coactivation of the hip adductors with the knee extensors should theoretically facilitate VMO activation. This can be accomplished by squeezing a ball or foam roller between the thighs before initiating (A) an open-chain SAQ or (B) a closed-chain wall glide. Placing biofeedback (MyoTrac by Thought Technology Ltd) over the VMO helps the patient to recruit the VMO.

Mobility/Ambulation Program. The patient obviously has difficulty in sit-to-stand transfers due to the pain. Avoiding low chairs, squatting activities, and floor-to-stand transfers is important at this stage.

An alteration of gait pattern has been found in patients with patellofemoral dysfunction. The patient ambulates with a reduced knee flexion angle[132(p21)] and a reduced ambulation velocity of 185 ft/min (56.5 m/min).[133(p1067)] The ambulation velocity is related to quadriceps strength. The patient should avoid walking on hilly terrain and

should take elevators instead of stairs whenever possible. Ambulation on even surfaces (albeit at a slower pace) is usually a pain-free activity that should be encouraged.

Activities of Daily Living Program. Pain on functional activities is one of the major reasons for the patient seeking help with this condition. Basic ADL of dressing and grooming are generally not affected. Getting on and off the toilet is painful, but raised toilet seats are usually not necessary. The patient should be encouraged to take showers instead of baths, as getting in and out of the tub can be hazardous. The patient should also be taught to hold onto a car door to unload the knee during car transfers. Lifting and carrying items should be kept to a minimum, especially if stair climbing is involved. The therapist should assess any recreational or sport activity to make sure that the patient is not exacerbating the condition. The patient must be reassured that these modifications in lifestyle are temporary, as patellofemoral pain tends to diminish quickly with adherence to the rehabilitation program.

External Support: Bracing, Taping, and Foot Orthotics. Although the use of a patellar tracking brace or patellar tape has been found to decrease pain and improve function, they are not the most vital components of the rehabilitation program. Patients will get better (although at a slower pace) by simply strengthening the quadriceps and stretching out the tight soft tissues.[134(p61)] In any event, the external supports should be viewed as temporary pain-reducing devices. They can be likened to training wheels on a bicycle. As the patient improves, the need for external help in tracking the patella diminishes.

Patellar braces come in a variety of off-the-shelf models. The basic type consists of a neoprene sleeve, with or without a patellar cutout. Some have pads on the lateral side to act as a buttress. Clinical studies consistently show that patients report decreased pain and increased stability with the brace on, yet there is minimal change in patella positioning, knee flexion angle, and conflicting data on changes in quadriceps isokinetic strength.[117(p337),135(p187),136(p133)] The OnTrack® brace by OrthoRX is designed to realign the patella in the intercondylar notch. This advanced brace consists of a neoprene sleeve and strap, which attaches to an underlying knee patch (Figure 6–29). Preliminary stud-

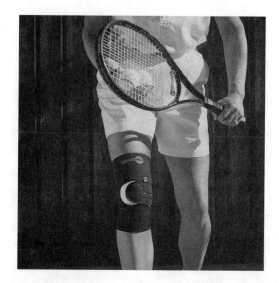

Figure 6–29 The OnTrack® patellofemoral brace. The neoprene strap attaches (by Velcro) to the underlying knee tape on the patella. The patient or therapist can pull the strap in the direction desired to centralize the patella. Courtesy of OrthoRX, San Diego, California.

ies show that the brace improves patellofemoral congruency[137]; however, further research needs to be done. Although high compliancy is usually seen with patellofemoral braces, elderly patients may have difficulty donning the neoprene sleeves.

Patellar taping, initially taught by McConnell, has also been successful in reducing knee pain and improving knee stability. In a recent study, the VMO activated earlier in a taped knee on step-ups and step-downs, possibly improving patellar tracking.[138(p31)] Somes et al found that taped knees had an improved patellar medial tilt as observed on radiograph.[139(p299)] Other researchers found no change in patellar alignment with tape. More research is needed to determine exactly how taping causes such a decrease in knee pain.

The technique for applying tape is straightforward. After assessing patellar alignment, the therapist determines which direction to pull the patella so that it will be centered. For example, if the therapist determines that the patella has a lateral glide orientation, the tape is applied to pull the patella in the medial direction (Figure 6–30). For the taping to be successful, the patient must perform a comparable sign test pain-free. In other words, the patient must perform a maneuver that usually sets off the knee pain, such as a squat or a step-up. If the patient can perform the activity with decreased pain or no pain, the tape is placed correctly. If the pain increases, it must be removed and reapplied. It is important to note that the criteria for successful taping are dependent on pain elimination, not on whether the patella alignment has been "corrected."

The biggest problem in using tape on the elderly patient is skin breakdown. The high-adhesive tape (e.g., Leukotape® P by Beiersdorf-Jobst or Rigid Strapping Tape by Smith & Nephew DonJoy) can cause severe skin reactions, especially in the more brittle skin of the elderly. For this reason, many therapists use Sween Prep first to prepare the skin of the elderly patient. In addition, other types of skin tape can be used with varying degrees of success. One of them, Kinesio Tex®, is

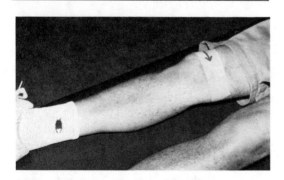

Figure 6–30 Patellar taping to control lateral glide. (Note: White underwrap tape is not necessary with Kinesio Tex® tape.)

cotton woven with an acrylic adhesive. This semi-elastic tape holds similarly to the more conventional patellar tapes, but the elderly patient tolerates the porous fabric better. For more information on these products, see the vendor listing at the end of this chapter.

Foot orthotics are sometimes prescribed to alleviate patellofemoral pain, thought to arise from excessive foot pronation. Although theoretically sound, research is scarce on the efficacy of foot orthotics in the treatment of this syndrome.

Phase II (Weeks 2 to 4)

During this intermediate phase, the pain level has already decreased significantly. The goals are to eliminate pain, increase strength, increase flexibility, and regain functional ability.

Exercise Program. Modalities can be used as needed to decrease swelling, inflammation, and pain. The patient must continue to strengthen the quadriceps, without aggravating the condition. All of the exercises in Phase I can now be done with weights or resistive tubing, and at varying speeds. The patient should avoid excessive exercise in the 20° to 50° range, due to the increased patellofemoral joint reaction forces and minimal patella contact area. However, it is imperative for the patient to work the knee gently in the 60° to 135° range for proper cartilage nutrition. This is best done in the open-chain, sitting, or prone-lying or through light stationary bicycle riding (closed-chain). The stretching program continues aggressively with emphasis on the ITB/TFL, hamstrings, rectus femoris, and Achilles tendon.

Mobility/Ambulation Program. The ability to rise from a chair should be improving, especially if the patient has a brace or tape on the knee. The therapist should still encourage the patient to avoid low chairs and floor-to-stand transfers when possible.

To promote more normal gait, the patient can begin low-level proprioception and balance activities in standing. Proprioception has been found to be diminished in patients with patellar pain.[140(p719)] The patient can stand on a foam mat, foam roller, or wobble-board in a door frame (Figure 4–9 in Chapter 4) to help restore proprioceptive input. In addition, walking backward and sideways will increase proprioception and maneuverability, with minimal shear forces at the knee. Stair climbing should still be kept to an absolute minimum.

Activities of Daily Living Program. Many ADL should be less painful to do, and the patient can use common sense in returning to his or her previous lifestyle. Excessive squatting, stair climbing, carrying, and lifting should still be avoided. However, the patient can be encouraged to try out activities to monitor the effects on the healing knee.

Phase III (PO Weeks 4 to 8)

The pain level at the knee should be significantly reduced or eliminated. Use of external support (i.e., patellar brace or tape) should be reserved for high-level activities only (i.e., work or sports). Gradual return to premorbid lifestyle may continue for 3 to 6 months.

Exercise Program. The need for modalities should be diminishing. The patient enters a more aggressive quadriceps strengthening program. The patient begins step-ups and step-downs on a 4-in aerobic step, initially with biofeedback on the VMO to ensure good firing. Lateral step-ups have been shown to be extremely quadriceps intensive[141(p113)] (Figure 6–31). In addition, the patient can work the squats lower, with emphasis on a 3-

second hold and rising up from the squat. This method of squatting has been shown to cause high activity in the VMO.[130(p40)] Stationary bicycle riding can be used for endurance training. The program should also emphasize speed work. (Many therapists fail to have elderly patients work the speed fibers [type II], even though research has clearly shown hypertrophy of these muscles with training regardless of age.) The patient may need to be taped or braced during these high-level exercise sessions.

Mobility/Ambulation Program. The patient should be able to perform all transfers with only minimal discomfort. Until the symptoms completely abate, kneeling and excessive squatting should be minimized. The gait program should emphasize maneuverability in all directions, the ability to negotiate uneven terrain (hills, ramps, stairs), and ambulation velocity. Normal ambulation velocity for the elderly is between 180 to 270 ft/min (55 to 82 m/min).[142(pp163–165),143(p88)]

Activities of Daily Living Program. The patient should be approaching independence in all areas of function and recreation. Any remaining deficits should be immediately addressed. Patellar taping and bracing can continue to be used for pain-free functional activities and sports.

Summary of Treatment of Patellofemoral Dysfunction

- *Weeks 1 to 2*
  1. Use modalities to reduce swelling, inflammation, and pain.
  2. Use massage, MFR, and patella mobilization to increase flexibility of soft tissues.
  3. Begin quadriceps exercises: quad sets, mini squats, wall glides, modified leg press.

Step-Ups and Step-Downs

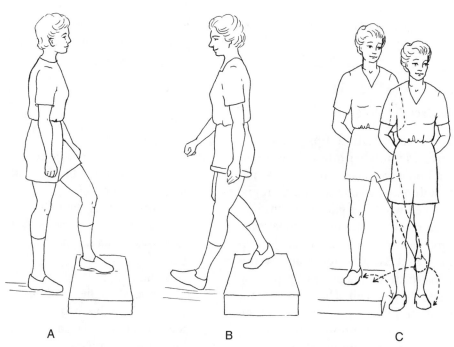

A   B   C

Figure 6–31 Step-ups and step-downs on a 4″ aerobic step. The patient performs forward and lateral step-ups and step-downs. The therapist may need to guard the elderly patient closely. In addition, the therapist must make sure that proper alignment is occurring and that the hips remain in neutral with the patellae tracking centrally. Biofeedback over the VMO can be used during this activity. *Source:* Adapted from T.S. Goldstein, *Functional Rehabilitation in Orthopaedics*, p. 98, © 1995, Aspen Publishers, Inc.

4. Use biofeedback to help recruit the VMO.
5. Stretch the lateral structures if needed: ITB/TFL, hamstrings, and lateral retinaculum.
6. Avoid deep squats, low chairs, and stair climbing.
7. Use patellar tape or brace to decrease pain and increase function.

• *Weeks 2 to 4*
1. Use modalities as needed.
2. Progress quadriceps strengthening in pain-free ROM, avoiding 20° to 50° range.

3. Gently increase knee ROM to full. Continue stretching lateral structures if needed.
4. Begin proprioceptive and balance training in standing.
5. Begin ambulation in all directions.
6. Avoid excessive stair climbing.
7. Begin to wean off patellar tape or brace.

• *Weeks 4 to 8*
1. Progress quadriceps strengthening full range in open and closed chain.
2. Increase resistance and speed of exercise.

3. All transfers should be independent and pain-free.
4. Progress gait training on uneven terrain and for speed.

5. All functional activities should be approaching independent and pain-free.
6. Use of patellar tape or brace should be restricted to high-level activity only.

DOCUMENTATION TIPS

Home Exercise Program

This documentation tips section is concerned mainly with how to write or draw a home exercise program that patients will use. In general, the therapist determines what the patient should do between physical therapy/ occupational therapy sessions (i.e., exercises, functional activities, pain logs) and writes these instructions on a piece of paper that is given to the patient. The written home program reinforces the verbal communication that occurs throughout all treatment sessions. Common sense dictates that the following documentation tips should be followed for a home program for an elderly patient:

- Print the patient's name and the date on the top of the paper.
- Print in large, clear letters. (Many elderly patients have vision problems.)
- Print the instructions clearly and briefly, including number of repetitions and frequency.
- Use large pictures to augment the text. Pictures are very helpful to visual learners. (See Figure 6–27 for an exercise sheet that is easy for an elderly patient to follow.)
- Print any precautions or contraindications, such as "Stop exercising if you feel any pain in the knee" or "Remove the patellar tape after a two-hour trial, slowly and carefully pulling the skin away from the tape."

- Print your name and work phone number so that the patient can call with any questions.
- Sign your name.
- Make a copy of the home program for the patient. Put the original in the medical record.
- Verbally go over the entire program with the patient, demonstrating any exercises the patient does not remember.
- Ask the patient if he or she has any questions about the program.
- Document in the medical record that the patient is "independent in the enclosed home program—see separate sheet."

Although writing a clear, concise exercise program is easy for the therapist, finding the time to write it is a major problem. There are many ways to decrease the amount of time needed to create an individual home program. Companies sell index cards of commonly used exercises, as well as books full of exercise sheets, made for the office copier.

After going through all the work to create the perfect, customized home program, the therapist may assume that the patient is, in fact, doing the exercises as written. This does not happen often. Therefore, simply writing the home program is only the first step. The therapist must then review the program in subsequent visits and reinstruct the patient in proper technique. This reinstruction must be documented in the medical record.

REFERENCES

1. Karpman RR, Del Mar NB. Supracondylar femoral fractures in the frail elderly. *Clin Orthop.* 1995;316:21–24.

2. Koval KJ, Zuckerman JD. *Fractures in the Elderly.* Philadelphia: Lippincott-Raven Publishers; 1998:193–215.

3. Meek RN, Boyle MR. Technique for the operative management of supracondylar and intracondylar fractures of the distal femur. *Techniques Orthop.* April 1986;1:39–43.

4. Cailliet R. *Knee Pain and Disability.* 3rd ed. Philadelphia: FA Davis Co; 1992.

5. Hohl M. Tibial condylar fractures. *J Bone Joint Surg.* 1967;49-A:1455–1467.

6. Collett P, Greenberg H, Terk MR. MR findings in patients with acute tibial plateau fractures. *Comput Med Imaging Graph.* 1996;20(5):389–394.

7. Tscherne H, Lobenhoffer P. Tibial plateau fractures. Management and expected results. *Clin Orthop.* 1993;292:87–100.

8. Touliatos AS, Xenakis T, Soucacos PK, Soucacos PN. Surgical management of tibial plateau fractures. *Acta Orthop Scand.* 1997;68(S275):92–96.

9. Canale ST. *Campbell's Operative Orthopaedics,* Vol 3. St. Louis, MO: Mosby-Year Book; 1998.

10. Braun W, Wiedemann M, Rutter A, Kundel K, Kolbinger S. Indications and results of nonoperative treatment of patellar fractures. *Clin Orthop.* 1993;289:197–201.

11. Exler Y. Patella fracture: Review of the literature and five case presentation. *J Orthop Sports Phys Ther.* 1991;13(4):177–183.

12. Albanese SA, Livermore JT, Werner FW, Murray DG, Utter RG. Knee extensor mechanics after subtotal excision of the patella. *Clin Orthop.* 1992;285:217–222.

13. Marder RA, Swanson TV, Sharkey NA, Duwelius PJ. Effects of partial patellectomy and reattachment of the patellar tendon on patellofemoral contact areas and pressures. *J Bone Joint Surg.* 1993;75-A(1):35–45.

14. Robinett CS, Vondran MA. Functional ambulation velocity and distance requirements in rural and urban communities. *Phys Ther.* September 1988;68(9):1371–1373.

15. Wixson RL. Status of joint reconstruction in the aged. *Top Geriatr Rehabil.* April 1989;4(3):40–51.

16. Panush RS. Exercise and arthritis. *Top Geriatr Rehabil.* April 1989;4(3):23–31.

17. Cyriax J. *Textbook of Orthopaedic Medicine.* 7th ed. London: Bailliere Tindall; 1978.

18. Messier SP. Osteoarthritis of the knee and associated factors of age and obesity—effects on gait. *Med Sci Sports Exerc.* 1994;26(12):1446.

19. Kohatsu ND, Schurman DJ. Risk factors for the development of osteoarthrosis of the knee. *Clin Orthop.* 1990;261:242–246.

20. Hulth A. Does osteoarthrosis depend on growth of the mineralized layer of cartilage? *Clin Orthop.* 1993;287:19–24.

21. Tsai CL, Liu TK. Estradiol-induced osteoarthrosis in ovariectomized rabbits. *Clin Orthop.* 1993;291:295–302.

22. Brittberg M, Lindahl A, Nilsson A, et al. Treatment of deep cartilage defects in the knee with autologous chondrocyte transplantation. *N Engl J Med.* 1994;331(14):889–895.

23. Iwata H. Pharmacologic and clinical aspects of intraarticular injection of hyaluronate. *Clin Orthop.* 1993;289:285–291.

24. Dieppe P, Altman R, Lequesne M, et al. Osteoarthritis of the knee: Report of a task force of the international league of associations for rheumatology and the osteoarthritis research society. *J Am Geriatr Soc.* 1997;45(7):850–852.

25. Brage ME, Draganich LF, Pottenger LA, Curran JJ. Knee laxity in symptomatic osteoarthritis. *Clin Orthop.* 1994;304:184–189.

26. Barrett DS, Cobb AG, Bemtley G. Joint proprioception in normal, osteoarthritic, and replaced knees. *J Bone Joint Surg.* 1991;73-B:53–56.

27. Marks R, Percy JS, Kumar S. Comparison between the surface electromyogram of the quadriceps surrounding the knees of healthy women and the knees of women with osteoarthritis. *Clin Exper Rheum.* 1994;12(1):11–15.

28. Wegener L, Kisner C, Nichols D. Static and dynamic balance responses in persons with bilateral knee osteoarthritis. *J Orthop Sports Phys Ther.* 1997;25(1):13–50.

29. Ettinger WH, Afable RF. Physical disability from knee osteoarthritis—the role of exercise as an

intervention. *Med Sci Sports Exerc.* 1994;26(12): 1435–1440.

30. Schilke JM, Johnson GO, Housh TJ, Odell JR. Effects of muscle strength training on the functional status of patients with osteoarthritis of the knee joint. *Nurs Research.* 1996;45(2):68–72.

31. Bohannon RW. Comfortable and maximum walking speed of adults aged 20–79 years—reference values and determinants. *Age Ageing.* 1997;26(1): 15–19.

32. Rantanen T, Avela J. Leg extension power and walking speed in very old people living independently. *J Geront.* Series A. 1997;52(4):M225–M231.

33. Sonn U. Longitudinal studies of dependence in daily-life activities among elderly persons—methodological development, use of assistive devices and relation to impairments and functional limitations. *Scand J Rehabil Med.* 1996;S34:1–35.

34. Kreindler H, Lewis CB, Rush S, Schaefer K. Effects of three protocols on strength of persons with osteoarthritis of the knee. *Top Geriatr Rehabil.* April 1989;4(3):32–39.

35. Fisher NM, Pendergast DR. Application of quantitative and progressive exercise rehabilitation to patients with osteoarthritis of the knee. *J Back Musculoskelet Rehabil.* 1995;5:33–53.

36. Fischer NM, White SC, Yack HJ, Smolinski RJ, Pendergast DR. Muscle function and gait in patients with knee osteoarthritis before and after muscle rehabilitation. *Disabil Rehabil.* 1997;19(2):47–55.

37. Brinkmann IR, Perry J. Rate and range of motion during ambulation in healthy and arthritic subjects. *Phys Ther.* July 1985;65(7):1055–1060.

38. Perry J. *Gait Analysis: Normal and Pathological Function.* Thorofare, NJ: Slack Inc, 1992.

39. Matsuno H, Kadowaki KM, Tsuji H. Generation II knee bracing for severe medial compartment osteoarthritis of the knee. *Arch Phys Med Rehabil.* 1997; 78:745–749.

40. Horlick SG, Loomer RL. Valgus knee bracing for medial gonarthrosis. *Clin J Sports Med.* 1993; 3:251–255.

41. Smith CA, Arnett FC. Epidemiologic aspects of rheumatoid arthritis. *Clin Orthop.* 1991;265:23–35.

42. Wilder RL, Crofford LJ. Do infectious agents cause rheumatoid arthritis? *Clin Orthop.* 1991;265: 36–41.

43. Sutej PG, Hadler NM. Current principles of rehabilitation for patients with rheumatoid arthritis. *Clin Orthop.* 1991;265:116–124.

44. Bell CL. Rheumatoid arthritis: current practices and rehabilitation. *Top Geriatr Rehabil.* April 1989:4(3):10–22.

45. Hakkinen A, Malkia E, Hakkinen K, et al. Effects of detraining subsequent to strength training on neuromuscular function in patients with inflammatory arthritis. *Brit J of Rheum.* 1997;36(10):1075–1081.

46. Ehrlich GE, ed. *Rehabilitation Management of Rheumatoid Conditions.* 2nd ed. Baltimore: Williams & Wilkins; 1986.

47. Knott M. Neuromuscular facilitation in the treatment of rheumatoid arthritis. *J Am Phys Ther Assoc.* August 1964;44:737–739.

48. Galloway MT, Joki P. The role of exercise in the treatment of inflammatory arthritis. *Bull Rheum Dis.* 1993;41(1):1–4.

49. Gerber LH, Hicks JE. Exercise in rheumatic disease. In: Basmajian JV, Wolf SL, eds. *Therapeutic Exercise.* 5th ed. Baltimore: Williams & Wilkins; 1990.

50. Nickel VL, Kristy J, McDaniel LV. Physical therapy for rheumatoid arthritis. *J Am Phys Ther Assoc.* March 1965;45:198–204.

51. Roberts SL, Falkenburg SA. *Biomechanics of Problem Solving for Functional Activity.* St. Louis, MO: Mosby-Year Book; 1992.

52. Bryan RS. Total knee arthroplasty revisited. In: Rand JA, Dorr LD, eds. *Total Arthroplasty of the Knee.* Rockville, MD: Aspen Publishers, Inc; 1987.

53. Sharma L, Sinacore J, Daugherty C. Prognostic factors for functional outcome of total knee replacement: a prospective study. *J Gerontol.* 1996;51A:M152–M157.

54. Tankersley WS, Hungerford DS. Total knee arthroplasty in the very aged. *Clin Orthop.* 1995;316: 45–49.

55. Hosick WB, Lotke MD, Baldwin A. Total knee arthroplasty in patients 80 years of age and older. *Clin Orthop.* 1994;299:77–80.

56. Laskin RS, ed. *Total Knee Replacement.* London: Springer-Verlag; 1991.

57. Scott WN, Stillwell WT, eds. *Arthroplasty: An Atlas of Surgical Technique.* Rockville, MD: Aspen Publishers, Inc; 1987.

58. McGann WA. Special surgical consideration in rehabilitation. Notes of a Lecture Given at Fourth Annual Knee Replacement Symposium; April 1989; Boston.

59. Savory C, Baker M. Current Concepts on Total Knee Arthroplasty. Lecture Notes from 1998 American

Physical Therapy Association Combined Sections Meeting, February 1998, Boston.

60. Kobs JK, Lachiewicz PF. Hybrid total knee arthroplasty. *Clin Orthop.* 1993;286:78–87.

61. Engh GA, Parks NL, Ammeen DJ. Influence of surgical approach on lateral retinacular releases in total knee arthoplasty. *Clin Orthop.* 1996;331:56–63.

62. Hofmann AA, Plaster RL, Murdock LE. Subvastus (southern) approach for primary total knee arthroplasty. *Clin Orthop.* 1991;269:70–88.

63. Masri BA, Laskin RS, Windsor RE, Haas SB. Knee closure in total knee replacement. *Clin Orthop.* 1996;231:81–86.

64. Lee AS, Kelly AJ, Ansari S, Prothero D, Newman JH. Flexion vs extension suturing of total knee replacement wounds—a randomized prospective study. *Knee.* 1997;4(2):65–67.

65. Emerson RH, Ayers C, Head WC, Higgin LL. Surgical closing in primary total knee arthroplasties. *Clin Orthop.* 1996;231:74–80.

66. Healy WL, Wasilewski SA, Takei R, Oberlander M. Patellofemoral complications following total knee arthroplasty—correlation with implant design and patient risk-factors. *J Arthrop.* 1995;10(2):197–201.

67. Andriacchi TP, Yoder D, Conley A, et al. Patellofemoral design influences function following total knee arthroplasty. *J Arthrop.* 1997;12(3):243–249.

68. Bourne RB, Rorabeck CH, Vaz M, et al. Resurfacing versus not resurfacing the patella during total knee replacement. *Clin Orthop.* 1995;321:156–161.

69. Bocell JR, Thorpe CD, Tullos HS. Arthroscopic treatment of symptomatic total knee arthroplasty. *Clin Orthop.* 1991;271:125–134.

70. Lynch NM, Trousdale RT, Ilstrup DM. Complications after concomitant bilateral total knee arthroplasty in elderly patients. *Mayo Clinic Proceedings.* 1997;72(9):799–805.

71. Swank M, Stulberg SD, Jiganti J, Machairas S. The natural history of unicompartmental arthroplasty. *Clin Orthop.* 1993;286:130–148.

72. Ivarsson I, Gillquist J. Rehabilitation after high tibial osteotomy and unicompartmental arthroplasty. A comparative study. *Clin Orthop.* 1991;266:139–144.

73. Carr A, Keyes G, Miller R, O'Connor J, Goodfellow J. Medial compartmental arthroplasty. *Clin Orthop.* 1993;295:205–213.

74. Thomas BJ, Cracchiolo A, Lee YF, et al. Total knee arthroplasty in rheumatoid arthritis. *Clin Orthop.* 1991;265:129–136.

75. Collins DN, Barnes CL, FitzRandolph RL. Cervical spine instability in rheumatoid patients having total hip or knee arthroplasty. *Clin Orthop.* 1991;272:127–135.

76. Elke R, Meier G, Warnke K, Morscher E. Outcome analysis of total knee replacements in patients with rheumatoid arthritis versus osteoarthritis. *Arch Orthop Trauma Surg.* 1995;114(6):330–334.

77. Rodriguez JA, Saddler S, Edelman S, Ranawat CS. Long-term results of total knee arthroplasty in class-3 and class-4 rheumatoid arthritis. *J Arthroscop.* 1996;11(2):141–145.

78. D'Lima DD, Colwell CW, Morris BA, Hardwick ME, Kozin F. The effect of preoperative exercise on total knee replacement outcomes. *Clin Orthop.* 1996; 326:174–182.

79. Scott CM, Gatti L. Physical therapy following total hip and total knee replacement. *Orthop Phys Ther Clin N Amer.* 1993;1(2):161–172.

80. Foster RR, Khalifa S. Total knee replacement rehabilitation. *Sports Med Arthrosc Rev.* 1996;4(1):83–91.

81. Enloe LJ, Shields RK, Smith K, Leo K, Miller B. Total hip and knee replacement treatment programs: A report using consensus. *J Orthop Sports Phys Ther.* 1996;23(1):3–17.

82. Pocquat S. MGH inpatient knee replacement management. Notes of a Lecture Given at Fourth Annual Knee Replacement Symposium; April 1989; Boston.

83. Basso DM, Knapp L. Comparison of two continuous passive motion protocols for patients with total knee implants. *Phys Ther.* March 1987;67(3):360–363.

84. Chiarello CM, Gundersen L, O'Halloran T. The effect of continuous passive motion duration and increment on range of motion in total knee arthroplasty patients. *J Orthop Sports Phys Ther.* 1997;25(2):119–127.

85. Ververeli PA, Sutton DC, Hearn SL, Booth RE, Hozack WJ, Rothman RR. Continuous passive motion after total knee arthroplasty. *Clin Orthop.* 1995;321:208–215.

86. Montgomery F, Eliasson M. Continuous passive motion compared to active physical therapy after knee arthroplasty. *Acta Orthop Scand.* 1996;67:7–9.

87. Johnson DP. The effect of continuous passive motion on wound-healing and joint mobility after knee arthroplasty. *J Bone Joint Surg.* 1990;72-A(3): 421–426.

88. Colwell CW, Morris BW. The influence of continuous passive motion on the results of total knee arthroplasty. *Clin Orthop.* 1992;276:225–229.

89. Jordan LR, Siegel JL, Olivo JL. Early flexion routine: an alternative method of continuous passive motion. *Clin Orthop.* 1995;315:231–233.

90. Kumar PJ, McPherson EJ, Dorr LD, Wan Z, Baldwin K. Rehabilitation after total knee arthroplasty. A comparison of 2 rehabilitation techniques. *Clin Orthop.* 1996;331:93–101.

91. Kim JM, Moon MS. Squatting following total knee arthroplasty. *Clin Orthop.* 1995;313:177–186.

92. Brimer MA. New clinical considerations in total knee arthroplasty rehab. *Clin Management Phys Ther.* January–February 1987;7:6–9.

93. Kuster MS, Wood GA, Stachowiak GW, Gachter A. Joint load considerations in total knee replacement. *J Bone Joint Surg.* 1997;79-B(1):109–113.

94. Hodge WA. Biomechanics of rehabilitation following TKA. Notes of a Lecture Given at Fourth Annual Knee Replacement Symposium; April 1989; Boston.

95. Smidt GL, Albright JP, Deusinger RH. Pre- and postoperative functional changes in total knee patients. *J Orthop Sports Phys Ther.* July/August 1984; 6:25–29.

96. Huang CH, Cheng CK, Lee YT, Lee KS. Muscle strength after successful total knee replacement: A 6 to 13 year followup. *Clin Orthop.* 1996; 328:147–154.

97. Jaramillo J, Worrell T, Ingersoll C. Effects of knee injury and surgery on hip muscle force development. Presentation at American Physical Therapy Association Annual Conference, June 1994.

98. Warren PJ, Olanlokun TK, Cobb AG, Bentley G. Proprioception after knee arthroplasty. The influence of prosthetic design. *Clin Orthop.* 1993;297: 182–187.

99. Holpit LA. Preoperative and postoperative physical therapy for the total shoulder, hip, and knee replacement patient. *Orthop Phys Therap Clin N Amer.* 1993;2(1):97–118.

100. MacDonald W, Owen JW. The effect of total hip replacement on driving reactions. *J Bone Joint Surg.* 1988;70-B:202–205.

101. Sinacore SL, Daugherty C, et al. Prognostic factors for functional outcome of total knee replacement: a prospective study. *J Gerontol.* 1996;51A: M152–M157.

102. Anouchi YS, McShane M, Kelly F, Elting J, Stiehl J. Range of motion in total knee replacement. *Clin Orthop.* 1996;331:87–92.

103. Skinner HB. Pathokinesiology and total joint arthroplasty. *Clin Orthop.* 1993;286:78–86.

104. Vail TP, Mallon WJ, Liebelt RA. Athletic activities after joint arthroplasty. *Sports Med Arthrosc Rev.* 1996;4(3):298–305.

105. Stone KR, Stoller D, Decarli A, Day R, Richnak J. The frequency of Baker's cysts associated with meniscal tears. *Am J Sports Med.* 1996;24(5):670–671.

106. Canale ST. *Campbell's Operative Orthopaedics,* Vol 2. St. Louis, MO: Mosby-Year Book; 1998.

107. Ihara H, Miwa M, Takayanagi K, Nakayama A. Acute torn meniscus combined with acute cruciate ligament injury. *Clin Orthop.* 1994;307:146–154.

108. Kimura M, Shirakura K, Hasegawa A, Kobuna Y, Niijima M. Second look arthroscopy after meniscal repair: factors affecting the healing rate. *Clin Orthop.* 1995;314:185–191.

109. Weiss CB, Lundberg M, Hamberg P, DeHaven KE, Gillquist J. Non-operative treatment of meniscal tears. *J Bone Joint Surg.* 1989;71-A(6):811–822.

110. Muscolo DL, Costapaz M, Makino A, Ayerza MA. Osteonecrosis of the knee following arthroscopic meniscectomy in patients over 50 years old. *Arthroscopy.* 1996;12(3):273–279.

111. O'Brien SJ, Ngeow J, Gibney MA, Warren RF, Fealy S. Reflex sympathetic dystrophy of the knee—causes, diagnosis, and treatment. *Am J Sports Med.* 1995;23(6):655–659.

112. Moffet H, Richards CL, Malouin F, Bravo G, Paradis G. Early and intensive physiotherapy accelerates recovery postarthroscopic meniscectomy: results of a randomized controlled study. *Arch Phys Med Rehabil.* 1994;75(4):415–426.

113. Silbey MB, Fu FH. *Knee Injuries in Sports Injuries: Mechanisms, Prevention, Treatment.* Fu FH, Stone DA, eds. Baltimore: Williams & Wilkins; 1994.

114. Shelbourne KD, Patel DV, Adsit WS, Porter DA. Rehabilitation after meniscal repair. *Clin Sports Med.* 1996;15(3):595–612.

115. Shankman GA. *Fundamental Orthopedic Management for the Physical Therapist Assistant.* St. Louis, MO: Mosby-Year Book; 1997.

116. Matthews P, St-Pierre DMM. Recovery of muscle strength following arthroscopic meniscectomy. *J Orthop Sports Phys Ther.* 1996;23(1):18–26.

117. Ingersoll CD. Rehabilitation of patellofemoral problems. *Orthop Phys Ther Clin N Amer.* 1994;3(3): 327–347.

118. Fulkerson JP, Shea KP. Current concepts review disorders of patellofemoral alignment. *J Bone Joint Surg.* 1990;72-A(9):1424–1429.

119. Simmons E, Cameron JC. Patella alta and recurrent dislocation of the patella. *Clin Orthop.* 1992; 274:265–269.

120. Heegaard J, Leyvraz PF, Van Kampen A, et al. Influence of soft structures on patella three-dimensional tracking. *Clin Orthop.* 1994;299:235–243.

121. Puniello MS. Iliotibial band tightness and medial patellar glide in patients with patellofemoral dysfunction. *J Orthop Sports Phys Ther.* 1993;17(3): 144–148.

122. Powers CM, Maffucci R, Hampton S. Rearfoot posture in subjects with patellofemoral pain. *J Orthop Sports Phys Ther.* 1995;22(4):155–160.

123. Grace K. *Patellofemoral Dysfunction Examination and Treatment Course Notes.* San Diego, CA: OrthoEd; 1996.

124. Harrison E, Magee D, Quinney H. Development of a clinical tool and patient questionnaire for evaluation of patellofemoral pain syndrome patients. *Clin J Sports Med.* 1996;6(3):163–170.

125. Winslow J, Yoder E. Patellofemoral pain in female ballet dancers: Correlation with iliotibial band tightness and tibial external rotation. *J Orthop Sports Phys Ther.* 1995;22(1):18–21.

126. Woodall W, Welsh J. A biomechanical basis for rehabilitation programs involving the patellofemoral joint. *J Orthop Sports Phys Ther.* 1990;11(11): 535–542.

127. Callaghan MJ, Oldham JA. The role of quadriceps exercise in the treatment of patellofemoral pain syndrome. *Sports Med.* 1996;21(5):384–391.

128. Doucette SA, Child DD. The effect of open and closed chain exercise and knee joint position on patellar tracking in lateral patellar compression syndrome. *J Orthop Sports Phys Ther.* 1996;23(2):104–110.

129. Steinkamp LA, Dillingham MF, Markel MD, Hill JA, Kaufman KR. Biomechanical considerations in patellofemoral joint rehabilitation. *Am J Sports Med.* 1993;21(3):438–444.

130. Gryzlo SM, Patek RM, Pink M, Perry J. Electromyographic analysis of knee rehabilitation exercises. *J Orthop Sports Phys Ther.* 1994;20(1):36–43.

131. Cerny K. Vastus medialis oblique/vastus lateralis muscle activity ratios for selected exercises in persons with and without patellofemoral pain syndrome. *Phys Ther.* 1995;75(8):672–683.

132. Nadeau S, Gravel D, Hebert LJ, Arsenault AB, Lepage Y. Gait study of patients with patellofemoral pain syndrome. *Gait & Posture.* 1997;5(1):21–27.

133. Powers CM, Perry J, Hsu A, Hislop HJ. Are patellofemoral pain and quadriceps femoris muscle torque associated with locomotor function? *Phys Ther.* 1997;77(10):1063–1075.

134. Kowall MG, Golk G, Nuber GW, Cassisi JE, Stern SH. Patellar taping in the treatment of patellofemoral pain—a prospective randomized study. *Am J Sports Med.* 1996;24(1):61–66.

135. Greenwald AE, Bagley AM, France P, Paulos LE, Greenwald RM. A biomechanical and clinical evaluation of a patellofemoral knee brace. *Clin Orthop.* 1996;324:187–195.

136. Gulling LK, Lephart SM, Stone DA, Irrgang JJ, Pincivero DM. The effects of patellar bracing on quadriceps EMG activity during isokinetic exercise. *Isokin Exerc Sci.* 1996;6(2):133–138.

137. Grace K, Rowe JG, Clark K, Slymen D. Use of the OnTrack® brace system in decreasing patellofemoral pain and recruiting the vastus medialis oblique muscle function. Unpublished clinical study, 1995.

138. Gilleard W, McConnell J, Parsons D. The effect of patellar taping on the onset of vastus medialis obliquus and vastus lateralis muscle activity in persons with patellofemoral pain. *Phys Ther.* 1998;78(1): 25–32.

139. Somes S, Worrell TW, Corey B, Ingersol CD. Effects of patellar taping on patellar position in the open and closed kinetic chain—a preliminary study. *J Sport Rehabil.* 1997;6(4):299–308.

140. Jerosch J, Schmidt K, Prymka M. Proprioceptive abilities of patients with a patellar pain syndrome with special reference to the effect of an elastic knee bandage. *Unfallchirurg.* 1997;100(9):719–723.

141. Cook TM, Zimmermann CL, Lux KM, Neubrand CM, Nicholson TD. EMG comparison of lateral step-up and stepping machine exercise. *J Orthop Sports Phys Ther.* 1992;16(3):108–113.

142. Himann JE, Cunningham DA, Rechnitzer PA, Paterson DH. Age-related changes in speed of walking. *Med Sci Sports Exerc.* 1988;20:161–166.

143. Bohannon RW, Andrews AW, Thomas MW. Walking speed: Reference values and correlates for older adults. *J Orthop Sports Phys Ther.* 1996;24(2): 86–90.

PRODUCT INFORMATION

For more information on the following products, please contact the companies listed below:

OnTrack® Patellar Tracking Brace
OrthoRx
8929 University Center Lane, Suite 200
San Diego, CA 92122
(800) 668-7258

Kinesio Tex® Tape
Summit Medical, Inc.
3100 Richmond Drive NE
Albuquerque, NM 87107-1921
(800) 759-7788

Leukotape® P Tape
Beiersdorf-Jobst
(800) 537-1063

7

The Ankle/Foot Complex

As the first body part to contact the ground during gait, the foot and surrounding structures play a vital role in everyday function. However, difficulties in defining "normal" still exist at the ankle/foot complex. Individual variations are so great within test populations that no conclusive averages for strength or range of motion (ROM) exist. There are also questions about the validity and reliability of the techniques to measure foot postural alignment.[1(p382)] Clinical observations often are unsupported by laboratory observations. The reader is forewarned that the following discussion of the ankle/foot complex contains discrepancies and that future research may support or refute some of the "facts" presented.

In addition, no standard nomenclature is used in the literature or in the clinic when the ankle and foot are discussed. This lack of standardization has caused further confusion for the student and the clinician in trying to understand the interactions of the various joints. Table 7–1 contains some of the more common names used to describe parts of the ankle and foot.

ANATOMY OF THE ANKLE AND FOOT

Twenty-six bones of the foot, along with the tibia and the fibula, comprise the ankle/foot complex. It is not within the scope of this book to describe in detail the surface features and axes of rotation of the many articulations of the ankle and foot. The reader is referred to the many anatomy and kinesiology texts for further information concerning the in-depth kinematics of these joints.

The Ankle (Talocrural Joint)

The ankle joint consists of the convex trochlear surface of the talus and the concave mortise of the tibia and fibula. The articular surface of the talus is wider anteriorly than posteriorly, thereby allowing only 10° to 20° of dorsiflexion to occur before the talus jams into the mortise in its close-packed position.[2(p247)] Dorsiflexion is the initial position from which all major thrusting movements are developed, such as walking, jumping, and running.[3(p461)] The primary dorsiflexor of the ankle is the tibialis anterior. Plantarflexion of up to 50° also occurs at this joint powered by the gastrocnemius and soleus muscles. (See Table 7–2 for a summary of all muscles and motions in the ankle and foot.) Studies of ankle ROM in the elderly population appear to indicate a loss of motion with age, with elderly persons averaging 10° of dorsiflexion and 34° of plantarflexion.[4(p921),5(p165)] However, in another study, by Chesworth and Vandervoort,[6(p221)] no significant difference

Table 7–1 Common Names for the Bones, Joints, and Movements of the Ankle/Foot Complex

Bones	
Forefoot	5 Metatarsals and 14 phalanges
Midfoot	Cuneiform, navicular, and 3 cuboids
Hindfoot	Talus and calcaneus (subtalar joint)
Joints	
Ankle joint =	Talocrural joint
Subtalar joint =	Talocalcaneal joint
	Hindfoot
Midtarsal joint =	Transverse tarsal joint
	Talonavicular and calcaneocuboid joints
	Talocalcaneonavicular joint
	Chopart joint
	(Joints between hindfoot and midfoot)
Movements	
Supination	Combined inversion and adduction
Pronation	Combined eversion and abduction

Note: Lack of a standard nomenclature for the ankle and foot causes unnecessary confusion.

in ankle joint stiffness was found between healthy 20- to 80-year-old subjects. Loss of dorsiflexion leads to a decrease in step length and walking speed, both common findings in the elderly.[7(p692)] In addition, unless 10° of dorsiflexion is present, heel-off will occur prematurely or the foot will have to pronate excessively during the stance phase of gait.[8(p186),9(p37)]

Many ligaments protect the integrity of the ankle joint (Figure 7–1). The mortise of the tibia and fibula is held together by the interosseous membrane and the anterior and posterior tibiofibular ligaments. The talus is locked into the mortise by the lateral collateral ligament and the deltoid ligament. The lateral collateral ligament, which is sprained often, consists of the anterior talofibular ligament, the calcaneofibular ligament, and the posterior talofibular ligament. The deltoid ligament, or medial collateral ligament, comprises four bands: the tibionavicular, the anterior talotibial, the calcaneotibial, and the

posterior talotibial ligaments. The deltoid is so strong that a severe eversion force will avulse the medial malleolus rather than tear the ligament.[10(pp6,7)]

The Subtalar and Midtarsal Joints

The subtalar, or talocalcaneal, joint involves the concave posterior facet of the talus and the convex posterior facet on the upper surface of the calcaneus (Figure 7–2). The midtarsal joint encompasses the articulations between the talus and the navicular and the calcaneus and the cuboid, i.e., the joints connecting the hindfoot to the midfoot (Figure 7–2). The major motions available at these joints are inversion (rearfoot varus) and eversion (rearfoot valgus).[11(p11)] The tibialis anterior and the tibialis posterior act to invert the foot, allowing an average of 30° in the elderly population. The peroneals evert the foot approximately 12°.[4(p922)] (See Table

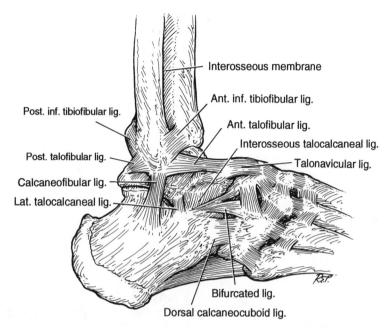

Figure 7–1 Ligamentous structures of the ankle (lateral view). *Source:* Reprinted with permission from T. Brosky et al., "The Ankle Ligaments: Consideration of Syndesmotic Injury and Implications for Rehabilitation," *Journal of Orthopaedic and Sports Physical Therapy*, Vol. 21, No. 4, p. 199, © 1995, Williams & Wilkins.

7–2.) Because of the obliquity of the axis of rotation, some adduction is associated with inversion. This combined motion is often called supination. Likewise, abduction is as-sociated with eversion and is termed prona-tion.[12(p371)] When the foot is on the ground transmitting weight and thrust, these move-ments are modified to maintain plantigrade

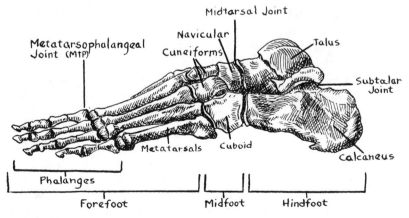

Figure 7-2 Bones and joints of the foot

Table 7–2 Geriatric Ankle and Foot Motions, Muscles, and Innervations

Motion*	Primary Muscles	Secondary Muscles	Innervation
Ankle			
dorsiflexion 0°–10°	Tibialis anterior		Deep peroneal: L4-5
		Extensor digitorum longus	Deep peroneal: L-5, S-1
		Extensor hallucis longus	Deep peroneal: L-5, S-1
		Peroneus tertius	Deep peroneal: L-5, S-1
Plantarflexion 0°–35°	Gastrocnemius		Tibial: S1-2
	Soleus		Tibial: S1-2
		Plantaris	Tibial: S1-2
		Tibialis posterior	Tibial: L4-5
		Flexor digitorum longus	Tibial: S2-3
		Flexor hallucis longus	Tibial: S2-3
Subtalar and midtarsal joints			
Inversion and adduction (supination) 0°–30°	Tibialis anterior Tibialis posterior		Deep peroneal: L4-5 Tibial: L4-5
Eversion and abduction (pronation) 0°–12°	Peroneus longus Peroneus brevis		Superficial peroneal: L-5, S1-2 Superficial peroneal: L-5, S1-2
MTP joints			
Dorsiflexion 0°–61°	Extensor digitorum longus		Deep peroneal: L-5, S-1
	Extensor hallucis longus		Deep peroneal: L-5, S-1
	Extensor digitorum brevis		Deep peroneal: S1-2
Plantarflexion 0°–6°	Flexor digitorum brevis		Medial plantar: S2-3
	Lumbricales and interossei		Lateral plantar: S2-3
		Flexors	
		Digitorum longus	Tibial: S2-3
		Hallucis longus	Tibial: S2-3
		Hallucis brevis	Tibial: S2-3
		Digiti minimi brevis	Lateral plantar: S2-3

continues

Table 7–2 continued

Motion*	Primary Muscles	Secondary Muscles	Innervation
MTP joints			
Adduction	Adductor hallucis		Lateral plantar: S2-3
	Plantar interossei		Lateral plantar: S2-3
Abduction	Abductor hallucis		Medial plantar: S2-3
	Abductor digiti minimi		Lateral plantar: S2-3
	Dorsal interossei		Lateral plantar: S2-3
Interphalangeal joints			
Dorsiflexion (to neutral)	Extensor digitorum brevis		Deep peroneal: S1-2
	Extensor digitorum longus		Deep peroneal: L-5, S-1
	Extensor hallucis longus		Deep peroneal: L-5, S-1
Plantarflexion 0°–50°	Flexor digitorum brevis		Medial plantar: S2-3
	Flexor digitorum accessorius		Lateral plantar: S2-3
	Flexor digitorum longus		Tibial: S2-3
	Flexor hallucis longus		Tibial: S2-3

Sources: Gray's Anatomy, ed 35 (pp 571–583), by R Warwick and PL Williams (eds), Churchill Livingstone, © 1973.
**Physical Therapy* (1984;64(6):921), Copyright © American Physical Therapy Association.

contact.[3(pp463,464)] (See "The Ankle/Foot Complex in Gait" for a description of the modified motion that occurs.)

Ligamentous stability (Figure 7–1) of the subtalar joint is provided by the joint capsule, the lateral and medial talocalcaneal ligaments, the interosseous talocalcaneal ligament, and the cervical ligament. The interosseous talocalcaneal ligament is taut on eversion, whereas the cervical ligament is taut on inversion, increasing the stability of the supinated foot.[3(pp463,464),13(p8)]

There are many interosseous ligaments connecting the various bones of the midtarsal joint; only two are discussed here. The long plantar ligament (Figure 7–3), connecting the calcaneus to the cuboid and metatarsal bones, helps to maintain the lateral longitudinal arch of the foot. The calcaneonavicular ligament, or spring ligament (Figure 7–3), connects the navicular to the calcaneus and supports the medial longitudinal arch of the foot.[3(pp464,465)]

The Metatarsophalangeal Joints

The metatarsophalangeal (MTP) joints consist of the five convex metatarsal heads and the concave proximal phalanges (Figure 7–2). The first MTP joint also articulates with two sesamoid bones, which assist the metatarsal head in gliding during propulsion activities.[9(pp54–60)] In the older foot, the ligaments of the MTP joint are commonly stretched, lowering the transverse arch. This

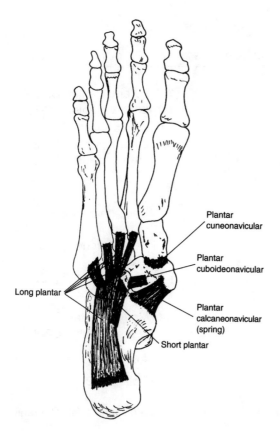

Plantar
cuneonavicular

Plantar
cuboideonavicular

Long plantar

Plantar
calcaneonavicular
(spring)

Short plantar

Figure 7–3 Right foot, ligaments on the plantar surface. *Source:* Reprinted from A.L. Logan, *The Foot and Ankle: Clinical Applications*, p. 8, © 1995, Aspen Publishers, Inc.

widening of the foot is due to years of weight bearing.[14(p25)] The primary plantarflexors of the MTP joints are the flexor digitorum brevis, the lumbricales, and the interossei muscles. Normally, 35° of plantarflexion is available at the MTP joint, but elderly persons average only 6° of this motion.[4(p921)] Fortunately, there is not much dysfunction associated with loss of plantarflexion. The primary dorsiflexors of the MTP joint are the extensors digitorum longus and brevis, and the extensor hallucis longus. Usually up to 90° of motion can occur at the MTP joint, but in a study by Walker et al[4(p921)] the elderly

population averaged only 61°. Unlike plantarflexion, dorsiflexion is integral to ambulation: 65° of minimal motion is necessary at heel-off.[9(p60)] Small amounts of abduction and adduction also occur at the MTP joints, powered by the intrinsic muscles of the foot (Table 7–2).

The Interphalangeal Joints

Each of the interphalangeal (IP) joints consists of the head of the more proximal phalanx and the base of the more distal phalanx. The great toe has only two phalanges, whereas the lesser toes have three each (Figure 7–2). All IP joints have a joint capsule and two collateral ligaments. Active motion occurs in the sagittal plane only; 50° to 90° of (plantar) flexion and 0° of extension are available.[15(p72)] Dorsiflexion normally does not occur at these joints. (See Table 7–2 for muscles that act on the IP joints.) The great toe acts to facilitate propulsion, providing the final toe-off during gait, while the lesser toes are concerned mainly with balance.[10(p10)]

Fat Pads

The fat pads of the heel and metatarsal heads are comprised of fat-filled microchambers that attenuate forces and dampen vibrations. They are held in place by a thick fibrous network. Along with ligaments and muscles, these plantar fat pads dissipate the enormous shock to which the feet are subjected with every step.[14(pp356,357)] With aging, the plantar fat pads may atrophy, allowing painful calluses to form under the metatarsal heads.[16(p25)]

Innervation

The ankle/foot complex receives its nerve supply from the tibial nerve (branching into the medial and lateral plantar nerves) and the common peroneal nerve (branching into the deep and superficial peroneal nerves). The tibial nerve supplies the plantarflexors of the foot, and the deep peroneal nerve supplies the dorsiflexors of the foot.[13(pp22–25)] (See Table 7–2 for specific muscular innervations.)

Sensory input from the ankle joint and the plantar surface of the foot is important in the feedback system for maintaining balance in the upright posture. Proprioceptive nerve fibers have been identified in ligaments and capsular tissues around the ankle.[14(p358)] This system often is impaired in elderly persons (as a result of peripheral neuropathies or diabetes) and may contribute to an increased incidence of falls. The tibial nerve innervates the ankle joint and the skin of the heel. Sensation in the medial aspect of the sole derives from the medial plantar nerve; sensation in the lateral aspect derives from the lateral plantar nerve.[3(p1058)]

Blood Supply

The popliteal artery branches into the anterior and posterior tibial arteries. The anterior tibial artery branches into the medial and lateral malleolar arteries that anastomose around and below the ankle joint. Below the ankle, the anterior tibial artery becomes the dorsal artery of the foot (dorsalis pedis), which terminates in the tarsal and metatarsal arteries.[3(pp681,682)]

The posterior tibial artery supplies the posterior muscles of the leg. At the plantar surface of the foot, it divides into the medial and lateral plantar arteries.[13(p26)] The branches of the posterior tibial artery anastomose with those of the anterior tibial artery to form many networks about the ankle and foot.

The superficial and deep veins of the lower limb return the blood to the heart through a system of valves and a system of muscular and fascial actions known as the "calf pump."[3(p705)]

In the older foot, sclerotic blood vessels cause increased resistance to blood flow. Combined with dry skin, fissures can easily form and progress to skin ulcers. Diminished blood supply can also lead to loss of bone density and predisposes the bones of the foot to fracture.[16(pp25,26)]

KINETICS OF THE ANKLE AND FOOT

Most of the kinetic studies of the ankle and foot concern the joint reaction forces of the ankle during ambulation. Since normal gait is one of the major mobility areas addressed by physical therapists, a review of the ankle and foot during gait is presented.

The Arches of the Foot

The three arches of the foot help the foot withstand and transmit large forces. They are dynamic, not static, structures supported by the ligaments and muscles of the foot.

The Medial Longitudinal Arch

The bones that form the medial longitudinal arch are

- the calcaneus
- the talus
- the navicular
- the cuneiforms
- the three medial metatarsals

During standing activities, the medial longitudinal arch sinks under the force of the body weight and relies mostly on ligaments to maintain its integrity. Immediately upon movement (walking), the following muscles actively support the arch:

- the tibialis posterior
- the flexor digitorum longus
- the flexor hallucis longus
- the intrinsic muscles of the foot[3(p469),17(p165)]

The Lateral Longitudinal Arch

The bones that comprise the lateral longitudinal arch are

- the calcaneus
- the cuboid
- the lateral two metatarsals

The lateral longitudinal arch appears to be built not to absorb the ground reaction forces, but to transmit weight and thrust to the ground. The ligaments are assisted by the peroneus longus and the intrinsic muscles of the fifth toe in maintaining this arch.[2(p469),17(p165)]

The Transverse Arch

The bony configuration of the metatarsals forms a transverse bow, which acts as a supporting beam. This flexible arrangement allows the transverse arch to support three to four times the body weight.[2(p250)] A rigid transverse arch is also formed more proximally by the three cuneiform bones and the cuboid bone.[13(p11)]

The Ankle/Foot Complex in Gait

Gait is divided into swing and stance phases. During the swing phase the leg rotates internally, the ankle dorsiflexes, and the subtalar and midtarsal joints invert and adduct (supinate). During the stance phase (heel strike, foot flat, and toe-off) the ankle and foot rotate and glide under the influences of body weight, skeletal structure, muscular contraction, and ground reaction forces. (See Figure 7–4 for a summary of the foot and ankle movements during the gait cycle.)

Heel Strike

As the unloaded foot prepares to accept weight at heel strike, it must be flexible enough to accommodate any terrain. Many elderly persons lack heel strike because of pain or loss of motion or strength. The following sequence normally occurs during this first part of the stance phase:

1. The entire leg rotates internally.
2. The ankle joint plantarflexes.
3. The subtalar and midtarsal joints pronate: the talus adducts and the calcaneus everts.
4. The body weight is borne on the lateral aspect of the heel.
5. The ankle joint reaction force is three times the body weight.

Foot Flat

During the foot-flat phase, the foot shifts from flexibility to rigidity in order to propel the body forward. The following sequence normally occurs:

1. The entire leg rotates externally.
2. The ankle joint dorsiflexes.
3. The subtalar and midtarsal joints supinate: the talus abducts and the calcaneus inverts.
4. The body weight is borne on the entire heel and on the metatarsal heads.
5. The ankle joint reaction force is three times the body weight.

Toe-Off

The foot is a rigid lever, propelling the body forward during toe-off to the next step. Many elderly persons lack a vigorous toe-off. The following sequence normally occurs during this last stage of the stance phase:

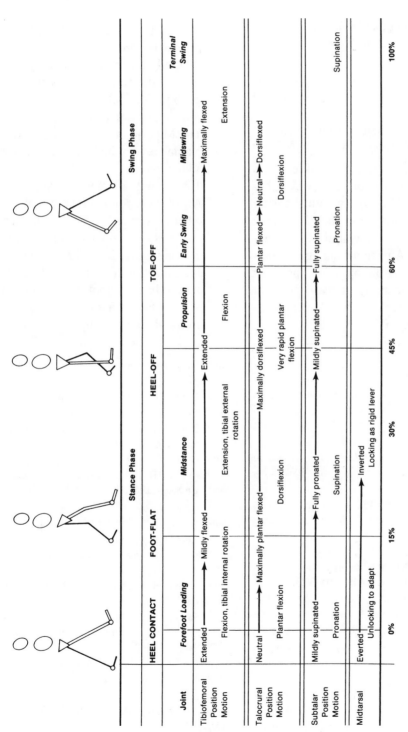

Joint		HEEL CONTACT	FOOT-FLAT		Midstance	HEEL-OFF	Propulsion	TOE-OFF	Early Swing	Midswing	Terminal Swing
		Forefoot Loading									
		Stance Phase							**Swing Phase**		
Tibiofemoral	Position	Extended →	Mildly flexed			Extended				Maximally flexed	
	Motion	Flexion, tibial internal rotation			Extension, tibial external rotation		Flexion			Extension	
Talocrural	Position	Neutral →	Maximally plantar flexed			Maximally dorsiflexed		Plantar flexed → Neutral → Dorsiflexed			
	Motion	Plantar flexion			Dorsiflexion		Very rapid plantar flexion		Dorsiflexion		
Subtalar	Position	Mildly supinated →		Fully pronated			Mildly supinated →	Fully supinated			Supination
	Motion	Pronation		Supination					Pronation		
Midtarsal		Everted →	Unlocking to adapt		Inverted Locking as rigid lever						
		0%	15%		30%	45%		60%			100%

Figure 7-4 Normal gait cycle. *Source:* Reprinted with permission from E. Mulligan, "Lower Leg, Ankle, and Foot Rehabilitation," in *Physical Rehabilitation of the Injured Athlete*, J.R. Andrews and G.L. Harrelson eds., p. 217, © 1991, W.B. Saunders Company.

1. The entire leg continues to rotate externally.
2. The ankle joint plantarflexes.
3. The subtalar and midtarsal joints continue to supinate.
4. The body weight is now borne medially, on the second and third metatarsal heads and the hallux.
5. The ankle joint reaction force peaks at 5½ times the body weight.[2(p255),9(pp129–131)]

During gait activities, the ankle bears enormous joint reaction forces; however, because there is such a large weight-bearing surface area, the loads transmitted across the joint per unit area are low, and little "wear and tear" occurs. Any small change in anatomical alignment (from an ankle sprain or fracture) can substantially increase the joint contact forces, possible leading to degenerative changes in the ankle.[18(pp157–159)]

SUMMARY

- The ankle joint allows dorsiflexion and plantarflexion.
- The subtalar and midtarsal joints primarily allow inversion with some adduction (supination), and eversion with some abduction (pronation).
- The MTP joints allow dorsiflexion and plantarflexion, and some abduction and adduction.
- The IP joints allow flexion and extension.
- All of these joints interact with one another to form a flexible foot that accommodates uneven terrain and a rigid foot that propels the body forward during gait.
- Joint reaction forces at the ankle greatly exceed body weight during ambulation, but the forces act over a large surface area and are normally well tolerated.

REFERENCES

1. McPoil TC, Hunt GC. Evaluation and management of foot and ankle disorders: Present problems and future directions. *J Orthop Sports Phys Ther.* 1995; 21(6):381–388.

2. Soderberg GL. *Kinesiology: Application to Pathological Motion.* Baltimore, Williams & Wilkins; 1986.

3. Warwick R, Williams PL, eds. *Gray's Anatomy.* 35th ed. Edinburgh, Scotland: Churchill Livingstone; 1973.

4. Walker IM, Sue D, Miles-Elkousy N, Ford G. Trevelyan H. Active mobility of the extremities in older subjects. *Phys Ther.* June 1984;64(6):919–923.

5. James B, Parker AW. Active and passive mobility of lower limb joints in elderly men and women. *Am J Phys Med Rehabil.* August 1989;68:165.

6. Chesworth BM, Vandervoort AA. Age and passive ankle stiffness in healthy women. *Phys Ther.* March 1989;69(3):217–224.

7. Mueller MJ, Minor SD, Schaaf JA, Strube MJ, Sahrmann SA. Relationship of plantar-flexor peak torque and dorsiflexion range of motion to kinetic variables during walking. *Phys Ther.* 1995;75(8): 684–693.

8. Perry J. *Gait Analysis.* Thorofare, NJ: SLACK Inc, 1992.

9. Root ML, Orien W, Weed J. *Normal and Abnormal Function of the Foot.* Los Angeles, Clinical Biomechanics Corp; 1977.

10. Mosely HF. Traumatic disorders of the ankle and foot. *Clin Symp.* 1965;17(1):3–30.

11. Logan AL. *The Foot and Ankle: Clinical Applications.* Gaithersburg, MD: Aspen Publishers, Inc; 1995.

12. Rocklar PA. The subtalar joint: anatomy and joint motion. *J Orthop Sports Phys Ther.* 1995;21(6): 361–372.

13. Cailliet R. *Foot and Ankle Pain.* Philadelphia: FA Davis; 1968.

14. Saltzman CL, Nawoczenski DA. Complexities of foot architecture as a base of support. *Phys Ther.* 1995;21(6):354–360.

15. Daniels L, Worthingham C. *Muscle Testing.* 3rd ed. Philadelphia: WB Saunders; 1972.

16. Edelstein JE. Physical therapy for elderly patients with foot disorders. *Top Geriatr Rehabil.* 1992; 7(3):24–35.

17. Thordarson DB, Schmotzer H, Chon J, Peters J. Dynamic support of the human longitudinal arch. *Clin Orthop.* 1995;316:165–172.

18. Frankel VH, Nordin M. *Basic Biomechanics of the Skeletal System.* 2nd ed. Philadelphia: Lea & Febiger; 1989.

8

Treatment of Common Problems of the Ankle/Foot Complex

Deformities of the ankle and foot can develop over time as a result of injury, disease, or the wearing of fashionable footwear. There is an extremely high prevalence (50% to 80%) of foot dysfunction in the elderly.[1(p219),2(p205)] Treatment of these problems requires an in-depth understanding of the complex anatomical relationships in the area. If left untreated, problems in the ankle/foot complex can worsen and lead to serious problems in the knee, hip, and back.

FRACTURES OF THE ANKLE/FOOT COMPLEX

Fractures about the ankle and foot in elderly persons can be the result of obvious trauma, such as sustained in an automobile accident, or the result of seemingly minor trauma, such as caused by stepping off a curb awkwardly. They are common in the elderly and tend to cause prolonged disability and diminished quality of life. Loss of bone stock and blood supply in the region makes both internal fixation and casting problematic for the orthopaedic surgeon.[3(p233)]

Fractures of the Ankle Joint

The diagnosis of ankle fracture usually indicates a fracture of the malleolus or of the fibula with disruption of the syndesmotic ligaments. Classifications of this type of fracture are confusing; some types are classified by eponym (e.g., Dupuytren, Maisonneuve), by mechanism of injury (e.g., Lauge-Hansen classification), or by morphology (e.g., Danis-Weber classification).[4(pp10,11)] It is not surprising, therefore, that therapy referrals often list the diagnosis simply as bimalleolar fracture, trimalleolar fracture, or just plain ankle fracture.

Medial Malleolus Fracture

The mechanism of injury in a medial malleolus fracture usually is a violent abduction or eversion force that normally would tear the deltoid ligament but avulses the medial malleolus instead.[5(p7)] Because medial malleolar fractures have a high rate of nonunion, surgical correction is usually required.[3(p236)] The orthopaedic surgeon opens the joint medially and repairs the fracture with 4.0-mm cancellous lag screws. Care must be taken to protect the saphenous vein and the posterior tibialis tendon.[4(pp13–15)]

Lateral Malleolus Fracture

A severe adduction or inversion force can fracture the distal fibula. This is the same type of force that causes the common ankle sprain of the lateral collateral ligament. If the fracture is stable, conservative treatment consists of closed reduction and weight bearing as tolerated in a short leg cast.[3(p235)] If open reduction is necessary, the joint is approached laterally and care is taken to protect the superficial peroneal nerve. Depending on the severity of the fracture, it is repaired with a single malleolar screw or with a lag screw-and-plate fixation (Figure 8–1).[4(pp12,15)]

Fractures of the Foot

Fractures of the foot are relatively uncommon in the elderly population and are usually the result of an accident or a fall.

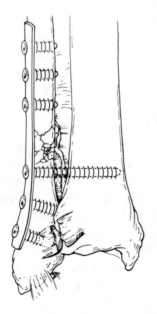

Figure 8–1 Fixation of a comminuted Danis-Weber type C fracture. A neutralization plate is used, being careful to maintain fibular length. Bone graft is added to the fracture site. A syndesmosis screw is placed through the plate. *Source:* Reprinted from *Techniques in Orthopaedics,* Vol. 2, No. 3, © 1987, Aspen Publishers, Inc.

Calcaneal Fractures

The calcaneus can suffer a crush fracture in a fall from a height. Since the calcaneus consists mostly of cancellous bone, this fracture requires 3 to 4 months to heal. Open reduction with screw and plate fixation may be necessary to stabilize the fracture.[6(p132)] Poor wound healing in elderly patients can be a problem following surgical correction. Often, the orthopaedic surgeon opts not to operate or even to cast the geriatric patient, to prevent the complications associated with prolonged immobilization, and treats the fracture as a soft tissue injury instead.

Talar Fractures

Although talar fractures are rare, they almost always contribute to a change in normal gait mechanics.[3(p239)] Fractures of the neck of the talus account for 50% of all talar fractures. This fracture is usually caused by excessive dorsiflexion of the ankle joint. Because the blood supply to this region is compromised easily by trauma, there is the danger that avascular necrosis will occur. If the fracture is displaced, the surgeon usually uses an anteromedial approach while carefully protecting the saphenous vein and nerve and the deltoid artery. The fracture is reduced and stabilized with compression screws, lag screws (Figure 8–2), or Kirschner wires.[3(p240),7(pp42–48),8(pp549,550),9(p136)]

Midfoot and Forefoot Fractures

A stress fracture of the navicular bone, which is the keystone of the medial arch of the foot, can occur in the active elderly. This overuse injury is usually treated conservatively with a short, non-weight bearing cast for 6 weeks.[3(pp240,241)]

The metatarsals are fractured more commonly than other bones of the foot. They can be fractured by a crushing force or by a low-

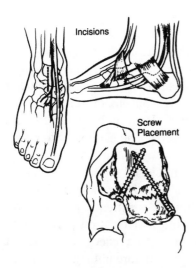

Figure 8–2 The surgical approach and technique of fixation of talar fractures with lag screws. At the top, the dorsolateral (left) and medial incisions are indicated by the dashed line. Screw placement is demonstrated on the bottom. One screw begins at the medial aspect of the talonavicular joint. The other is the sinus tarsi. *Source:* Reprinted with permission from B.J. Sangeorzan, et al., "Intraarticular Fractures of the Foot: Talus and Lesser Tarsals," *Clinical Orthopaedics and Related Research,* Vol. 292 No. 137, © 1993, Lippincott-Raven Publishers.

grade, repetitive force (e.g., prolonged walking). They may be considered postmenopausal osteoporotic fractures.[10(p558)] Although these fractures generally heal well, the patient can develop metatarsalgia, which can limit functional ability. The phalanges usually are injured by a crushing force or by "stubbing" a toe. Open reduction is rarely indicated for these types of fractures, and even casting is not often required.

Treatment of Fractures of the Ankle/Foot Complex

During the initial evaluation, the therapist should ascertain the following information in addition to the standard assessment presented in Chapter 2: the location of the fracture(s), the method of reduction and stabilization, and the weight-bearing orders. If possible, the therapist also needs to measure (circumferentially or volumetrically) the edema present at the forefoot, midfoot, and ankle.

Control of Edema

The accumulation of fluid in the foot and ankle region is common after any injury to the foot/ankle complex. This edema slows the healing process, blocks full range of motion (ROM), is painful, and may contribute to reflex sympathetic dystrophy. One of the primary goals of therapy is to eliminate edema to restore the foot and ankle to normal function.

Even before the cast is removed, the patient must be instructed in ways to minimize edema in the lower leg. While resting, the patient should elevate the casted leg as much as possible and flex and extend the toes to help pump out the fluid.

After the cast is removed, more aggressive therapy can be used to combat the edema, such as

- ice application
- contrast baths
- massage
- electrical stimulation
- sequential intermittent compression
- active exercise
- compression bandages (e.g., Malleotrain by Bauerfeind).

With the exception of contrast baths, all of the above methods for reducing edema can be augmented by elevating the limb. Standard whirlpool treatments tend to increase edema as a result of the heat and the dependent position of the lower leg and are not recommended.

Exercise Program

If the leg is casted, the patient still can perform isometrics within the cast as well as active exercise for the surrounding joints. When the cast is removed (usually 6 to 8 weeks postfracture), the patient should begin gentle active exercises for the entire ankle/foot complex. Light manual resistance or exercise tubing also can be used. The patient begins proprioceptive retraining in sitting position by manipulating a small balance board (Figure 8–3). Use of a rocking chair can also provide proprioceptive input to the foot/ankle complex.

When the bone is healed completely and the edema is minimal, the patient can begin a more aggressive therapy program to restore lost ROM. Restricted ROM at the ankle joint hampers the performance of chair-to-stand and floor-to-stand transfers, forcing the patient to use compensatory strategies that may be dangerous in the elderly population.[11(pp961,962)] Joint mobilization should be performed gently and cautiously to restricted joints to restore vital accessory motions in patients with closed reduction. Figures 8–4 and 8–5 show two basic mobilizations for the ankle joint. For patients who had open-reduction internal fixation performed, the therapist must first check with the orthopaedic surgeon before initiating joint mobilization techniques.

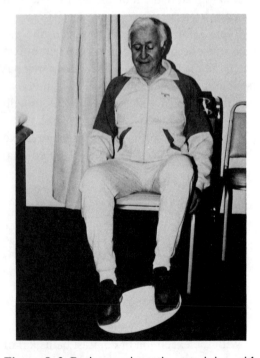

Figure 8–3 Basic proprioceptive retraining with use of a round balance board for dorsiflexion/plantarflexion and inversion/eversion in the sitting position. Other benefits of this exercise include increased ankle/foot strength, ROM, and coordination.

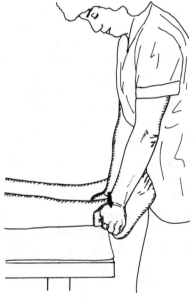

Figure 8–4 Posterior glide of the fibula on the tibia. This mobilization technique increases the general mobility of the mortise when dorsiflexion is restricted. *Source:* Adapted with permission from C. Kisner and L.A. Colby, Peripheral Joint Mobilization, *Therapeutic Exercise: Foundations and Techniques,* 3 ed., p. 229, © 1996, F.A. Davis Company.

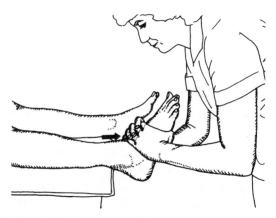

Figure 8–5 Joint traction of the ankle joint to promote general mobility. *Source:* Adapted with permission from C. Kisner and L.A. Colby, Peripheral Joint Mobilization, *Therapeutic Exercise: Foundations and Techniques,* 3 ed., p. 229, © 1996, F.A. Davis Company.

Passive stretching at the end of range helps restore the normal length of other soft tissue structures. Stretching is more effective when done frequently; therefore, the therapist should teach the patient self-stretching techniques to be done independently (Figure 8–6). The patient strengthens the extrinsic and intrinsic muscles of the foot and ankle by grasping a towel with the toes (Figure 8–7) and picking up small objects, such as pencil erasers or marbles, with the toes. In addition, the patient performs resisted isotonics with exercise tubing, for the muscles of the midtarsal, subtalar, and ankle joints. The patient must perform both concentric and eccentric work. As the foot and ankle are weight-bearing joints, they also must be strengthened in their position of function. Standing heel-offs and proprioceptive work on both the rectangular and round balance boards while the patient is supported in a doorway are important activities for gait retraining (Figures 8–8 and 4–9).

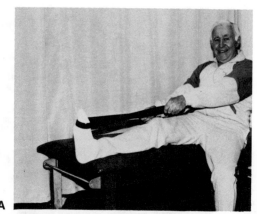

A

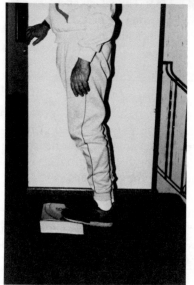

B

Figure 8–6 Self-stretching techniques for the Achilles tendon. **A.** The patient places a belt around the forefoot while sitting with the knee extended and gently pulls the ankle into dorsiflexion. **B.** The patient places the balls of the feet on the bottom stair or on a telephone book and gently lowers the heels, allowing gravity to stretch the ankles into dorsiflexion.

Mobility/Ambulation Program

If the patient is casted, the therapist must teach bed and bathroom transfers, as well as walking with crutches on level surfaces and

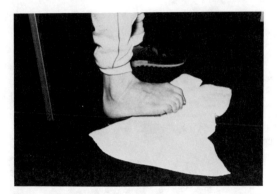

Figure 8–7 Towel-grasping exercise for intrinsic muscles of the foot. The patient attempts to bunch up the towel by flexing the toes. The smoother the towel, the more difficult the exercise.

With the exception of forward or "normal" walking, the patient progresses from 1 or 2 steps to up to 20 steps in each of the above activities. The patient then learns to ambulate on outdoor surfaces such as sidewalks, grass, and gravel; and on uneven surfaces such as slopes, curbs, and stairs. Finally, as the gait pattern normalizes, the therapist must be sure that the patient is ambulating at a functional velocity of 150 to 208 ft/min (44.5 to 63.5 m/min) for a functional distance of about 1,000 feet to ambulate safely in the community.[13(pp1372,1373)]

stairs. Strict weight-bearing precautions (sometimes as long as 12 weeks) must be maintained to prevent avascular necrosis of a tarsal fracture or further progression of a crush fracture of the calcaneus.[12(p377)]

When the bones and soft tissues have healed sufficiently to allow full weight bearing (FWB), the patient begins advanced balance, proprioceptive, and gait training, consisting of

- one-legged balancing (5 to 10 seconds)
- two-legged balancing on a foam mat or air disc (e.g., SitFit™) (Figure 8–9)
- forward walking
- backward walking
- side-stepping
- toe-walking (tiptoeing)
- heel-walking
- agility stepping (e.g., cross-overs, cutting maneuvers)
- step-ups and step-downs on 4″ aerobic step
- mini-trampoline marching (Figure 8–10)
- light jogging

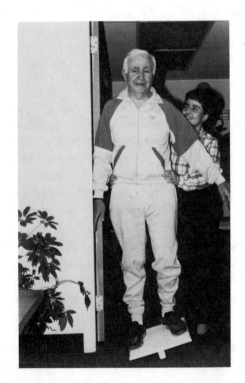

Figure 8–8 Advanced proprioceptive retraining that progresses from a rectangular wobbleboard (shown above), which allows motion in one plane only, to a round wobbleboard (see Figure 4–9 in Chapter 4) in a protected standing position. Strength, ROM, balance, and coordination also improve with this type of exercise.

Activities of Daily Living Program

Elderly patients tend to have a long, painful recovery from ankle and foot fractures that severely affect daily functioning. In the majority of cases, they are casted for 2 to 6 weeks, requiring complete assistance in basic and instrumental activities of daily living (ADL). Their activity level, including ambulation distance, is reported to be only two-thirds of the activity level of age-matched controls up to 2 years postfracture.[14(p106)]

If pain persists, the therapist should evaluate the patient for orthotics. Often the patient's anatomical alignment does not return to prefracture status, and a properly fitted orthotic may allow for a more functional result. Tomaro and Butterfield[12(p377)] recommend beginning with a temporary device, which allows for modifications, before fabricating a permanent orthotic.

Summary of Treatment of Fractures of the Ankle/Foot Complex

- Know the location of the fracture, the method of reduction, and the weight-bearing order.
- During the first 6 weeks postfracture
  1. elevate the casted foot
  2. begin active exercises to surrounding joints
  3. begin isometric exercise to affected joints
  4. teach crutch-walking on level surfaces and stairs.
- As the fracture heals
  1. reduce edema in lower limb aggressively
  2. maximize foot and ankle ROM by using joint mobilization and passive stretching

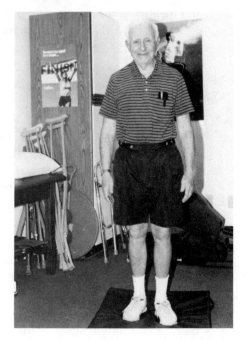
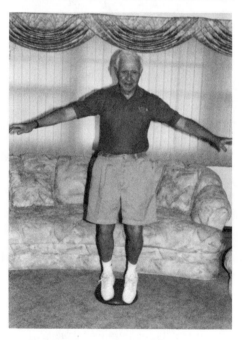

Figure 8–9 Two-legged standing balance on a variable surface such as (A) a foam exercise mat or (B) an air-filled disc. Depending on the patient's frailty and activity level, this activity can be assisted or challenged by the therapist.

3. improve concentric and eccentric strength by using resisted isotonics
4. retrain the ankle and foot in a weight-bearing posture
5. retrain balance and proprioception
6. begin advanced gait training on all surfaces in all directions
7. assess the patient for possible foot orthotics.

RHEUMATOID ARTHRITIS OF THE ANKLE/FOOT COMPLEX

Rheumatoid arthritis (RA) often affects the foot and ankle early in the progression of the disease. Almost all patients with RA eventually report symptomatic involvement

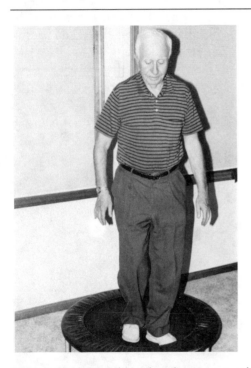

Figure 8–10 Marching in place on a mini-trampoline is an advanced balance and proprioceptive activity for high-level patients. This activity can be performed with the patient holding onto a support. The therapist must assist the patient in getting on and off this equipment.

of their feet. These problems primarily involve the forefoot where the metatarsophalangeal (MTP) joints are particularly vulnerable.[15(p1)] Five major foot deformities occur as a result of the disease process itself combined with the forces associated with ambulation.

1. **Hallux valgus:** Synovial proliferation stretches out the joint capsule of the first MTP joint. Lateral deviation of the proximal phalanx of the great toe occurs, assisted by the bowstring pull of the unbalanced flexors and extensors.[16(p1149),17(p2)]

2. **Depression of the lesser metatarsal heads:** As the hallux valgus deformity progresses, more weight is shifted to the lesser metatarsal heads. The lesser MTP joints become inflamed and unstable. The plantar plate and surrounding ligaments erode, resulting in a dislocation of the MTP joints. The plantar fat pad thins and displaces distally.[15(p1),17(p2)]

3. **Hammer and claw toe deformities:** As the MTP joints dislocate, the long flexors and extensors lose their balanced positions. Claw toe deformity occurs with dorsiflexion of the MTP joint and flexion of the interphalangeal (IP) joints; hammertoe deformity occurs with dorsiflexion of the MTP and distal IP joint and flexion of the proximal IP joint.[16(p1150)]

4. **Foot pronation:** To unload the painful metatarsal heads, patients with RA alter their gait pattern, everting the foot on weight bearing. The adapted gait pattern, although successful in decreasing pain in the forefoot, places exaggerated pronation forces on a weakened subtalar joint causing a

hindfoot valgus deformity over time. This deformity is also associated with later genu valgum deformity in the knee.[17(p2),18(p600),19(pp246,247)]

5. **Heel pain:** RA causes inflammation of the insertion of the Achilles tendon. The tendon shortens, causing a decreased ability to dorsiflex the ankle.[16(p1150),20(p121)] In addition, rheumatoid nodules can develop on the calcaneus or bone spurs can develop in the plantar fascia due to calcaneal erosion, causing more heel pain.[21(p282)]

Treatment of Rheumatoid Arthritis of the Ankle/Foot Complex

Ideally, the therapist would treat the patient at the onset of RA in order to prevent the progressive destruction of the entire foot complex, as well as later damage to the ipsilateral knee. Preventive measures such as bracing, orthotics, or corrective footwear may be effective in this regard.[19(p245)] However, the patient usually does not seek medical attention until the deformities have begun and gait is extremely painful. In these cases, therapy may be able to restore some function but cannot correct the damage done.

Early Intervention

If the patient presents with only foot pronation and some knee instability, the following treatment program often is helpful in preventing progression of the disease and obtaining pain relief. Depending on the patient, some of the exercises may be too difficult and may require modifications:

- strengthening of the posterior tibialis, gastrocnemius, and quadriceps muscles
- strengthening of toe intrinsic muscles: towel exercise (Figure 8–7), picking up erasers with toes, etc.

- progressive weight bearing to FWB as muscle strength improves
- one-legged balancing while raising the medial arch simultaneously (when FWB only)
- ROM exercising for all joints
- passive stretching of peroneal muscles to regain inversion
- wearing of shoes with solid medial counters and wearing of orthotics to prevent foot pronation[15(pp4,5)]

Treatment of Patients with Fixed Deformities

If the patient presents with greater damage to the foot or knee (e.g., hallus valgus, genu valgum, forefoot deformities), the early intervention program can prevent greater progression of the disease, but it cannot reverse any of the damage. Some of the exercises shown above may be too difficult or even harmful for the patient with painful deformities to perform. The therapist needs to carefully assess the patient's current status and weigh the benefits of exercising against the risks, on an individual basis. The clinical signs and gait deviations observed with the five common foot deformities associated with RA, as well as therapeutic treatment goals for each condition, are described in Table 8–1.

Prosthetic Replacement and Arthrodesis

Before 1973, arthrodesis was the only surgical option for treating the painful, degenerative foot or ankle. With the success of other joint replacement procedures, it was hoped that prosthetic implants at the ankle/foot complex would offer greater functional ability. At the ankle joint, this did not happen. High long-term failure rates of the prosthetic ankle joint have caused a return to arthrodesis.[22(p232)] Unfortunately, arthrodesis at the

Table 8–1 Gait Deviations, Physical Examination Findings, and Treatment Goals Associated with the Five Common Foot Deformities Caused by Rheumatoid Arthritis

Gait Deviation	Physical Examination Findings	Treatment Goals
Pronated Foot		
Shuffled progression	Tenderness over subtalar-midtarsal area	Relieve subtalar and midtarsal joint stresses
Decreased step length	Limited inversion range	Increase ankle inversion
Initial contact with medial border of foot	Weak and painful posterior tibialis muscle	Strengthen posterior tibialis muscle
Decreased single-limb balance	Pronated weight-bearing posture of foot	Stabilize hypermobile joints with rigid orthosis
Prolonged double-support phase	Lax medial collateral ligament of knee	Maintain neutral alignment in stance by foot positioning
Late heel rise		
Plantar flexion of ipsilateral limb in swing		
Genu valgum with weight bearing		
Hallux Valgus		
Lateral and posterior weight shift	Lateral deviation of great toe	Accommodate foot with wide-toe box shoe
Late heel rise	Swelling of first MTP joint	
Decreased single-limb balance	Shortening of flexor hallucis brevis muscle	Increase extension of great toe
	Tenderness of great toe	Relieve weight-bearing stresses
	Weakness of great toe abduction	
Metatarsophalangeal Joint Subluxation		
Diminished roll-off	Painful MTP heads with weight bearing	Redistribute pressure with metatarsal bar
Decreased single-limb stance	Callus formation over MTP heads	Relieve pressure with soft cutout shoe insert
Apropulsive progression	Ulcerations over MTP heads	
Decreased single-limb balance	Limited MTP flexion	Increase flexion mobility of MTP joints
	Prominent MTP heads	Accommodate foot with extra-depth shoe

continues

Table 8–1 continued

Gait Deviation	Physical Examination Findings	Treatment Goals
Hammertoes or Claw Toes		
Diminished roll-off	Posture of MTP joint hyperextension with proximal and distal interphalangeal joint flexion	Improve toe alignment with metatarsal bar
Decreased single-limb stance		Accommodate foot with extra-depth shoe
Apropulsive progression		
Decreased single-limb balance	Posture of MTP and distal interphalangeal joint hyperextension with proximal interphalangeal flexion	
	Callus formation at plantar tips and dorsum of proximal interphalangeal joint	Diminish pressure with soft insert
	Limited MTP flexion	Increase toe mobility
Painful Heel		
Toe-heel pattern	Painful active plantarflexion	Decrease inflammation with steroid injection or modalities
No heel contact in stance	Painful passive and active dorsiflexion	
Decreased stride length		
Decreased velocity	Swelling and pain at Achilles insertion	Relieve weight-bearing stress
Plantarflexion of ankle in swing	Tenderness over spur	Decrease pressure over spur with soft shoe insert
Increased hip flexion in swing	Decreased ankle dorsiflexion range	Maintain ankle mobility
Decreased step length of contralateral limb		

Source: Reprinted from P. Dimonte and H. Light, *Physical Therapy,* Alexandria, Virginia, American Physical Therapy Association, 1982, Vol. 62, No. 8, p. 1152, with permission of the American Physical Therapy Association.

ankle joint in patients with RA also has a high failure rate.[23(pp907,908)]

Prosthetic replacement of the first MTP joint with silicone spacers continues to be a successful operation.[24(p1695)] A single- or double-stemmed implant is used to correct the deformity. A longitudinal incision is made on the mediolateral aspect of the joint. Complete release of contractures, tendon tension readjustment, and realignment of the toes are important for optimal results. The patient is then placed in a splint to maintain alignment.[25(pp30–32)]

Rehabilitation consists of edema control and frequent, active toe flexion and extension beginning on postoperative Day 2. As healing occurs, the dynamic splint is replaced with an ambulatory type splint. Partial weight bearing (PWB) in a splint and a nonconstrictive shoe begins no later than 3 weeks postoperatively.[25(p32)]

Summary of Treatment of Rheumatoid Arthritis of the Ankle/Foot Complex

- During the acute stage
  1. limit weight bearing on affected limb
  2. stretch peroneal muscles gently
  3. prescribe short-duration isometric exercise of the quadriceps, gastrocnemius, and posterior tibialis muscles (to be done five times daily)
  4. prescribe ambulation devices that do not strain the wrists and hands.

- During the chronic stage
  1. progress to PWB-FWB as muscle strength allows
  2. progress to resisted exercise
  3. strengthen the toe intrinsic muscles, including arch exercises
  4. work on one-legged balance with medial arch raised, if appropriate
  5. continue stretching of peroneal muscles
  6. prescribe, or refer patient for, proper footwear.

ANKLE SPRAIN

The most common injury to the elderly ankle is a sprain of the lateral collateral ligament (anterior talofibular or the calcaneofibular ligament) caused by an inversion force (Figure 8–11). With increased age, there is a surprisingly decreased incidence in ankle injury from walking, hiking, running, tennis, and golf.[26(p214)] In general, elderly patients rarely suffer a complete tear of the ligament with subsequent ankle instability (Grade III).[27(p75)] Injury to the deltoid ligament also is a rare occurrence.

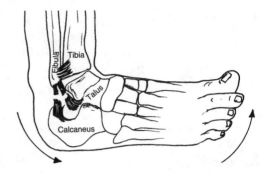

Figure 8–11 Inversion sprain showing disruption of the anterior talofibular and calcaneofibular ligaments. In the elderly, a partial tear of these ligaments is most common, but complete healing can still take up to 3 months. *Source:* Adapted from A.L. Logan, Conditions and Their Treatment, *The Foot and Ankle: Clinical Applications,* p. 153, © 1995, Aspen Publishers, Inc.

Treatment of Ligament Sprain

The treatment of ankle sprains includes edema control; an exercise program to restore proprioception, ROM, and strength; gait training; and functional training. This injury can take up to 3 months to heal fully in the elderly population.[27(p75)]

Edema Control

In treating an acute ligament sprain, the ankle is usually treated by the RICE method (rest, ice, compression, and elevation). However, in a study by Wilkerson and Horn-Kingery, increased frequency and duration of cryotherapy did not enhance the rate of recovery from this injury.[28(p240)] Therefore, ice therapy should be avoided in patients with any sensory loss, peripheral neuropathy, or diabetes, as the risks far outweigh the benefits of this modality. General compression can be achieved by fitting the patient with an Air-Stirrup brace (Aircast Inc., Summit, NJ), which allows dorsiflexion and plantarflexion, but limits inversion and eversion. The Air-Stirrup brace is worn inside an athletic shoe.

Exercise Program

The patient immediately can begin active ankle dorsiflexion and plantarflexion exercises with the Air-Stirrup to prevent any accidental inversion. Gradually, the patient begins active inversion and eversion exercises and progresses to resisted exercise as tolerated. Rubber tubing or Theraband™ works well to provide graduated resistance (Figure 8–12). A closed-chain press exercise can be performed on the Shuttle MiniClinic (Figure 6–20 in Chapter 6) if the Air-Stirrup is in place. This allows the entire lower quarter to act as one unit, but with less force than a standing squat. The patient should also begin to stretch the Achilles tendon, as this is often tight in the elderly and inhibits recovery. As the injury heals, exercising or swimming in the pool environment enhances ROM, decreases swelling, and allows for normal gait pattern.

Although strengthening is important, several studies prove that restoration of proprioception or passive movement sense is the key to restoring function in the ankle.[28(p206),29(p605)] Because mechanoreceptors respond to changes in direction and speed, the exercise program must focus on these aspects. Training on either a Biomechanical Ankle Platform System™ board or a standard wobbleboard (such as a Rockboard or Xerboard) has been shown to improve passive position sense and decrease instability in both normal and sprained ankles.[30(p90),31(p332)] The patient can begin standing dorsiflexion and plantarflexion exercises on the rectangular wobbleboard (supported in a doorway) and sitting inver-

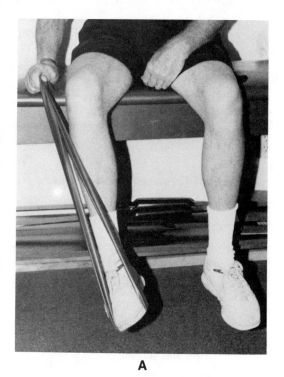

A

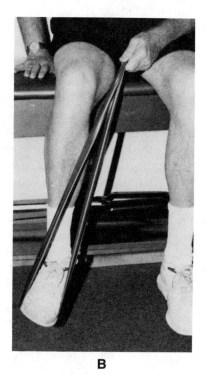

B

Figure 8–12 Resisted ankle inversion (A) and eversion (B) with elastic band

sion/eversion exercises. The patient then progresses to standing inversion/eversion exercises (Figure 8–8). To further retrain proprioception and strength, the patient progresses to the round wobbleboard and performs "circles" and other advanced footwork in both sitting and supported standing positions. An even more difficult proprioceptive exercise is standing on an inflated air disc (Figure 8–9).

Gait Training

An integral first step in gait training is restoration of balance deficits. There is growing evidence that an ankle sprain can alter proximal muscular function[32(p17)] and decrease the ability to balance on the affected leg.[33(p969)] Fortunately, many of the standing proprioception exercises can double for balance activities. Simple one-legged standing activities on level surfaces and foam surfaces may be sufficient for many elderly patients. (It should be noted that the ability to balance on one leg has not been found to necessarily improve walking balance.)

Gait training on level surfaces includes the advanced skills of toe-walking and heel-walking, as well as side-stepping and cross-over stepping. For many elderly patients, pregait warm-up exercises of toe-offs and heel-offs (with support for balance) may be necessary before initiating such high-level gait activities. (Caution: Care must be taken during heel-walking, because many elderly patients tend to lose balance backwards!) The patient can also progress to ambulating on a foam mat placed on the floor and maneuvering around an obstacle course. The patient must also be able to negotiate uneven surfaces such as stairs, ramps, and grassy hills with confidence. Lastly, the patient must be able to walk at a safe speed (over 150 ft/min)[13(pp1372,1373)] for community ambulation. High-level patients trying to return to sports need to progress to jogging and running, as well as speed and agility drills.

Activities of Daily Living Program

Basic functional tasks are usually only impaired for the first week after injury, especially if the patient needs a walker to unload the foot. Instrumental ADL and recreational or sports activities are often affected up to 3 months in the elderly. In order to determine if the patient is fully recovered, the following functional tests should be done. The patient should be able to:

1. squat (dorsiflexion)
2. stand on toes (plantarflexion)
3. stand on one foot
4. stand on toes of one foot (if returning to sports)
5. negotiate stairs
6. walk on heels and toes
7. run straight and cut (if returning to sports)
8. jump and hop on one leg (if returning to sports)[34(p8)]

As the reader can plainly see, many of the functional tests are in fact the functional exercises already described. If any symptoms occur during one of the activities, more work is needed in that specific area.

Summary of Treatment of a Sprained Ankle

- decrease edema through RICE
- restore strength, ROM, and proprioception through
  1. active to resistive ankle and foot exercises
  2. Achilles tendon stretching
  3. closed-chain wobbleboard work in sitting and standing
- train balance and gait

- restore ADL, work, sports, and recreation activities to normal with functional exercises

TENDINITIS

Most tendon injuries in the geriatric population are insidious in onset and result from chronic conditions rather than from acute injury. The two tendons most commonly involved in the elderly are the Achilles and the posterior tibialis tendons.[27(p77)]

Achilles Tendinitis

The patient with Achilles tendinitis usually presents with pain located 3 to 6 cm proximal to the calcaneus. This is the area where the gastrocnemius and soleus muscles intertwine with each other, forming a region of concentrated stress.[35(p171)] This area of the tendon also has the poorest blood supply and is subjected to torsional forces during walking or running.[36(p444)] Histological changes usually occur in the tendon itself and not the paratenon (or covering sheath). With increasing age, there is a more advanced and widespread tendon histopathology than in younger patients.[37(p151)] The following factors can contribute to Achilles tendinitis:

- prolonged pronation during the stance phase of gait
- Achilles tendon tightness
- gastrocnemius and/or soleus weakness
- running or walking on excessively hilly terrain
- improper footwear: inflexible sole or inadequate rearfoot stabilizers[35(p173),] [36(p446), 38(p54)]

Posterior Tibialis Tendinitis

Posterior tibialis tendinitis presents with pain over the medial aspect of the ankle that is exacerbated by ambulation. The patient usually has a flatfoot deformity and an inversion weakness. Other factors that contribute to this condition are footwear that has an inflexible sole or inadequate arch support, and walking or running on a surface that is either too hard or too soft.[36(pp454,455)] If untreated, the posterior tibialis tendon may rupture, leading to progressive hindfoot disorders.[27(pp78,79)]

Treatment of Tendinitis

As with all overuse injuries, the therapist must try to identify and correct the cause of the tendinitis to prevent its recurrence. Patients usually respond well to conservative treatment consisting of

- oral nonsteroidal anti-inflammatory medication (on physician's orders)
- ultrasound
- massage
- muscle stretching: maintaining the medial arch during stretch
- strengthening exercises (including eccentric exercise)
- modification of walking surface
- orthotics
- alterations of footwear, such as a heel lift for Achilles tendinitis or a 2° or 4° medial wedge for posterior tibialis tendinitis
- proprioceptive retraining on the small balance board

Summary of Treatment for Tendinitis

- Evaluate the ankle/foot complex, including the patient's footwear.
- Identify the cause of injury.
- Treat the soft tissues with a combination of therapeutic exercise, treatment mo-

dalities, and advanced proprioceptive training.

- Prescribe, or refer the patient for, alterations in footwear to help correct any mechanical abnormalities that may have contributed to excessive soft tissue stresses.

PLANTAR FASCIITIS

Plantar fasciitis refers to an inflammation or microtear of the plantar fascia (plantar aponeurosis) at its insertion on the medial tubercle of the calcaneus. It is an overuse injury, commonly seen in runners. Other contributing factors include:

- prolonged standing
- flat feet or high-arched feet
- improper footwear
- tight Achilles tendon
- decreased motion at the first MTP joint
- an overweight patient
- a sudden increase in activity level. [36(pp459,460),39(p252),40(p367)]

The patient complains of heel pain on the plantar aspect of the foot of insidious origin. The pain is worst during the first steps in the morning and gradually lessens as the plantar fascia and muscles stretch out. [38(p54),41(p509)] The gait pattern may display any or all of the following deviations:

- no heel contact
- plantarflexion in swing phase
- short stride lengths
- decreased ambulation velocity [42(p22)]

Treatment of Plantar Fasciitis

Treatment of this overuse injury includes reduced activity and protection of the injured site from excessive stresses. Since the heel is constantly in use for everyday activities and walking, some doctors even recommend no weight bearing for a few days. [41(p509)] The inflammation can be reduced with modalities, including ice massage and cross-friction massage. Patients generally report good relief with ultrasound, but a study by Crawford and Snaith found this modality (set at 0.5 W/cm^2, 3 MHz, pulsed) to be no more effective than placebo for decreasing plantar heel pain. [43(p265)] Pulsed phonophoresis with 10% cortisone may be helpful. [41(p509)] Joint mobilization to the first MTP joint can be used to restore normal mobility to this joint. These modalities must be done in conjunction with an exercise program to strengthen the foot intrinsics, such as towel grasping. It is also imperative to gently stretch out the Achilles tendon. This must be done with the heel in contact with the floor and a small towel roll under the foot to maintain the arch. [38(p55),40(p368)] Standing with the ball of the foot on a step or phone books and letting the heel drop (as shown in Figure 8–6B) places too much stress on the plantar fascia and should not be done for this condition.

Stresses to the plantar fascia can also be reduced through taping, orthotics, or alterations in footwear. LowDye taping is the most common method used for treating plantar fasciitis in the athlete. Orthotics and footwear need to be evaluated on an individual basis because plantar fasciitis has multiple causes. A temporary heel lift (made of sponge rubber) may be used to unload the plantar fascia. A sole or heel counter that is too flexible may cause too much pronation. A sole that is too hard may not absorb sufficient stresses and can also contribute to the problem. [36(p460)]

Summary of Treatment of Plantar Fasciitis

- Decrease the inflammation at the site.
- Reduce the activity level.

- Use modalities as needed (ice, massage, joint mobilization).
- Strengthen the toe intrinsics.
- Stretch out the Achilles tendon with the medial arch supported.
- Evaluate and prescribe proper orthotics or footwear.

PROBLEMS OF THE FOREFOOT

Many problems occur in the forefoot of the elderly person. These abnormalities can affect gait and ADL. A brief review of some of the more common disorders and their treatment is presented.

Hallux Valgus (Bunion)

Hallux valgus is the term used to describe a progressive deformity of the first ray, causing a lateral deviation of the great toe. As the first MTP joint subluxes, a dorsal medial bunion and a hammertoe-like deformity of the second toe can occur. More weight is born on the lesser metatarsal heads, possibly leading to metarsalgia, calluses, corns, and stress fractures. The major causes of this condition are heredity and ill-fitting footwear.[24(pp1621–1624)]

Hallux Rigidis

Hallux rigidus refers to limitation of motion of the first MTP joint. Although the cause is unknown, cartilage damage is believed to cause the synovitis, which than destroys the cartilage and subchondral bone. The initial cartilage damage may be caused by trauma, disease, arthritis, or an osteochondral fracture.[24(p1693)] The patient complains of pain at the first MTP joint, loss of MTP extension, and painful gait at terminal stance phase.[40(p372)]

Lesser Toe Abnormalities

Hammertoe and claw toe deformities are common in the elderly patient, and result in an abnormal flexion position of the proximal IP joint. Claw toe is usually caused by a neuromuscular disease and involves all the lesser toes. In addition, it always involves an extension deformity of the MTP joint and a flexion deformity at the distal interphalangeal (DIP) joint. Hammertoes appear to be the result of wearing shoes that have extremely tight toe-boxes or from trauma. The MTP joint may be extended or in neutral, and the DIP joint is usually extended.[44(p1750)]

Mallet toe refers to a flexion deformity of the DIP and usually involves the second toe. It is common in patients with diabetes and/or peripheral neuropathy. A corn may form at the distal end beneath the nail. In a diabetic patient, this corn can ulcerate and become infected.[44(pp1759,1760)]

Treatment of Problems of the Forefoot

Many of the problems are treated surgically. Conservative treatment consists of decreasing inflammation and pain through modalities, manual treatment, muscle strengthening of the toe intrinsics, and alterations in footwear. See Tables 8–2 and 8–3 for treatment ideas and shoe modifications.

OTHER FOOT PROBLEMS

Many elderly persons complain of foot problems that concern their toenails and skin. With aging, nails can become dry, thick, and brittle. Loss of total body flexibility can make it difficult to even trim the toenails. Nails can become ingrown and infected, causing severe pain. If the patient also has diabetes or peripheral neuropathy, the infection can become catastrophic.

Table 8–2 Review of Etiology and Treatment of Toe Deformities

Findings	Location	Description	Etiology	Treatment	Diagram
Hallux Abductor Valgus (HAV)	1st MTP (usually both feet)	painful bump or prominent exostosis med side of foot, lat deviation & pronation of hallux, 1st met adducts, hallux abducts, dislocation/sublux of 1st met head from sesmoid sling, attenuation of med MTP jnt capsule, contracture add hallucis ms, associated 2nd digit deformities.	metatarsus primus varus predisposes women to it, imbalance of soft tissues & intrinsics & extrinsic ms of hallux, abnormal bony configuration of 1st cune/MTP jnt, ill-fitting shoes, short achilles, pes planus, hypermobility of cunel/meta jnts, lat displacement of long flex/ext tendons.	chevron osteotomy, mcbride, keller, arthrodesis, correct shoe gear, bunion last shoes, stretch shoes, ms strengthening, orthotics.	
Hallux Rigidus (Limitus)	1st MTP	deg jnt dis of 1st MTP, causes pain & decreased ROM, painful osteophyte formation on dorsal aspects of met heads & base prox phalanx.	stub toe, fall, kick hard object, infection, arthritis, severe form of periarticular fibrositis, tight shoes press on flat-shaped met head more common than round head.	chellectomy, arthrodesis, arthroplasty w/silastic implant, change shoe gear, orthotics.	
Mallet	Lesser toes (single)	deformity of lesser toe(s), DIP is flexed, PIP & MTP normal, feels painful callus on tip of toe.	ill-fitting shoes—too short	release flex dig longus tendon & volar capsule, excise distal end of prox phalanx, correct shoe gear, jnt mob.	

Table 8–2 continued

Findings	Location	Description	Etiology	Treatment	Diagram
Hammer	Lesser toes (single)	usually 3rd or 4th digit, PIP flexed, DIP in extension, MTP in neutral or hyperextension, can be flexible or static.	congenital, heredity or acquired, ill-fitting shoes—too short	detach flex dig brevis or excise distal end of prox phalanx, transfer flex dig long tendon, toes, sleeves, stretch shoes, orthotics, pads.	
Claw	Lesser toes (multiple)	hyperflexion of PIP & DIP & hyperextension of MTP, callus over PIP jnt & tip of toe, excessive pressure on met head.	restrictive shoes, contracture of long flexors & extensors of lesser toes, ms imbalance, intrinsic ms weakness of flexor & interosseous ms, neurologic involvement, diabetes, RA.	release of dorsal capsule of MTP, lengthen extensor tendon, tendon transfer, toe sleeves, ROM ex, correct shoe gear.	
Overlapping/ Underriding Toes	All toes	disloc of MTP jnts or PIP jnts w/med/ lat/ flex/ext displacement, hallux under or over 2nd digit, 4th rotates on long axis & under 3rd, problem of corns & nails.	imbalance of soft tissue, abnormal config of MTP jnts, ill-fitting shoes, trauma, contractures of add hallucis, jnt capsule & articular lig.	capsulotomy, tendon transfers, budin splint toe crests, orthotics, stretch shoes.	

Source: Adapted from H. Herman and J.M. Bottomley, "Anatomical and Biomechanical Considerations of the Elder Foot," *Topics in Geriatric Rehabilitation*, Vol. 7, No. 3, p. 6, © 1992, Aspen Publishers, Inc.

Corns are skin problems that are caused by mechanical stresses usually due to faulty foot mechanics, bony deformities, or tight-fitting shoewear. Calluses are a hypertrophy of the keratinized layer of skin caused by shear forces and pressures from ambulation.[21(pp280,281)]

These nail and skin lesions need to be referred to a podiatrist or dermatologist for proper treatment. Although not "orthopaedic" problems per se, these disorders are extremely painful and often lead to deviations in gait pattern as well as loss of function.

Table 8–3 Shoe Characteristics of Adaptions for Common Foot Problems

Foot Problem	Shoe Characteristic
Instability	Firm heel counters
	Shankpiece or wedge
	Four to six pairs of eyelets
	Board lasted
Excessive Pronation	Extended medial counter
	Rear-foot stabilizer
	Straight lasted
Excessive Supination	Flexible heel counter
	Relatively softer midsole material
	Slip lasted or curve lasted
Hammertoes or claw toes	Extradepth shoe
Edema	Resilient outsole (crepe or rubber)
Hyper/hyposensitive foot	Metatarsal bar
Hallux valgus	Bunion shield
	Resilient outsole
	Internal metatarsal bar
	Bunion last
Metatarsalgia	Full-length insole
	Soft insert
	Extended medial counter
	Resilient outsole
	Metatarsal bar
Plantar callus	Cushioned insole/soft insert
	Resilient outsole

THE ANKLE/FOOT COMPLEX AND FALL PREVENTION

Thirty to forty percent of elderly people living at home fall at least once each year. Twenty-five percent of those who fall suffer serious injury. A study by Tinetti et al[45(pp1701–1705)] demonstrated that the risk of falling increases linearly with the number of risk factors present, suggesting that the predisposition to fall may result from the accumulated effect of multiple disabilities. One of the major risk factors cited involves foot problems. The authors concluded that the risk of falling might be reduced by modifying even a few factors through medical, surgical, rehabilitative, and environmental intervention. The following discussion deals only with the relationship between the ankle/foot complex and falling. For more detailed information on fall prevention, the reader is referred to Chapter 17 on Balance Intervention for the Orthopaedic Patient.

Preventive Treatment of Falls

To best serve the needs of the elderly clientele, therapists routinely should screen all patients referred to therapy for balance problems. Although many of the causes of falling have nothing to do with the status of the foot/ankle complex, it is important to eliminate this area as a potential risk factor.

In brief, balance involves both a response to a stimulus, such as reacting to a push, and an anticipation of a stimulus, as in leaning forward to negotiate a steep hill. For everyday activities, the balance response is anticipatory and is not a reaction to an event. It is therefore more beneficial to measure functional balance rather than balance reactions. Two common methods of measuring balance objectively are the one-legged balance test

with eyes open or closed and the "get up and go" test. In the "get up and go" test, the clinician assesses the quality of movement (i.e., slowness, hesitancy, or stumbling) as the patient rises from a chair, walks 10 feet, turns around and walks back to the chair, and turns around and sits back down in the chair. The clinician grades the balance on a scale of 1 to 5, with 1 being normal and 5 being severely abnormal with risk of falling. (Other balance assessment tools are presented in Chapter 17.)

In general, one of the major ways that people maintain balance is by a distal-to-proximal motor response called the ankle strategy. Forward postural sway causes the soleus to fire, while backward sway causes the dorsiflexors to fire to maintain balance. In order for the somatosensory feedback loop to work properly, the elderly person must have sufficient

- sensation on the soles of the feet to feel pressure
- ankle ROM to bias the muscle spindle system and activate the joint receptors
- ankle strength to control the balance response[46(p3)]

In a study of falls occurring in the nursing home setting, Whipple et al[47(p13)] discovered severe strength deficits in the knees and ankles of people who had fallen; the greatest strength loss occurred in ankle dorsiflexion. This is consistent with the fact that most elderly tend to lose their balance backward.[46]

Preventive treatment consisting of passive stretching to the Achilles tendon, ankle mobilization, dorsiflexion-strengthening exercises, and proprioceptive retraining on the small balance board may have a major impact in restoring the somatosensory system and in preventing some falls in the elderly population.

FOOTWEAR

The importance of proper footwear for the elderly patient cannot be overemphasized. Commercially available footwear and inserts can accommodate many of the common problems experienced by the geriatric foot. In general, soft inserts are recommended for the elderly patient because of loss of the plantar fat pads, but they do not provide the same correction that more rigid inserts do. For complex foot problems, customized shoes or inserts can be fabricated. A list of companies providing prescription orthotics for elderly persons appears at the end of this chapter.

The different components of athletic and nonathletic footwear are identified in Figures 8–13 and 8–14. A brief overview of shoe adaptations for some of the most common elderly foot problems is given in Table 8–3. Running or walking shoes possess many of the characteristics needed by the geriatric patient with foot pain. Most of the "good" athletic shoes possess

- rear-foot stabilizers
- extended medial counters
- reinforced counters
- removable insoles for orthotic use
- resilient midsole[48(p1862)]

Despite its good qualities, the athletic shoe may not be the answer for all elderly patients. Although the traction provided is excellent for outdoor walking or for walking on tile floors, it can be dangerous to a patient with a shuffling-type gait (e.g., as in Parkinson's disease). In addition, the athletic shoe and walking shoe provide less proprioceptive input and foot stability as compared to shoes with harder and thinner midsoles.[49(p66)] This can be important in fall prevention.

Heel Height in Footwear

Designers of women's footwear have (until recently) been more concerned with fashion than with comfort. Pointy, narrow toe-boxes have contributed to the forefoot deformities mentioned earlier. High-heeled shoes also have a profound effect on posture and gait pattern. A decreased lumbar lordosis has been found in women wearing a 2″ (5.1 cm) heel and may contribute to low back pain.[50(p99)] Heel heights greater than 2″ alter the position

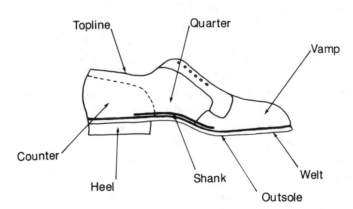

Figure 8–13 Sections and components of a nonathletic shoe. *Source:* Reprinted from T.G. McPoil, *Physical Therapy,* Alexandria, Virginia, American Physical Therapy Association, 1988, Vol. 68, No. 12, p. 1858, with permission of the American Physical Therapy Association.

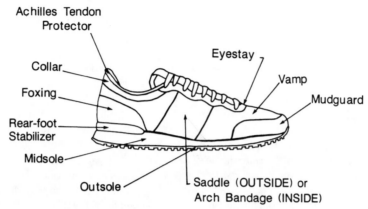

Figure 8–14 Sections and components of an athletic shoe. *Source:* Reprinted from T.G. McPoil, *Physical Therapy,* Alexandria, Virginia, American Physical Therapy Association, 1988, Vol. 68, No. 12, p. 1859, with permission of the American Physical Therapy Association.

of the ankle and the center of mass, increase the ground reaction force, increase the energy cost of walking, and theoretically pose a greater risk of injury.[51(p190),52(p568)]

DOCUMENTATION TIPS: DEMONSTRATING SAFETY

One of the most effective and least used tactics in demonstrating a need for physical or occupational therapy services is the documentation of patient safety issues. Neither health care providers nor third-party payees wish to leave their patients or clients at risk for further injury; therefore, in order to illustrate the patient at risk performing functional activities, the therapist can document the:

1. ability to safely cross the street. In a study by Robinett and Vondran, the average ambulation velocity required to cross a street safely in a moderate sized city was determined to be 190 ft/min.[13(p1373)] Does the patient meet or exceed that minimum safety speed for the width of the street?
2. ability to exit a nursing home in a fire. Can the patient safely negotiate the fire stairs (not the main stairs) in the nursing facility? Fire stairs usually have a higher rise than standard stairs for faster egress.
3. ability to telephone for emergency assistance.
4. ability to perform ADL while manipulating ambulation devices (i.e., functional ambulation) rather than simply documenting the gait deviations and level of assistance.
5. ability to get in and out of bed.
6. ability to get on and off the floor.

As can easily be seen, documenting safety is akin to documenting functional ability. By documenting safety, the therapist recognizes that the main purpose of rehabilitation is to allow the patient to interact with the environment with a minimum of risk. And *that* is covered under all insurance benefits.

REFERENCES

1. Elton PJ, Sanderson SP. A chiropodial survey of elderly persons 65 years in the community. *Pub Health.* 1986;100:219–222.

2. Jessett DF. Foot problems. In: Pathy MSJ, Finucan P, eds. *Geriatric Medicine: Problems and Practice.* Berlin: Springer-Verlag; 1989.

3. O'Malley MJ, DeLand JT. Foot and ankle. In: Koval KJ, Zuckerman JD, eds. *Fractures in the Elderly.* Philadelphia: Lippincott-Raven Publishers; 1998.

4. Morris M, Chandler RW. Fractures of the ankle. *Techniques in Orthop.* October 1987;2:10–19.

5. Mosely HF. Traumatic disorders of the ankle and foot. *Clin Symp.* 1965;17(1):3–30.

6. Benirschke SK, Sangeorzan BJ. Extensive intraarticular fractures of the foot. Surgical management of calcaneal fractures. *Clin Orthop.* 1993;292:128–134.

7. Mayo KA. Fractures of the talus: principles of management and techniques of treatment. *Techniques Orthop.* October 1987;2:42–54.

8. Swanson TV, Bray TJ, Holmes GB. Fractures of the talar neck: a mechanical study of fixation. *J Bone Joint Surg.* 1992;74-A(4):544–551.

9. Sangeorzan BJ, Mayo KA, Hansen ST. Intraarticular fractures of the foot: talus and lesser tarsals. *Clin Orthop.* 1993;292:135–141.

10. Varenna M, Binelli L, Zucchi F, Beltrametti P, et al. Is the metatarsal fracture in postmenopausal women an osteoporotic fracture? A cross-sectional study on 113 cases. *Osteoporosis Intern.* 1997;7(6):558–563.

11. King LA, VanSant AF. The effect of solid ankle-foot orthoses on movement patterns used in a supine-to-stand rising task. *Phys Ther.* 1995;75(11):952–964.

12. Tomaro JE, Butterfield SL. Biomechanical treatment of traumatic foot and ankle injuries with the use of foot orthotics. *J Orthop Sports Phys Ther.* 1995;21(6):373–380.

13. Robinett CS, Vondran MA. Functional ambulation velocity and distance requirements in rural and urban communities. *Phys Ther.* September 1988;68(9):1371–1373.

14. Gelcher GL, Radomisli TE, Abate JA, Stabile LA, Trafton PG. Functional outcome analysis of operatively treated malleolar fractures. *J Orthop Trauma.* 1997;11(2):106–109.

15. Freiberg RA, Moncur C. Arthritis of the foot. *Bull Rheum Dis.* 1991;40(1):1–8.

16. Dimonte P, Light H. Pathomechanics, gait deviations, and treatment of the rheumatoid foot. *Phys Ther.* August 1982;62:1148–1156.

17. Marks RM, Merson MS. Foot and ankle issues in rheumatoid arthritis. *Bull Rheum Dis.* 1997; 46(5):1–3.

18. Shields MN, Ward JR. Treatment of related knee-ankle-foot deformities in rheumatoid arthritis. *Phys Ther.* June 1966;46:600–605.

19. Keenan MA, Peabody TD, Gronley JK, Perry J. Valgus deformities of the feet and characteristics of gait in patients who have rheumatoid arthritis. *J Bone Joint Surg.* 1991;73-A(2):237–247.

20. Sutej PG, Hadler NM. Current principles of rehabilitation for patients with rheumatoid arthritis. *Clin Orthop.* 1991;265:116–128.

21. McPoil T. Foot disorders in the elderly. *Orthop Phys Ther Clin N Amer.* 1993;2(3):277–287.

22. Guyton JL. Arthroplasty of ankle and knee. In Canale ST, ed. *Campbell's Operative Orthopaedics,* 9th ed, Vol. 1. St Louis: Mosby-Year Book; 1998.

23. Cracchiolo A, Cimino WR, Lian G. Arthrodesis of the ankle in patients who have rheumatoid arthritis. *J Bone Joint Surg.* 1992;74-A(6):903–909.

24. Richardson EG, Donley BG. Disorders of the hallux. In: Canale ST, ed. *Campbell's Operative Orthopaedics,* 9th ed, Vol. 2. St Louis: Mosby-Year Book; 1998.

25. Swanson AB. Reconstructive surgery in the arthritic hand and foot. *Clin Symp.* 1979;31(6):2–32.

26. Requa RK, McCormick J, Garrick JG. Age-related injury patterns in a sports medicine outpatient clinic. *Sports Med Arthroscopy Rev.* 1996;4(3):205–220.

27. Ouzounian TJ, Shereff MJ. Common ankle disorders of the elderly: diagnosis and management. *Geriatrics.* December 1988;43:73–80.

28. Lentell G, Baas B, Lopez D, McGuire L, et al. The contributions of proprioceptive deficits, muscle function, and anatomic laxity to functional instability of the ankle. *J Orthop Sports Phys Ther.* 1995;21(4):206–215.

29. Lentell GL, Katzman LL, Walters MR. The relationship between muscle function and ankle stability. *J Orthop Sports Phys Ther.* 1990;11(12):605–611.

30. Hoffman M, Payne VG. The effects of proprioceptive ankle disk training on healthy subjects. *J Orthop Sports Phys Ther.* 1995;21(5):90–99.

31. Wester JU, Jespersen SM, Nielen KD, Neumann L. Wobble board training after partial sprains of the lateral ligaments of the ankle: a prospective randomized study. *J Orthop Sports Phys Ther.* 1996;23(5): 332–336.

32. Bullock-Saxton JE. Local sensation changes and altered hip muscle function following severe ankle sprain. *Phys Ther.* 1994;74(1):17–28.

33. Goldie PA, Evans OM, Bach TM. Postural control following inversion injuries of the ankle. *Arch Phys Med Rehabil.* 1994;75(9):965–975.

34. Lemak LJ, Ellis EA. Acute and chronic ankle sprains: assessment and management. *Sports Med Update.* 1993;8(3):6–11.

35. Reynolds NL, Worrell TW. Chronic Achilles peritendinitis: etiology, pathophysiology, and treatment. *J Orthop Sports Phy Ther.* 1991;13(4):171–176.

36. Winkel D. *Diagnosis and Treatment of the Lower Extremities.* Gaithersburg, MD: Aspen Publishers, Inc; 1997.

37. Astrom M, Rausing A. Chronic Achilles tendinopathy. A survey of surgical and histopathologic findings. *Clin Orthop.* 1995;316:151–164.

38. Knortz K. Lower extremity overuse injuries in the older athlete. *Top Geriatr Rehabil.* 1991;6(4):47–55.

39. Mulligan E. Lower leg, ankle, and foot rehabilitation. In: Andrews J, Harrelson GL, eds. *Physical Rehabilitation of the Injured Athlete.* Philadelphia: WB Saunders Company; 1991.

40. Bottonley JM, Herman H. Foot injuries: A rehabilitation perspective. In: Lewis CB, Knortz KA, eds. *Orthopedic Assessment and Treatment of the Geriatric Patient.* St Louis: Mosby-Year Book; 1993.

41. Travell JG, Simons DG. Myofascial pain and dysfunction. *The Trigger Point Manual.* Vol 2. Baltimore: Williams & Wilkins; 1983.

42. Edelstein JE. The aging lower extremity: Foot section. Course Notes. Dallas, Texas; March 1998.

43. Crawford F, Snaith M. How effective is therapeutic ultrasound in the treatment of heel pain? *Ann Rheum Dis.* 1996;55:265–267.

44. Murphy GA, Richardson EG. Lesser toe abnormalities. In: Canale ST, ed. *Campbell's Operative Orthopaedics,* 9th ed, Vol. 2. St Louis: Mosby-Year Book; 1998.

45. Tinetti ME, Speechley M, Ginter SF. Risk factors for falls among elderly persons living in the community. *N Engl J Med.* December 1988;319:1701–1707.

46. Daleiden S. Aging, balance, and falling. Course Notes, April 1989.

47. Whipple RH, Wolfson LI, Amerman PM. The relationship of knee and ankle weakness to falls in nursing home residents: an isokinetic study. *J Am Geriatr Soc.* January 1987;35:13–20.

48. McPoil TG. Footwear. *Phys Ther.* December 1988;68(12):1857–1865.

49. Robbins S, Waked E, Allard P, McClaran J, Krouglicof N. Foot position awareness in younger and older men: the influence of footwear sole properties. *JAGS.* 1997;45(1):61–66.

50. Franklin ME, Chenier TC, Brauninger L, Cook H, Harris S. Effect of positive heel inclination on posture. *J Orthop Sports Phys Ther.* 1995;21(2):94–99.

51. Ebbeling CJ, Hamill J, Crussemeyer JA. Lower extremity mechanics and energy cost of walking in high-heeled shoes. *J Orthop Sports Phys Ther.* 1994; 19(4):190–196.

52. Snow RE, Williams KR. High heeled shoes: their effect on center of mass position, posture, three-dimensional kinematics, rearfoot motion, and ground reaction forces. *Arch Phys Med Rehabil.* 1994;75(5): 568–576.

For more information on prescription foot orthotics contact:

PAL Health Technologies, Inc.
293 Herman Street
Pekin, IL 60554
1-800-447-0151 or (in Illinois)
1-800-223-2957

Sole Supports, Inc.
835 Fairview Boulevard West
Fairview, TN 37062
1-888-650-7653

9

The Spine

Changes in the spine caused by aging, trauma, and degeneration have an impact on the entire body. By the seventh decade, a vast majority of elderly persons will have suffered through some form of disabling back pain. A brief overview of anatomy, biomechanics, and the aging process as they specifically relate to the spine is presented in this chapter. The reader is encouraged to refer to the many excellent detailed anatomical texts for more information on the structure and function of the spine. A basic understanding of these concepts and the spine's relationship to the rest of the body helps the therapist to plan an optimal program for the elderly patient with back pain or dysfunction.

ANATOMY OF THE SPINE

The vertebral column consists of 7 cervical, 12 thoracic, 5 lumbar, 5 fused sacral, and approximately 4 fused coccygeal vertebrae. The column functions to protect the spinal cord, support the thorax, and maintain upright posture.[1(p722)]

The Vertebrae

A typical vertebra possesses a body and a vertebral arch (Figure 9–1). The vertebral arch consists of

- a spinous process
- two pedicles
- two laminae
- two transverse processes
- two superior articular processes (facets)
- two inferior articular processes (facets)
  [2(pp733–734)]

In each area of the spine, the vertebrae possess specific characteristics, such as short, bifid spinous processes in the cervical region; heart-shaped bodies in the thoracic region; and large, thick bodies in the lumbar region. The orientation of the facet joints is 45° to the horizontal in the cervical spine (up to T-2), preventing forward slippage of the vertebrae and providing support for the head and neck.[3(p14)] The facets of the thoracic and lumbar spine are more vertically oriented, restricting movement, especially rotation. The forces attenuated by the bones dictate trabecular alignment. In the low back region, the alignment of the trabecular bone seems to indicate that the activity of walking primarily determines the internal structure of the lumbar vertebrae.[4(p2823)]

Blood to the vertebral body and arch is supplied by the radicular arteries and the periarticular plexus of the vertebral artery supplies the facet joints.[5(p62)] Mechanoreceptors that provide position sense have been lo-

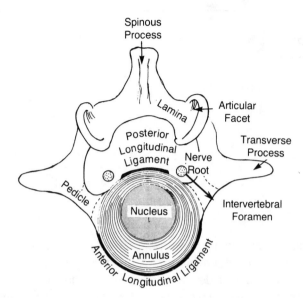

Figure 9–1 Superior view of a lumbar vertebra with its intervening disc. *Source:* Reprinted with permission from R. Cailliet, *Low Back Pain Syndrome*, 4 ed., p. 13, © 1998, F.A. Davis Company.

cated in the facet joint capsules and discs of the cervical and lumbar spine.[3(p15),6(p653)]

Every decade there is a 3% loss of cortical bone and a 6% to 8% loss of trabecular bone. Bone strength decreases even more rapidly than does bone quantity. By the fourth decade, the vertebral body's load-bearing capacity diminishes from 55% to only 35%.[7(p1)]

The Ligaments

Two longitudinal track systems connect the vertebrae—the multisegmental and the unisegmental systems (Figure 9–2). The multisegmental system consists of the anterior and posterior longitudinal ligaments and the supraspinous ligaments. Interestingly, the posterior longitudinal ligament narrows to half its width at the level of the third lumbar vertebra,[8(p13)] thereby offering less support to the discs of the lower lumbar spine.

The unisegmental system consists of the

- interspinous ligaments
- ligamentum flavum
- intertransverse ligaments

Ligaments on the posterior aspect limit flexion, while those on the anterior aspect function to limit trunk extension.[1(p738)]

The Intervertebral Discs

The intervertebral discs make up 20% of the total height of the spinal column.[2(p412)] They permit movement while equalizing and dispersing the forces and stresses placed on the spine.[9(p850)] Each disc consists of the cartilaginous end-plate, the nucleus pulposus, and the annulus fibrosus (Figure 9–2).

The Cartilaginous End-Plate

The cartilaginous end-plate is composed of hyaline cartilage and separates the nucleus and the annulus from the vertebral bodies.[10(pp765,766)] In the neonate there are blood vessels in the end-plate, but they are almost completely closed down by cartilaginous

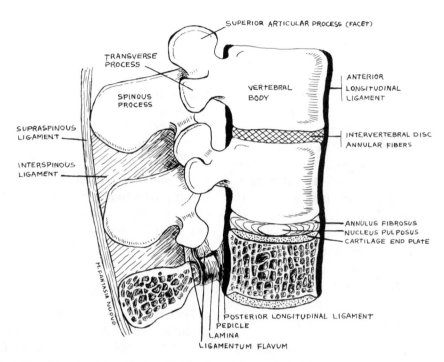

Figure 9–2 Combination lateral and sagittal view of the articulations of three vertebrae of the lumbar spine

tissue during the teenage years.[11(p1209)] In a study of cervical vertebrae, Oda et al[11(pp1206–1211)] found that 7% of the end-plate was calcified by the third decade. In the fourth and fifth decades, over 50% of the end-plate was calcified. By the eighth decade, 93% of the end-plate was calcified. As long as the bone formation remained inside the end-plate, they found no serious degenerative changes in the nucleus. Any bone formation outside the end-plate appeared to induce degeneration of the nucleus.

The Nucleus Pulposus

At birth, the nucleus is a gel-like substance in which notochordal cells are suspended in a ground substance made up of 88% water and a meshwork of collagen fibrils and protein polysaccharide complexes.[7(p2)] Within this matrix are many nega-

tive acid radicals that act to bind water. As the disc ages, the polysaccharide complexes degenerate, allowing the matrix to absorb but not retain water.[8(pp4,12)] By the end of the seventh decade, the nucleus contains only 70% water and has a 20% increase in collagen content.[7(p2)] As the disc becomes drier, it gradually loses its ability to store energy and distribute stresses.[12(p186)]

As the cervical and lumbar discs are thicker anteriorly, they contribute to the natural lordoses in these regions.[2(p412)] The loss of water content therefore is also responsible for some of the flattening observed in these curves in the elderly.

The Annulus Fibrosus

The annulus fibrosus is a fibrocartilaginous structure encapsulating the nucleus with bundles of collagen fibers arranged in a crisscross pattern. It attaches to adjacent vertebral bodies and serves to hold the nucleus in place. The posterior fibers of the annulus offer less support than do the anterior fibers, because they are thinner and are arranged in a more parallel fashion. Nerve fibers with free nerve endings, as well as mechanoreceptors, have been found within the annulus, raising the possibility of a proprioceptive function for this structure. [6(p653),13(p29)] With time, there is fragmentation and degeneration of the collagen fibers of the annulus, resulting in total annular lamellar disorganization by the age of 80 years. [10(pp765,766),14(pp523,524)] The annulus also suffers a minor loss of water content (78% to 70%). [7(p2)]

Phases of Degeneration

Degenerative changes in the spine are the result of the body's attempts to heal itself, albeit unsuccessfully, from a traumatic insult. Although similar to the changes that occur from normal aging, the degeneration of the spinal unit is a pathological entity.

Dysfunctional Phase

Trauma usually affecting the capsule or synovium of the facet joints results in synovitis, which can stretch the joint capsule further or initiate cartilage damage. Trauma to the disc region can cause circumferential tears in the annulus, which can lead to radial tears into the nucleus. [7(p2)] Sether et al [15(p385)] consider the radial tear to be the most significant indicator of pathological degeneration of the spine. Interestingly, it is not completely clear that the presence of a tear actually contributes to back pain. [16(p71)]

Instability Phase

The stretched joint capsule can lead to a permanent laxity or even a facet-joint subluxation. If damage to the nucleus occurs, the disc will lose some height, causing the annulus to bulge. The bulge can stretch out the anterior and posterior longitudinal ligaments and result in disc instability. [7(p3)] Excessive movement occurs at the zygapophyseal joints with an inability to optimally bear loads. [13(p124)]

Restabilization Phase

The body responds to the ligamentous instability with increased subperiosteal bone, which results in osteophyte and bone spur formation. [7(p3)] Both desirable and undesirable motions are now restricted by bony blocks.

Muscles and Motion

The orientation and shape of the posterior articular facets determine the available motion of the vertebrae. In the cervical region, forward flexion, extension, lateral flexion (45°), and rotation (90°) occur freely. In the thoracic spine, mostly lateral flexion and rotation occur, but these motions are limited by the rib cage. The lumbar spine allows more extension than forward flexion, some lateral flexion, but only minimal rotation. [2(pp413,414)]

Fitzgerald et al [17(p1779)] found great individual variability in the range of motion (ROM) of the lumbar spine in the elderly population. The motions of lateral flexion and extension decreased in 20-year intervals, with the elderly participants achieving only half the motion of the young adults (Table 9–1). Motion in the cervical spine also decreases with advancing age, with men losing more neck movement than women. [18(p286)]

Although the amount of movement available between two vertebrae can be measured, the ability to determine "normal" ROM for the spine as a whole is very difficult to establish. Despite the use of the trunk for the most basic activities of daily living, no functional ROM data presently exist.

Table 9–1 Means and Standard Deviations in 10-Year Intervals for Lumbar Range of Motion

Age (yr)	Shöber (cm)			Extension (°)			Right Lateral Flexion (°)			Left Lateral Flexion (°)		
	$\bar{X}$	s	CV	n*	$\bar{X}$	s	CV	n	$\bar{X}$	s	CV	n	$\bar{X}$	s	CV	n
20–29	3.7	0.72	19.5	31	41.2	9.6	23.3	31	37.6	5.8	15.4	31	38.7	5.7	14.7	31
30–39	3.9	1.00	25.6	42	40.0	8.8	22.0	44	35.3	6.5	18.4	44	36.5	6.0	16.4	44
40–49	3.1	0.81	26.1	16	31.1	8.9	28.6	16	27.1	6.5	24.0	16	28.5	5.2	18.2	16
50–59	3.0	1.10	36.7	43	27.4	8.0	29.2	43	25.3	6.2	24.5	44	26.8	6.4	23.9	44
60–69	2.4	0.74	30.8	26	17.4	7.5	43.1	27	20.2	4.8	23.8	27	20.3	5.3	26.1	27
70–79	2.2	0.69	31.4	9	16.6	8.8	53.0	10	18.0	4.7	26.1	10	18.9	6.0	31.7	10

*Different numbers appear in some age groups because of the difficulty in measuring patients with various medical conditions (e.g., rash). CV = coefficient of variation.

Source: Reprinted from G.K. Fitzgerald, K.J. Wynveen, W. Rheault, and B. Rothschild, *Physical Therapy*, Alexandria, Virginia, 1983, Vol. 63, No. 11, p. 1778, with permission of the American Physical Therapy Association.

The interactions of the lumbopelvic muscles with the thoracolumbar fascia, the fascia lata, and the abdominal fascia are important in the stabilization and function of the lumbar spine.[13(p61)] The muscles act as movers, stabilizers, and shock absorbers. Three layers of muscles influence spinal motion. The deepest layer consists of the shortest muscles: the multifidi, the rotators, the interspinales, and the intertransversarii. The large intermediate layer consists of the erector spinae. The superficial layer is composed of the latissimus dorsi and the gluteus maximus posteriorly and the transversus abdominis and the internal and external obliques anteriorly.[19(p557)] Because of the intricate relationship of the spine to the pelvis and hip, all the hip muscles affect posture and motion at the spine. The actions of individual muscles of the neck and trunk are summarized in Table 9–2.

Innervation

The ventral rami of the spinal nerves innervate the anterior vertebral musculature; the dorsal rami innervate the deep muscles of the neck and back. These spinal nerves exit the spinal cord through the intervertebral foramina and can be compressed or irritated as a result of disc degeneration, vertebral body disease, osteoarthritis of the facet joint, or disc protrusion.[2(pp509–525,1031)] As mentioned earlier, nociceptive and proprioceptive fibers have been found in the facet joints as well as in the annulus fibrosus.

KINETICS OF THE LUMBAR SPINE

Nachemson's study[20(pp59–71)] of L-3 disc pressure showed that posture greatly affects the load on the lumbar spine. He found the compression force on the L-3 disc was

- least in hook-lying
- about equal to body weight in relaxed standing
- greater than body weight in sitting

The load measurements at the L-3 disc during various everyday activities are shown in Table 9–3.

In addition to guiding the direction of segmental movement, the facet joints protect the disc from destructive torsional forces, especially during trunk rotation. They appear to unload the disc during extension activities, such as standing and walking. When degenerative changes occur in the spine, significantly greater compressive forces are supported by the facet joints.[12(pp186,187),21(pp111,119)]

Limb and pelvic position, maintenance of lumbar lordosis, muscle activation, availability of other support (chair with armrests, lumbar curve, etc), and any external forces affect the loads on the lumbar spine.[12(p203)]

SUMMARY

- The spine comprises 33 vertebrae and acts to protect the spinal cord and to maintain upright posture.
- The intervertebral discs allow movement and dispersion of forces placed on the spine.
- Degenerative changes occur in the spine as a result of trauma and aging.
- The elderly lumbar spine possesses only half the available motion of the younger spine.
- The muscles act in conjunction with three fascial systems for normal movement as well as stability of the lumbar spine.
- Loads exceeding body weight commonly are placed on the lumbar spine during everyday activities.

Table 9–2 Summary of Muscle Actions on the Spine

Motion	*Area*	*Muscle*	
Flexion	Head and neck	Sternocleidomastoideus	Rectus capitis anterior and lateralis
		Scaleni	
		Longus colli and capitis	Suprahyoid and infrahyoid muscles
	Trunk	Rectus abdominis	External and internal oblique
Extension	Head and neck	Splenius capitis and cervicis	Multifidi
		Upper trapezius	Rotatores
		Obliquus capitis inferior and superior	Interspinales
		Rectus capitis major and minor	
		Sacrospinalis and semispinalis (capitis and cervicis portions)	
	Trunk	Sacrospinalis and semispinalis (other than capitis and cervicis portions)	Rotatores
			Interspinales
		Multifidi	
Lateral flexion	Neck	Sternocleidomastoideus	Sacrospinalis and semispinalis (cervicis and capitis portions)
		Scaleni	
		Upper trapezius	
		Rectus capitis lateralis and anterior	Obliquus capitis inferior
			Intertransversarii
		Splenius capitis and cervicis	
	Trunk	External and internal oblique	Quadratus lumborum
		Sacrospinalis and semispinalis (other than capitis and cervicis portions)	Intertransversarii
Rotation	Head and neck (same side)	Splenius capitis and cervicis	Rectus capitis major
		Rectus capitis posterior major and minor	Sacrospinalis (capitis and cervicis portions)
		Obliquus capitis inferior and superior	
	Head and neck (opposite side)	Sternocleidomastoideus	Multifidi
		Semispinalis (capitis and cervicis portions)	Rotatores
		Upper trapezius	

continues

Table 9–2 continued

Motion	Area	Muscle	
	Trunk (same side)	Sacrospinalis (except capitis and cervicis portions)	External oblique
	Trunk (opposite side)	Semispinalis (except capitis and cervicis portions) Multifidi	Internal oblique Rotatores

Source: Reprinted from B.E. Kent, *Physical Therapy,* Alexandria, Virginia, American Physical Therapy Association, 1980, Vol. 54, No. 7, p. 743, with permission of the American Physical Therapy Association.

Table 9–3 Load Measurements in the L-3 Disc of a 70-kg Individual during Various Everyday Activities

Activity	Load (kg)
Supine in traction	10
Supine	30
Erect with corset	30
Erect standing	70
Walking	85
Twisting (erect)	90
Bending sideways	95
Upright sitting with no support	100
Isometric abdominal exercises	110
Coughing	110
Jumping	110
Straining	120
Laughing	120
Bending forward 20°	120
Bilateral straight leg raising in supine position	120
Hyperextension exercise (prone)	150
Sit-up exercises (knee extended)	175
Sit-up exercises (supine with knees bent)	180
Bending forward 20° with 10 kg	185
Lifting 20 kg with back straight and knees bent	210
Lifting 20 kg with back bent but knees straight	340

Source: Reprinted with permission from R. Cailliet, *Low Back Pain Syndrome,* 4 ed., p. 199, © 1988, F.A. Davis Company.

REFERENCES

1. Kent BE. Anatomy of the trunk: a review, Part I. *Phys Ther.* July 1974;54:722–744.

2. Warwick R, Williams, PL, eds. *Gray's Anatomy,* 35th ed. Edinburgh, Scotland: Churchill Livingstone; 1973.

3. Paris SV. Cervical symptoms of forward head posture. *Top Geriatr Rehabil.* 1990;5(4):11–19.

4. Smit TH, Odgaard A, Schneider E. Structure and function of vertebral trabecular bone. *Spine.* 1997; 22(24):2823–2833.

5. Paris SV. The Spine. Course Notes for S-I Introduction to Spinal Evaluation and Manipulation; 1979.

6. McCarthy PW, Carruthers B, Martin D, Petts P. Immunohistochemical demonstration of sensory nerve fibers and endings in lumbar intervertebral discs of the rat. *Spine.* 1991;16(6):653–655.

7. Dupuis PR. The natural history of degenerative changes in the lumbar spine. In: Watkins RG, Collis JS Jr, eds. *Lumbar Discectomy and Laminectomy.* Rockville, MD: Aspen Publishers, Inc; 1987.

8. Cailliet R. *Low Back Pain Syndrome.* 4th ed. Philadelphia: FA Davis Co; 1988.

9. Kent BE. Anatomy of the trunk: a review, Part II. *Phys Ther.* August 1974;54:850–860.

10. Jensen GM. Biomechanics of the lumbar intervertebral disc: a review. *Phys Ther.* June 1980;60:765–773.

11. Oda J, Tanaka H, Tsuzuki N. Intervertebral disc changes with aging of human cervical vertebra. *Spine (Jpn ed.).* November 1988;13:1205–1211.

12. Lindh M. Biomechanics of the lumbar spine. In: Frankel VH, Nordin M, eds. *Basic Biomechanics of the Skeletal System.* 2nd ed. Philadelphia: Lea & Febiger; 1989.

13. Porterfield JA, DeRosa C. *Mechanical Low Back Pain.* 2nd ed. Philadelphia: WB Saunders Co; 1998.

14. Bernick S, Walker JM, Paule WJ. Age changes to the anulus fibrosus in human intervertebral discs. *Spine.* 1991;16(5):520–524.

15. Sether LA, Yu S, Haughton VM, Fischer M. Intervertebral disk: Normal age-related changes in MR signal intensity. *Radiology.* 1990;177:385.

16. Ross JS, Modic MT. Current assessment of spinal degenerative diseases with magnetic resonance imaging. *Clin Orthop.* 1992;279:68–81.

17. Fitzgerald GK, Wynveen KJ, Rheault W, Rothschild B. Objective assessment with establishment of normal values for lumbar spine range of motion. *Phys Ther.* November 1983;63:1776–1781.

18. Schops P, Kober L, Schenk M, Rinckpfister S. Functional anatomy and range of motion of the cervical spine. *Physikal Med Rehabil Kurotmed.* 1997; 7(6):286–290.

19. Saudek CE, Palmer KA. Back pain revisited. *J Orthop Sports Phys Ther.* June 1987;8:556–566.

20. Nachemson AL. The lumbar spine: an orthopaedic challenge. *Spine.* January 1976;1:59–71.

21. Jackson RP. The facet syndrome: myth or reality? *Clin Orthop.* 1992;279:110–121.

10

Treatment of Common Problems of the Spine

It is a rare human being who enters the seventh decade of life without ever having complained of a backache. The current lifestyle of cars, computers, desk jobs, television sets, and remote controls particularly abuses the vertebral column. The combination of degeneration, disease, and lifestyle causes some of the typical postural changes found in the elderly:

- forward head
- increased kyphosis of the thoracic spine
- loss of normal lumbar lordosis
- round shoulders
- increased flexion at the elbows, wrists, hips, and knees.[1(pp15–18)]

These energy-wasting postural changes not only affect the flexibility of the peripheral joints, but also have an impact on the ability to breathe. The effects of these postural changes will be discussed throughout this chapter. Almost all patients can benefit from postural reeducation, trunk flexibility exercises, and strengthening exercises. Because of the enormous effect of the spine on the entire body, even small postural corrections can lead to major benefits in breathing, gait, and functional level.

OSTEOPOROSIS

Osteoporosis is the most common bone disease in elderly women, affecting at least 8 million white women in the United States.[2(p1100)] Nearly 40% of all elderly women will suffer an osteoporotic fracture[3(p3)]; however, elderly women are not the only ones to suffer this disease. In the United States alone, osteoporosis affects nearly 25 million people—annually causing 1.5 million fractures, a third of which are vertebral fractures.[4]

As discussed in Chapters 1 and 9, Type II involutional osteoporosis involves a gradual decrease in the density of both trabecular and cortical bone that is associated with the aging process itself. Type II osteoporosis becomes clinically significant after age 70 and affects twice as many women as men. The cause is still unknown, but it is probably related to a complex series of age-related changes that affect both sexes. It can cause vertebral wedge fractures and femoral neck fractures of the hip, as well as fractures of the proximal humerus, distal femur, pubic ramus, and ribs (Table 10–1).[5(pp935,936),6(pp1,2)]

In postmenopausal women, Type I involutional osteoporosis is characterized by a 3% to 10% loss of trabecular bone and 1% to 2%

of cortical bone per year.[7(p33)] The loss of estrogen (which increases bone sensitivity to parathyroid hormone) causes the postmenopausal woman to resorb calcium from the bones at twice the rate as before menopause, with no accompanying increase in bone reformation. It also decreases the body's ability to absorb calcium from the intestines.[8(pp1533,1534),9(p73)] More bone loss occurs in the first 5 years after menopause than in the subsequent 15 years.[3(p3)] Type I osteoporosis is associated with compression fractures of the vertebrae, intertrochanteric hip fractures, and Colles' fractures (Table 10–1).[9(p73),10(p55)]

The exact mechanism for developing osteoporosis is still unknown. Despite the strong association of menopause with bone loss, only one quarter of all postmenopausal women actually have osteoporosis.[11(p138)] Additional risk factors for osteoporosis include sedentary lifestyle, poor diet (insufficient calcium, protein, and vitamin C and vitamin D intake), drugs (steroids, alcohol), cigarette smoking, genetic disorders, cancer, rheumatoid arthritis (RA), diabetes mellitus, and endocrine abnormalities.[12(p216),13(p4)] During a life span, osteoporosis will result in a bone loss of 20% to 30% in men and 40% to 50% in women.[6(p2)]

Treatment of Osteoporosis

Because the deformities that result from osteoporotic fractures of the spine are irre-

Table 10–1 Comparison of Primary Types of Osteoporosis

Characteristics	Type I: Postmenopausal	Type II: Age Related
Age	Begins after menopause Lasts 5–8 years	Begins > 40 years Clinically significant > 70 yrs
Sex Ration (F:M)	8:1	2:1
Type of Bone Loss	Mostly trabecular	Trabecular and cortical
Associated Fractures	Vertebral compression fractures Intertrochanteric hip fractures Distal radial fractures	Multiple vertebral wedge fractures Femoral neck fractures of hip Proximal humeral fractures Distal femur fractures Pubic ramus fractures Rib fractures
Mechanism of Bone Loss	• Diminished estrogen causes increased sensitivity to PTH* • PTH recruits osteoclasts • Osteoclasts cause bone resorption	Unknown, but probably related to a complex series of age-related physiological changes in both sexes

*PTH = parathyroid hormone

Sources: Data from *Bulletin on the Rheumatic Diseases* (1993:42[5]:1–3), Copyright © 1993, The Arthritis Foundation; and *Orthopaedic Physical Therapy Clinics of North America* (1996;5[1]:73).

versible, prevention of this metabolic bone disorder is the best treatment. Prevention should focus on three main goals:

1. attaining optimal peak mass in adolescence
2. maintaining peak bone mass through middle age
3. slowing the rate of bone loss from osteoporosis[13(p5),14(pp15–17)]

During childhood and adolescence, emphasis should be on maintaining a minimum calcium intake of approximately 1,000 mg, exercising, and not smoking. During adulthood, excessive alcohol intake should also be discouraged. Various pharmacological strategies have been tried to slow the rate of bone loss in perimenopausal and postmenopausal women.[9(pp74–78),13(p5)]

Hormone replacement therapy (HRT) is effective in preventing bone loss in postmenopausal women if taken within the first 5 years after menopause, but it cannot reverse any bone atrophy that has already occurred.[11(p138),13(p5)] Controversy exists over the increased risk of cervical and breast cancer versus the benefits of this treatment.[14(p16)] Table 10–2 lists the characteristics of persons who would absolutely benefit from HRT and who should not take HRT. Fluoride treatment supplemented with calcium appears to increase bone formation by increasing the number of osteoblasts; however, the efficacy of this treatment is still controversial. Serious side effects are associated with fluoride therapy and include peripheral pain, nonvertebral fractures, gastrointestinal complications, and possible toxicity.[15(pp264,271,272),16(pp28,29)] Other drugs, such as calcitonin, bisphosphonates, and bone-derived growth factors are also being studied for use in osteoporosis.[14(pp16–17),16(p22),17(p7),18(pp43–45)] Research is ongoing in this area.

The one prophylactic treatment that has been proven effective in preventing bone loss with only minimal side effects is physical activity, consisting of weight bearing and aerobic exercises, resistance training, postural training, and balance training.[19(p49),20(pp7–8),21(p33)] Tai Chi is recommended as a beneficial exercise for the prevention of osteoporosis, because it combines weight bearing, flexibility, and balance training and is enjoyable to perform.[20(p8)] There appears to be no upper age limit to the effectiveness of physical activity on gains in bone mass[7(p33)]; however, exercise appears to increase skeletal mass only in areas where the forces are applied.[2(p1102)] Therefore, walking may help to maintain bone density in the lower extremities and spine, but it will not prevent bone loss in the distal radius.[22(p2809),23(p253)]

To maintain the integrity of the vertebral column, the therapist faces a paradox in the exercise prescription: The type of bone-loading activity required to maximize bone gain (twisting and high-impulse loading) is also the type of activity most likely to cause a vertebral fracture.[7(p33)] Based on the amount of bone loss and the degree of the patient's symptoms, the therapist can determine a suitable level of activity. The resistive exercise program can be as advanced as a complete Nautilus regimen or can be a simple walking program. Because a large amount of bone loss can occur asymptomatically, the therapist should cautiously prescribe a preventive program for osteoporosis.

An additional goal of therapy is to improve spinal alignment through patient education, manual techniques, and postural exercises. It is imperative for the therapist to teach the patient about osteoporosis and the need to maintain good posture through improved awareness and exercise. Myofascial release (MFR) and scapular mobilization

Table 10–2 Indications and Contraindications for Hormone Replacement Therapy (HRT)

Indications for HRT	Contraindications for HRT
Menopausal symptoms	Thrombophlebitis
Hysterectomy or early menopause	Myocardial infarction
Sedentary lifestyle	Cerebrovascular accident
Paget's Disease	Diabetes with vascular involvement
History of steroid use or alcohol use	Lymphedema
Osteogenesis imperfecta	Gallbladder disease
Family history of osteoporosis	Large uterine fibroids
Loss of height/kyphosis	Extensive endometriosis
Malnutrition	Brease cancer (or family history of)
Heavy smokers	Heart disease

Women with the above symptoms or histories need to discuss the benefits versus the risks of HRT with their doctors. Women who do not have symptoms or histories on either list fall into the "gray zone" and also must discuss treatment strategies for osteoporosis with their physicians.

HRT = hormone replacement therapy

Source: Data from *Clinical Orthopaedics and Related Research* Vol. 269, pp. 138–139, © 1991, J.B. Lippincott Company.

can help to restore normal alignment and flexibility. The emphasis of the postural exercise program is on improving the strength and endurance of the back extensors, the abdominals, and the scapular retractors[24(pp17,18)] and depressors (Figure 10–1). Flexion exercises should be avoided, as they appear to cause anterior wedging or compression fractures of the vertebrae.[8(p1539),23(p2809),25(p593)]

The therapist also should analyze the patient's movement patterns during activities of daily living and recommend any changes needed in technique or posture.[24(p17)] In addition, bending and lifting activities have been found to generate loads that exceed the strength of osteoporotic vertebrae. Therapists need to caution patients with osteoporo-sis about the dangers of lifting-type activities.[26(pS25)]

Summary of Prevention of Osteoporosis

- Refer patient appropriately to physician for medical consultation on pharmacological options.
- Load the spine to minimize bone loss through weight-bearing exercises, such as walking or Tai Chi.
- Improve posture through patient education, exercise, MFR, and scapular mobilization.
- Improve the strength and endurance of the back extensors, abdominals, and scapular retractors and depressors through exercise.

- Avoid exercising in flexed postures.
- Improve balance (see Chapter 17 for balance training).

VERTEBRAL COMPRESSION FRACTURES

The high incidence of fractures in the elderly is associated more with lower bone density (osteoporosis) than with other age-related factors, such as an increased frequency of falling and a decreased ability to reduce the impact of those falls.[3(p4)] Because the vertebrae are composed mostly of trabecular bone, they are susceptible to damage from Type I osteoporosis. A compression fracture of the vertebra generally occurs in the thoracic or upper lumbar region of the spine, usually while performing a mundane activity such as rising from a chair, coughing, or reaching for an object.[12(p218),27(p1)] The patient complains of severe back pain from paraspinal muscle spasms. The quality of trunk motion is poor, with "catches" occurring on minimal movement. Range of motion (ROM) is extremely limited. Severe postural changes result. Radiographic evidence usually confirms the diagnosis.

Treatment of Vertebral Compression Fractures

During the initial evaluation, the therapist should be sure to ascertain whether the patient is having any bowel or bladder dysfunction. Either symptom could indicate a cauda equina disorder, which must be reported to a physician immediately. If such a symptom is present, the therapist should not administer any further treatment until the patient is checked medically. (This condition may require emergency surgery to correct.)

Acute Phase

During the acute phase, the patient is in severe pain and is confined to bed rest. Local application of ice to the vertebral column may help to reduce pain and swelling. Hydrocollator packs and massage are beneficial in reducing the painful paravertebral muscle spasms. As the pain subsides, the patient can begin walking and sitting for about 10 minutes out of every hour. The patient must avoid flexion activities and kyphotic postures, as these cause additional wedging deformities that can lead to new compression fractures. The therapist also begins teaching the patient about osteoporosis, posture, and exercise to prevent further injury.[2(p1102),28(p152)]

Subacute Phase

During the subacute phase, the therapist should teach the patient isometric exercises to strengthen the abdominals and isotonic exercises to strengthen the back extensors and scapular retractors (Figure 10–1). Because a fracture has already occurred, trunk flexion exercises are absolutely contraindicated. The therapist should continue to teach the patient about good posture. The therapist also should recommend that the patient take short rest periods throughout the day until the muscular endurance of the postural muscles returns to normal. The gait pattern should be evaluated and any deviations corrected. Low-heeled, soft-soled shoes may help to cushion some of the forces to the spine resulting from ambulation. The patient usually is pain free and can return to normal activity 6 to 8 weeks after the fracture.[8(p1539)] Lifting items over 10 lbs is usually restricted indefinitely, due to the excessive forces this places on the osteoporotic vertebrae.[27(p2)]

Supine in Hook-Lying Position

1. Abdominal strengthening
   With hands behind head, lift head off plinth but not shoulders. Tighten abdominals. Hold for 5 seconds. Relax and repeat.

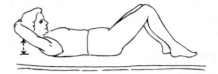

2. Scapular adduction
   With hands behind head, pull elbows down to plinth while pulling shoulder blades together. Hold for 2 seconds Relax.

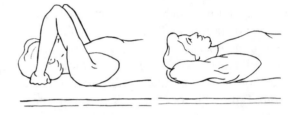

Prone

3. Back extension
   While lying prone on a pillow (with hands behind head if possible), lift head and upper body off pillow, keeping neck in neutral.
   Hold for 2 seconds. Relax.

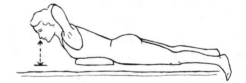

Sitting

4. Butterflies
   With hands behind head, pull elbows backward. Hold for 5 seconds and relax. Repeat.

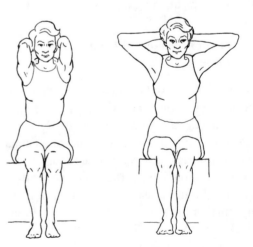

Figure 10–1 Preventive exercises for osteoporosis of the spine

continues

Figure 10–1 continued

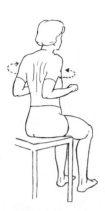

5. Scapular adduction
   With elbows bent and shoulders abducted, pinch shoulder blades together.

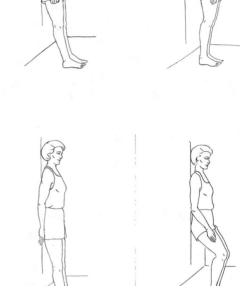

6. Upper trunk rotation
   With arms crossed in cradle position, slowly and rhythmically rotate the whole upper trunk and neck to both sides. (Erect posture must be maintained during this exercise.)

Standing

7. Wall bridge
   Stand one foot from the wall with back, shoulders, and head flush to the wall. Arch the back, lifting the back and shoulder–but not the head–off the wall. Slowly return to the start position. Relax and repeat.

8. Wall slide
   With feet comfortably apart, stand one foot from the wall, with the back, shoulders, and head flush to the wall. Perform a quarter squat, sliding the back down the wall. (Make sure the knees are not in valgus during this activity.) Slowly return to the standing position. Relax and repeat.

Summary of Treatment of Vertebral Compression Fractures

- During the acute phase
  1. treat with bed rest and modalities
  2. teach postural awareness.
- During the subacute phase
  1. begin strengthening of abdominals, back extensors, and scapular retractors
  2. avoid flexion activities and exercises
  3. avoid lifting over 10 lbs
  4. continue patient education.

CERVICAL ARTHRITIS

Arthritis is probably the most common cause of neck pain in the elderly. Nearly all persons over the age of 70 years have roentgenographic evidence of osteoarthritis (OA) at the apophyseal joints, the joints of Luschka, or the discs. The patient will report some of the following symptoms when the osteophytes impinge on a neural or vascular structure:

- local pain
- paresthesia
- stiffness
- joint crepitance
- radicular symptoms (sharp shooting pains in neck and arm)
- loss of motion[29(p66),30(p71)]

More than 50% of patients with RA report involvement at the neck, and they present with signs and symptoms similar to those of patients with OA. These patients also may have atlanto-axial subluxation, which causes the additional symptom of pain in the neck, occiput, forehead, or shoulder—and possible signs of spinal cord compression.[29(p67)] In many instances, atlanto-axial subluxation is asymptomatic. The subluxation may progress to upward migration of the odontoid process. In a small number of patients, these conditions may cause brainstem compression and death.[31(pp1055,1056)]

Treatment of Cervical Arthritis

In addition to the standard musculoskeletal assessment, the therapist must check for any neurological involvement (Table 10–3). If radicular signs are present, the cervical spine may require temporary immobilization to prevent further traction or impingement on the affected nerve root. In general, modalities and massage are used to alleviate muscle spasms and to reduce pain. Fascial restrictions can be freed with MFR techniques. Gentle manual traction can be beneficial in patients with OA, but is absolutely contraindicated in patients with RA because of the high possibility of vertebral subluxation in this patient population.

The therapist should instruct the patient in active pain-free neck exercises, including modified axial extension to neutral.[32(p241)] The easiest way to prescribe the exercises is with a $7 \times 7 \times 7$ program: seven repetitions of seven neck motions, performed seven times a day. (Caution: The therapist should rule out vertebral artery syndrome before prescribing backward bending.) The therapist also should teach the patient to self-stretch the upper trapezius, levator scapula, scalene, and pectoral muscles, as they usually are tight. As ROM improves, the patient can begin resisted isometric neck exercises in addition to the active exercises. The therapist also must instruct the patient in the importance of proper posture. Although the exercises technically are easy to perform, the changing of a lifetime habit of poor posture can be an impossibility.

Table 10–3 Cervical Radiculopathy Symptoms and Findings

Disk Level	Nerve Root	Symptoms and Findings
C2-3	C3	*Pain:* Back of neck, mastoid process, pinna of ear *Sensory change:* Back of neck, mastoid process, pinna of ear *Motor deficit:* None readily detectable except by EMG *Reflex change:* None
C3-4	C4	*Pain:* Back of neck, levator scapulae, anterior chest *Sensory change:* Back of neck, levator scapulae, anterior chest *Motor deficit:* None readily detectable except by EMG *Reflex change:* None
C4-5	C5	*Pain:* Neck, tip of shoulder, anterior arm *Sensory change:* Deltoid area *Motor deficit:* Deltoid, biceps *Reflex change:* Biceps
C5-6	C6	*Pain:* Neck, shoulder, medial border of scapula, lateral arm, dorsal forearm *Sensory change:* Thumb and index finger *Motor deficit:* Biceps *Reflex change:* Biceps
C6-7	C7	*Pain:* Neck, shoulder, medial border of scapula, lateral arm, dorsal forearm *Sensory change:* Index and middle fingers *Motor deficit:* Triceps *Reflex change:* Triceps
C7-T1	C8	*Pain:* Neck, medial border of scapula, medial aspect of arm and forearm *Sensory change:* Ring and little fingers *Motor deficit:* Intrinsic muscles of hand *Reflex change:* None

Source: Reprinted with permission from H.N. Herkowitz, Management of Syndromes Related to Spinal Stenosis, in *Essentials of the Spine*, J.N. Weinstein, B.L. Rydevik, V.K.H. Sonntag, eds., p. 178, © 1995, Lippincott-Raven Publishers.

Summary of Treatment of Cervical Arthritis

- Use modalities and massage for symptomatic relief.
- Prescribe active pain-free neck exercises and progress to resistive isometric exercises.
- Teach the patient to self-stretch the upper trapezius, scalene, levator scapulae, and pectoral muscles.
- Teach the importance of restoring the cervical lordosis in order to prevent further degeneration.

SPINAL STENOSIS

Spinal stenosis is an anatomic narrowing of the spinal canal, which can cause significant symptoms in older persons. Aside from the rare cases of congenital (or primary) stenosis, most spinal stenosis occurs due to degenerative changes in the vertebral bodies, facet joints, and intervertebral discs. Encroachment by osteophytes, a thickened joint capsule, infolding of an inelastic ligamentum flavum, or a bulging annulus can reduce the spinal canal size at the segmental level and compress the spinal cord or the spinal roots.[33(p40),34(p188),35(p86)] Spinal stenosis can also be acquired after spinal surgery (discectomy or fusion) or as a result of a metabolic bone disease, such as Paget disease or osteoporosis.[36(p263)]

Clinically, there are two types of stenotic syndromes: root entrapment syndrome and neurogenic claudication. Patients with root entrapment syndrome have severe and constant pain down the leg to the foot. The pain is not aggravated by coughing, sneezing, or sitting; and they have limited spinal extension.[33(p41)] Patients with neurogenic claudications present with one or more of the following symptoms:

- deep ache that begins in the buttocks and radiates down the thighs, often going below the knee
- long history of intermittent low back pain (LBP)
- decreased spinal extension
- paresthesias (tingling, burning, or numbness) in the saddle area or anywhere in the lower extremities
- sensations of leg "falling asleep" or "giving way" or "feeling rubbery"
- nonspecific disturbances in sensory and motor function

- impairment of bowel and bladder control[33(p41),34(pp188–189),37(p4),38(pp269,270)]

Walking or standing aggravates the symptoms, and only forward flexion or sitting alleviates the symptoms.

It is important to differentiate neurogenic claudication from vascular claudication. In general, patients with neurogenic claudication can exercise vigorously as long as they maintain a flexed trunk posture (as in bicycle riding), whereas patients with vascular claudication have difficulties with lower extremity activity regardless of trunk position. Table 10–4 describes other clinical findings that differentiate neurogenic from vascular claudication.

Conservative Treatment of Spinal Stenosis

Conservative measures usually do not alleviate this mechanical problem of bony origin; however, most patients opt not to have surgery and are referred to therapy. The therapist can use modalities (e.g., hot packs, ultrasound, massage) to decrease paravertebral muscle guarding. Because lumbar extension exacerbates the symptoms, the therapist should prescribe a program of (Williams') flexion exercises to increase both flexibility and strength (Figure 10–2). These exercises also open up the intervertebral foramen, decreasing nerve root compression.[38(p271)] In addition, lumbar stabilization exercises, performed with a reduced lumbar lordosis (i.e., a posterior pelvic tilt), are beneficial for this condition.[38(p272)] However, a lumbar stabilization program can be difficult for some patients to learn. The therapist should also prescribe an appropriate conditioning program, such as stationary bike riding, for this patient population.

The therapist should teach the patient to avoid extension postures such as prolonged walking, standing, and prone-lying.[36(p267)]

Table 10–4 Clinical Findings To Differentiate Neurogenic from Vascular Claudication

	Vascular Claudication	*Neurogenic Claudication*
Exercise	Worsened pain	Variable
Stationary bicycle	Worsened pain	Can ride with comfort
Lying flat	Relief of pain	Variable
Standing	Relief of pain	Worsened
Sensory deficits	Stocking-glove distribution	Poorly localized
Pulses	Decreased with bruits	Normal
Back motion	No change in pain	Worsened pain with hyperextenstion
Genitourinary	Impotence	Urinary retention or frequency

Source: From the *Bulletin on the Rheumatic Diseases,* Volume 45, Number 4, copyright 1996. Used by permission of the Arthritis Foundation. For more information, please call the Arthritis Foundation's information line 1-800-283-7800.

The therapist must be alert to the symptoms of cauda equina compression, such as loss of bowel or bladder control or saddle paresthesia. If these symptoms occur, the therapist must contact the physician immediately, as permanent damage can occur without emergency surgery.

Surgical Treatment of Spinal Stenosis

Patients undergoing surgical decompression have a good short-term prognosis for relief of symptoms, with 64% having good to excellent results.[39(p1)] The removal of the lamina and the spinous process (total laminectomy) relieves the mechanical narrowing of the spinal canal and prevents damage to the nerve roots. The positive results from the decompression deteriorate significantly with time.[40(p2938)]

Surgical Approach

With the patient prone, the surgeon removes the paraspinal muscles, the multifidi, and the erector spinae from the spinous process and the lamina. In a total laminectomy, the posterior elements of the vertebra are removed, leaving the dura mata exposed.[41(pp1004,1005)] Often a laminectomy patch is used to form a barrier between the paraspinal muscles and the contents of the spinal canal. This thin, nonadherent material reduces the inevitable scar formation and can help stop epidural bleeding.[42(p187)] The muscles on both sides are sutured together and the incision is closed.[41(p1005)]

Rehabilitation

Postlaminectomy patients can mobilize rapidly. The decompression of the nervous system affords these patients more ambulatory ability immediately after surgery than was available before surgery.[41(p1005)]

The patient begins a gentle, active exercise program in the pain-free range to regain strength and ROM and also works on ambulation endurance. Rest periods should be scheduled. The patient should continue with flexion or lumbar stabilization exercises, as other vertebral segments may also be affected by the stenosis. Developmental sequence helps restore functional mobility in

Supine Lying

1. Posterior pelvic tilt

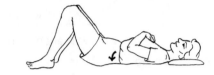

2. Single knee to chest stretch

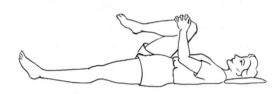

3. Bilateral knee to chest stretch

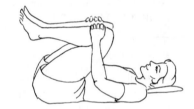

4. Curl-ups (abdominal strengthening)

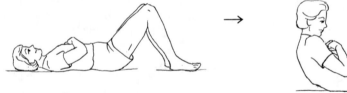

5. Active hip flexion with knees bent

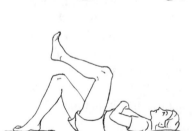

Figure 10–2 Examples of flexion exercises for patients with spinal stenosis. These types of exercises open up the intervertebral foramen, alleviating pressure on the nerve roots. In addition, they improve strength and flexibility in a pain-free posture.

continues

Figure 10–2 continued

6. Gentle lower trunk rotation. With knees together, rhythmically rock legs side to side.

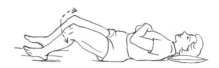

7. Butterflies (hip rotations). Bring knees together and pull apart.

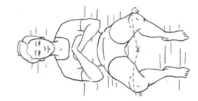

Sitting

8. Hamstring and low back stretch. Gently reach forward, keeping back flat.

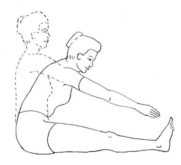

9. Marching

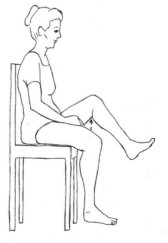

continues

Figure 10–2 continued

10. Kicking

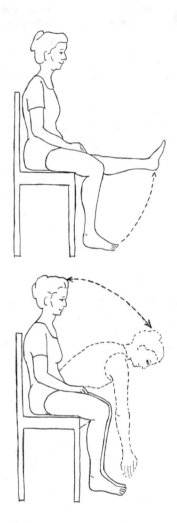

11. Trunk stretch

different positions. The therapist should educate the patient on avoiding hyperextension of the spine. Most patients do not require formal outpatient therapy and can return to normal functional status independently.

Summary of Treatment of Spinal Stenosis

- Prescribe flexion exercises or lumbar stabilization exercises in posterior pelvic tilt.

- Educate the patient to avoid extension postures and prolonged extension activities, such as walking, standing, or prone-lying.
- Be alert for symptoms of cauda equina compression.
- Postlaminectomy
  1. prescribe active (flexion) exercises to tolerance;
  2. increase ambulation endurance;

3. restore mobility through a developmental sequence program.

LOW BACK PAIN

Low back pain is not as common a complaint in the elderly population as it is in the younger population. It is important to remember that LBP is a symptom, not a diagnosis.[33(p27)] The mechanical causes of LBP include:

- disc protrusion (most common)
- spinal stenosis
- degeneration of the apophyseal joint
- muscle fatigue or strain
- ligament fatigue or sprain
- sacroiliac joint dysfunction
- spondylolisthesis (defect in the pars interarticularis)[33(pp29–32)]

Determining the cause of LBP is extremely difficult for physician and therapist alike and requires a good patient history and physical examination. At present, the "high tech" imaging tests (magnetic resonance imaging, computed tomography scans) are far from perfect, resulting in many false-positive and false-negative findings.[43(p67)] Table 10–5 depicts the commonly seen symptoms of classic discogenic LBP and pain from spinal stenosis. The two most important physical signs observed in lumbar disc herniation are a decreased lumbar ROM and a crossed Lasegue sign.[44(p192)] (The crossed Lasegue sign refers to a straight leg raise on the uninvolved leg causing neurological symptoms in the involved leg.) The therapist must also assess hip ROM, as loss of motion there can contribute to movement dysfunction in the low back.[45(p1508)] For more information on the assessment of the spine, the reader is referred to any of the excellent assessment texts on the market. If there is any suspicion of nonspinal causes, such as gynecologic, renal, or intestinal disorders, the patient must be referred back to the physician.

Conservative Treatment of Low Back Pain

The only conservative measures that have scientific studies validating their effectiveness are back schools, mobilization or manipulation, exercises, and epidural blocks. Of the different exercise protocols available in the treatment of LBP, several studies have found the one described by McKenzie to be greatly beneficial.[46(pp136,137),47(pp30,31),48(pS206)] This so-called "extension program" in fact

Table 10–5 Mechanical Relationships in Low Back Pain

Position	Discogenic Low Back Pain	Pain from Spinal Stenosis
Standing/walking	Decreased	Increased
Sitting	Increased	Decreased
Valsalva maneuver	Increased	No change
Bending	Increased	No change or decreased
Lifting	Increased	No change
Bed rest	Decreased	Variable

Source: From the *Bulletin on the Rheumatic Diseases*, Volume 45, Number 4, p. 4, copyright1996. Used by permission of the Arthritis Foundation. For more information, please call the Arthritis Foundation's information line 1-800-283-7800.

incorporates all trunk motions, but in a very individualized manner. The patient cooperates eagerly, as the exercises reduce pain and increase function immediately.

Although some modifications in technique may be needed, McKenzie's fundamental principles apply to treating the older population.

- The evaluation provides clues to the mechanical cause of the injury and the pain.
- The therapist prescribes exercises and postures to correct the injury and to eliminate the pain.
- The therapist progresses the program to restore full ROM.
- The patient learns proper posture and self-care of the back (back school).

Extension versus Flexion Exercises

In the classic case of discogenic LBP, the patient complains that the pain is worse in flexed postures or activities, such as sitting, driving, bending, or lifting. Extension activities, such as standing, walking, or lying down, alleviate the symptoms. On evaluation, the therapist finds that repeated forward bending worsens the symptoms and that repeated backward bending (extension) either decreases the pain or causes it to "centralize." "Centralization" refers to a lessening of peripheral symptoms (radiating pain), which may or may not cause an increase in central back pain.

Treatment consists of educating the patient about proper posture and body mechanics, and a progression of extension postures and exercises (Figure 10–3) until the pain is eliminated. The therapist can kill two birds with one stone by treating the soft tissue structures while the patient is maintaining a prone position. The therapist can easily apply heat, massage, and MFR techniques to sore muscles or fascial restrictions. However, the therapist must emphasize the curative powers of posture and exercise over the temporary "nice feeling" associated with hot packs and massage. In the acute stage, the patient should perform the exercise program independently every 2 hours or as needed to alleviate the symptoms. Sufka et al report that patients who show "centralization" of their pain have improved functional outcome and quality of life.[49(p205)] As the symptoms subside, the therapist discontinues the palliative treatment and gradually adds flexion and rotation exercises into the program to restore normal motion and function. The importance of restoring normal pain-free ROM, including flexion, cannot be overemphasized. The patient cannot return to normal function without the ability to move freely in all directions.

When extension activities exacerbate the patient's pain, McKenzie advocates flexion exercises initially, previously shown in Figure 10–2. (This means McKenzie and "extension" exercise are not really synonymous.) As the symptoms subside, extension and rotation exercises become incorporated into the program.

Motor Control Exercises

Regardless of its initial mechanical or postural cause, chronic LBP can also be considered a movement disorder of the neuromuscular system. Mannion et al discovered a greater proportion of Type IIB (fast-twitch glycolytic) muscle fibers in the paraspinal muscles of patients with LBP as compared to normals. They concluded that the low back muscles of people with LBP would become fatigued easier than the muscles of healthy

1. Prone-lying

    Lie prone to tolerance (20 seconds to 20 minutes). If necessary, place pillow(s) under pelvis. Remove pillow(s) gradually (over days or weeks) to tolerance. If you cannot tolerate prone-lying at all, begin with back bends in standing position.

2. Prone-on-elbows

    Use this developmental sequence position to increase the lumbar lordosis. You may tolerate it more easily than prone-lying.

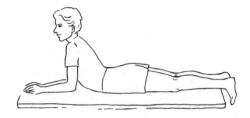

3. Modified press up

    Place hands ahead of shoulders as shown. Push upper body but not pelvis off plinth using arms only. This is a *passive* back exercise! Repeat until symptoms decrease or are eliminated. Number of press ups is limited by upper extremity strength and endurance.

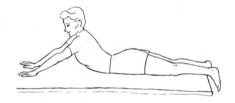

4. Standing back bends

    Place feet shoulder-width apart. Place hands in the small of back. Lift upper torso up and over hands, while keeping neck in neutral and knees straight.

5. Walking

    Walk, Walk, Walk!

    Do not sit for more than 45 minutes at a time without getting up and walking around. Begin a daily walking program. Gradually build up endurance.

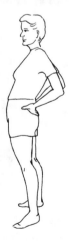

Figure 10–3 Modified extension postures and exercise

people.[50(p881)] Hodges and Richardson found delayed muscle contraction in the transversus abdominus, rectus abdominus, erector spinae, and oblique abdominal muscles in patients with LBP, which altered their postural control of their trunk.[51(p46)]

Lumbar stabilization exercises can therefore be used successfully to correct faulty movement patterns and restore pain-free motion. The term *stabilization* does not mean to keep the spine completely rigid, but to use the trunk muscles (abdominals and gluteus maximus primarily) as an internal brace to help guide movement in coordinated, fluid patterns. The therapist teaches the patient to control excessive movement in the spine while the peripheral joints move. For example, during arm elevation, the patient must ensure that the back does not hyperextend to complete the range. Lumbar stabilization exercises are extremely functional and are performed in all positions, including standing. Some examples of low-level stabilization exercises are shown in Figure 10–4. Since these exercises require good proprioception and motor awareness, many patients have difficulty performing them successfully.

Another motor control "exercise" is the martial art form Tai Chi, which can be performed by patients of all ability levels. Tai

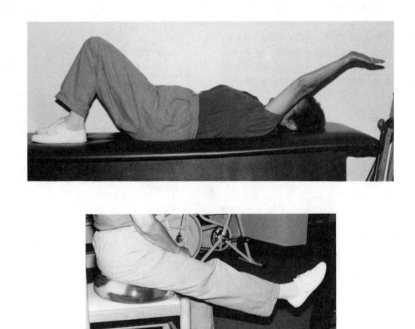

A

B

Figure 10–4 Examples of lumbar stabilization exercises. (A) Supine-lying arm elevation. Patient must concentrate on holding lumbopelvic position with abdominals. (B) Sitting on an air disc, knee extension (kicking). Advanced patients can progress to a physioball instead of the air disc. Patient must maintain erect position of spine and not "slump" to achieve knee extension.

Chi has been found to increase lumbar and thoracic flexibility by 11° in community dwelling elderly persons.[52(p345)] Other gains include increased cardiorespiratory function, knee strength, balance, and feeling of well-being.[53(p380),54(p505),55(p1222)] Recently, many health care professionals and their elderly patients have begun to appreciate the many benefits of this ancient Chinese martial art. Promising research continues in this area.

Other Conservative Treatment

Other types of exercise have also been successful in the treatment of LBP. Regaining flexibility in tight structures are key adjunct treatments to flexion, extension, and lumbar stabilization exercising. Resisted strength training as well as aerobic conditioning have all been effective in reducing pain and improving function.

Modalities, such as moist heat and ultrasound, are commonly used in the treatment of LBP.[56(p361)] In addition, flexion, extension, and lumbar stabilization exercises can be performed in the therapeutic pool.[57(pp192–196)]

Exercise and physical agents cannot always correct a mechanical problem in the back. Manual therapy consisting of joint mobilization,[58(p28)] muscle energy, massage, strain-counterstrain, and MFR can be used safely on elderly patients by skilled clinicians.

Surgical Management of Low Back Pain

Although disc herniation is not common in elderly persons, surgical management should not be ruled out on the basis of age alone. In a study by Maistrelli et al,[59(pp63–64)] 32 elderly patients (aged 60 to 79) with unrelenting back pain and sciatica underwent surgery (after conservative treatment had failed). Of the 32 patients, 16 had complete herniation, 10 had incomplete herniation, and 6 had bulging of the L4-5 disc. After removal of the disc and partial removal of the vertebral arch, all patients had immediate pain relief. After 6 months, 90% reported complete relief from sciatica and 71% had complete relief of lumbar and sciatic pain.

Summary of Treatment of Low Back Pain

- Evaluate the patient and determine an individual treatment program.
- Use modalities and manual therapy to reduce muscle guarding.
- Restore proper flexibility to hypomobile regions and stabilize hypermobile regions.
- Teach extension exercises initially for patients with discogenic pain.
- Teach flexion exercises initially for patients with pain from lumbar stenosis.
- Restore all spinal motions as symptoms subside.
- Use other effective forms of exercise: lumbar stabilization exercises, Tai Chi, resistive training, and aerobic conditioning.
- Teach and reinforce the need for proper posture.
- Teach the patient to be independent in back care.

DOCUMENTATION TIPS: SETTING GOALS

Within the past decade, there has been a change in documenting treatment goals. The therapist's weekly goals for the patient used to be labeled short-term goals, and the therapist's goals for discharge were called long-term goals. Now that patients are being discharged faster, the distinction between the two types of treatment goals has become blurred. The documentation of those goals needs to remain clear.

By setting clear and concise goals with the patient, the therapist can better direct the treatment plan. The therapist determines what the patient should reasonably be able to accomplish in a set amount of time (i.e., a week). The goal should be specific (i.e., decrease lbp) and measurable (i.e., decrease lbp to level 4/10). If the goal is not achieved in the time predicted, the therapist needs to figure out the reason. This includes a reevaluation of the treatment plan itself. Has the treatment worked? How can it be modified to be more effective? Do the goals reflect the patient's goals, hopes, and desires? Are they the therapist's goals only?

Although the primary purpose for setting treatment goals is to help design a treatment plan, the companies paying the bills are very interested in the "appropriateness" of those goals. In other words, are the limited health care dollars being spent wisely? At present, wisdom is practically synonymous with function; therefore, it is important for physical therapists to document functional goals for their patients. (Occupational therapists have obviously always documented functional goals.) Some examples of functional goals for patients with LBP include the ability to lift and carry (in lbs) certain loads, ambulation endurance (e.g., in feet, blocks, miles), driving endurance (in time), brushing teeth, etc. It is also important when documenting goals to use proper semantics (or current "buzzwords") and avoid certain terminology (such as the word "maintenance"). See Documentation Tips in Chapter 14 on Buzzwords.

REFERENCES

1. Kaufmann T. Posture and age. *Top Geriatr Rehabil.* July 1987;2:13–26.

2. Aisenbrey JA. Exercise in the prevention and management of osteoporosis. *Phys Ther.* July 1987;67(7):1100–1104.

3. Barden HS, Mazess RB. Bone densitometry of the appendicular and axial skeleton. *Top Geriatr Rehabil.* January 1989;4:1–110.

4. National Institutes of Health: Consensus Development Conference Statement—Optimal Calcium Intake. Bethesda, MD: NIH; 1994.

5. Babbitt A. Osteoporosis. *Orthoped.* 1994; 17: 935–941.

6. Simon L. Pathogenesis of osteoporosis. *Bull Rheum Dis.* 1993;42(5):1–3.

7. Martin AD, Brown E. The effect of physical activity on the human skeleton. *Top Geriatr Rehabil.* January 1989;4:25–35.

8. MacKinnon JL. Osteoporosis: a review. *Phys Ther.* October 1988;68(10):1533–1540.

9. Pomerantz EM. Osteoporosis and the female patient. *Orthop Phys Ther Clin N Amer.* 1996;5(1): 71–84.

10. Rosenthal RE. Osteoporosis. *Arch Amer Acad Orthop Surg.* 1998;2(1):52–59.

11. Forbes AP. Fuller Albright: His concept of postmenopausal osteoporosis and what came of it. *Clin Orthop.* 1991;269:128–141.

12. Netter FH. The CIBA Collection of Medical Illustrations. *The Musculoskeletal System, Part I.* Summit, NJ: CIBA-GEIGY Corp; 1987.

13. Scott JC. Prevention of osteoporosis. *Bull Rheum Dis.* 1993;42(5):4–5.

14. Silver JJ, Einhorn TA. Osteoporosis and aging. Current Update. *Clin Orthop.* 1995;316:10–20.

15. Gruber HE, Bayling DJ. The effects of fluoride on bone. *Clin Orthop.* 1991;267:264–277.

16. Rosen CJ. The role of bisphosphonates and fluorides in the prevention and treatment of osteoporosis. *Top Geriat Rehabil.* 1995;10(5):19–34.

17. Martin AD. Osteoporosis: a geriatric public health issue. *Top Geriatr Rehabil.* 1995;10(4):1–11.

18. Edwall D, Mohan S, Baylink DJ. Growth factors: potential treatment of osteoporosis. *Top Geriatr Rehabil.* 1995;10(4):35–47.

19. MacKinnon JL. The role of physical therapy in the prevention and treatment of osteoporosis. *Top Geriatr Rehabil.* 1995;10(4):48–54.

20. Vargo MM, Gerber LH. Exercise strategies for osteoporosis. *Bull Rheum Dis.* 1993;42(5):6–9.

21. Katz WA, Sherman C. Osteoporosis—the role of exercise in optimal management. *Phys and Sportsmed.* 1998;26(2):33.

22. Swezey RL. Exercise for osteoarthritis—is walking enough? The case for site specificity and resistive exercise. *Spine.* 1996;21:2809–2813.

23. Ebrahim S, Thompson PW, Baskaran V, et al. Randomized placebo-controlled trial of brisk walking in the prevention of postmenopausal osteoporosis. *Age Ageing.* 1997;26:253–260.

24. Cirullo JA. Osteoporosis. *Clin Manage Phys Ther.* January/February 1989;9:15–19.

25. Sinaki M, Mikkelsen BA. Postmenopausal spinal osteoporosis: flexion versus extension exercises. *Arch Phys Med Rehabil.* 1984;65:593–596.

26. Myers ER, Wilson SE. Biomechanics of osteoporosis and vertebral fracture. *Spine.* 1997;22(24 Suppl):S25–S31.

27. Yacyshyn E, Evans JM. Case management study: osteoporotic vertebral compression fracture. *Bull Rheum Dis.* 1998;47(1):1–2.

28. Main WK, Cammisa FP, O'Leary PF, et al. The spine. In: Koval KJ, Zuckerman JD, eds. *Fractures in the Elderly.* Philadelphia: Lippincott-Raven Publishers; 1998.

29. Maricic MJ, Gall EP. Cervical arthritis: which therapy for your patient? *J Musculoskel Med.* October 1989;6:66–76.

30. Zigler JE, Capen DA, Rothman SLG. Spinal disease in the aged. *Clin Orthop.* 1995;316:70–79.

31. Rana NA. Natural history of atlanto-axial subluxation in rheumatoid arthritis. *Spine.* 1989;14(10):1054–1056.

32. Enwemeka CS, Bonet IM, Ingle JA, et al. Postural correction in persons with neck pain. *J Orthop Sports Phys Ther.* November 1986;8(11):240–242.

33. Porter RW. Pathology of spinal disorders. In: Weinstein JN, Rydevik BL, Sonntag VKH, eds. *Essentials of the Spine.* New York: Raven Press; 1995.

34. Nowakowski P, Delitto A, Erhard RE. Lumbar spinal stenosis. *Phys Ther.* 1996;76(2):187–190.

35. Salcido R. Pre-existing conditions and the aging spine. *Top Geriatr Rehabil.* 1998;13(3):84–87.

36. Cailliet R. *Low Back Pain Syndrome.* 4th ed. Philadelphia: FA Davis Co; 1988.

37. Moreland LW. Spinal stenosis. *Bull Rhem Dis.* 1996;45(4):3–6.

38. Fiebert IM, Lebwohl NH. Rehabilitation for patients with lumbar spinal stenosis. *Orthop Phys Ther Clin N Amer.* 1993;2(3):265–276.

39. Turner JA, Ersek M, Heroon L, Deyo R. Surgery for lumbar spinal stenosis: Attempted meta-analysis of the literature. *Spine.* 1992;17(1):1–8.

40. Jonsson B, Annertz M, Sjoberg C, Stromqvist B. A prospective and consecutive study of surgically treated lumbar spinal stenosis—Part II—5-year follow-up by an independent observer. *Spine.* 1997;22(24):2938–2944.

41. Mooney V. Surgery and postsurgical management of the patient with low back pain. *Phys Ther.* 1979;59:1000–1006.

42. Collis JS, Jr. The laminectomy patch. In: Watkins RG, Collis JS Jr, eds. Lumbar Discectomy and Laminectomy. Rockville, MD: Aspen Publishers, Inc; 1987.

43. Deyo RA. Understanding the accuracy of diagnostic tests. In: Weinstein JN, Rydevik BL, Sonntag VKH, eds. *Essentials of the Spine.* New York: Raven Press; 1995.

44. Vucetic N, Svensson O. Physical signs in lumbar disc hernia. *Clin Orthop.* 1996;333:192–201.

45. Porter JL, App M, Wilkinson A. Lumbar-hip flexion motion—a comparative study between asymp-

tomatic and chronic low back pain in 18 year old to 36 year old men. *Spine.* 1997;22(13):1508–1513.

46. Ponte DJ, Jensen GJ, Kent BE. A preliminary report on the use of the McKenzie protocol versus Williams protocol in the treatment of low back pain. *J Orthop Sports Phys Ther.* September/October 1984;6:130–139.

47. DiMaggio A, Mooney V. Conservative care for low back pain: what works? *J Musculoskel Med.* September 1987;4:127–139.

48. Donelson R, Grant W, Kamps C, Medcalf R. Pain response to sagittal end-range spinal motion. *Spine.* 1991;16(6S):S206–S212.

49. Sufka A, Hauger B, Trenary M, Bishop B, et al. Centralization of low back pain and perceived functional outcome. *J Orthop Sports Phys Ther.* 1998; 27(4):205–212.

50. Mannion AF, Weber BR, Dvorak J, Grob D, Muntener M. Fiber-type characteristics of the lumbar paraspinal muscles in normal healthy-subjects and in patients with low back pain. *J Orthop Res.* 1997; 15(6):881–887.

51. Hodges PW, Richardson CA. Delayed postural contraction of transversus abdominus in low back pain associated movement of the lower limb. *J Spinal Disord.* 1998;11(1):46–56.

52. Lan C, Lai JS, Chen SY, Wong MK. 12-month Tai Chi training in the elderly—its effect on health

and fitness. *Med Sci Sports Exer.* 1998;30(3): 345–351.

53. Wolf SL, Barhart HX, Ellison GL, Coogler CE. The effect of Tai Chi Quan and computerized balance training on postural stability in older subjects. *Phys Ther.* 1997;77(4):371–381.

54. Wolfson L, Whipple R, Derby C, Judge J, et al. Balance and strength training in older adults: intervention gains and Tai Chi maintenance. *J Am Geriatr Soc.* 1996;44(5):498–506.

55. Lai JS, Lan C, Wong MK, Teng SH. Two year trends in cardiorespiratory function among older Tai Chi Chuan practitioners and sedentary subjects. *J Am Geriatr Soc.* 1995;43(11):1222–1227.

56. Sullivan MS, Kues JM, Mayhew TP. Treatment categories for low back pain: a methodological approach. *J Orthop Sports Phys Ther.* 1996;24(6):359–364.

57. Cirullo JA. Aquatic physical therapy approaches for the spine. *Orthop Phys Ther Clin N Amer.* 1994; 3(2):179–208.

58. Koes BW, Bouter LM, Van Mameren H, Essers AHM, et al. The effectiveness of manual therapy, physiotherapy, and treatment by the general practitioner for nonspecific back and neck complaints. *Spine.* 1992; 17(1):28–35.

59. Maistrelli GL, Vaughan PA, Evans DC, Barrington TW. Lumbar disc herniation in the elderly. *Spine.* January/February 1987;12:63–66.

11

The Shoulder Complex

Shoulder pain is one of the most common musculoskeletal complaints in the elderly.[1(p129)] Many older patients do not seek medical attention until function has been grossly impaired. The therapist has to sift through years of accumulated disease process and injury to identify the damaged structures. In order to treat this patient successfully, the therapist must possess a complete understanding of the anatomy and biomechanics of the individual joints that comprise the shoulder complex, as well as an understanding of their intricate interactions.

ANATOMY OF THE SHOULDER COMPLEX

The scapula, clavicle, and humerus articulate with each other to create four separate joints:

1. the glenohumeral (GH) joint
2. the sternoclavicular (SC) joint
3. the acromioclavicular (AC) joint
4. the scapulothoracic (ST) joint

Together these joints afford the shoulder incredible mobility in all planes of motion, but at the expense of GH stability. Although instability is not a common complaint in the elderly, the effects of prior instability may manifest in later years as arthritis.[1(p129)]

The Glenohumeral Joint

The GH joint is a ball-and-socket joint that relies on muscular integrity and capsuloligamentous structures rather than bony conformation for its stability. The glenoid fossa of the scapula is pear-shaped and faces laterally, anteriorly, and superiorly. Hyaline cartilage covers the fossa and is thinnest at the center. The glenoid labrum, a fibrocartilaginous rim, stabilizes the GH joint by deepening the articular surface of the glenoid and also assists in joint lubrication.[2(pp424,425)] It has a similar morphology to knee meniscal tissue (i.e., a triangular cross-section) and is vascularized throughout its peripheral attachment to the joint capsule.[3(pp48,52)] The head of the humerus has three to four times the surface area of the glenoid and faces medially, posteriorly, and superiorly.[4(p226)] Hyaline cartilage covers the humeral head as well and is thickest at the center. The joint capsule is loose and lax and is supported by the GH ligaments, the coracohumeral ligament, and the insertions of the rotator cuff tendons (Figure 11–1). Stability of the GH joint is enhanced by the airtight seal of the capsule, creating a relative vacuum between the joint surfaces; therefore, any injury to the capsule, ligaments, or labrum will "pop the seal" and cause the joint to sublux.[5(p372),6(pp346–347)] The

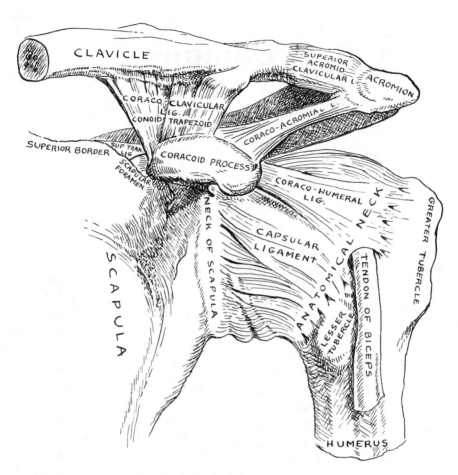

Figure 11–1 Glenohumeral and acromioclavicular joints

inferior capsule is the least protected and is a common site for dislocations.[2(pp424,425)] Table 11–1 shows the active and passive factors contributing to GH joint stability.

Approximately nine bursae are interspersed between the various soft tissue and bony structures of the joint. The subdeltoid (also called the subcoracoid or subacromial) bursa is the largest bursa in the body. The deep layer overlies the rotator cuff and humeral head and the superficial layer adheres to the anterior two-thirds of the acromion, forming a giant curtain over the joint.[7(p153)] This bursa contributes signifi-

cantly to smooth GH joint motion, but when it becomes inflamed, major losses in joint movement occur (Figure 11–2).[8(p39)]

Muscles and Motions

While standing with the arm hanging dependently by the side, the normal muscle tone of the supraspinatus along with the upward orientation of the glenoid fossa maintains the joint's integrity.[2(p426)] The rotator cuff muscles connecting the scapula to the humeral tubercles consist of the supraspinatus, the infraspinatus, the subscapularis, and the teres minor. The long head of the biceps

Table 11–1 Stability of the Glenohumeral Joint

Factors Limiting Anterior Translation

Coracohumeral and superior glenohumeral ligament	Limit external rotation between 0 and 60° elevation[a]
Subscapularis muscle and middle glenohumeral ligament	Effective stabilizers between 0 and 90° elevation[a]
Anterior band of the inferior glenohumeral ligament	Primary stabilizer above 90° elevation[a]
Infraspinatus and teres minor muscles	Prevent anterior translation of humeral head in abducted, externally rotated position[b]

Factors Limiting Posterior Translation

Infraspinatus and teres minor muscles	Static stabilizers in all positions of abduction[c]
Subscapularis muscle	Prevents posterior translation of humeral head on glenoid[c]
Inferior glenohumeral ligament	Most effective stabilizer at 90° abduction[d]
Anterior superior capsule	Disruption necessary for posterior dislocation to occur[c]
Retrotilt of the glenoid fossa	Excessive retrotilt implicated in posterior subluxation[e]

Factors Limiting Inferior Translation

Superior joint capsule and superior glenohumeral ligament	Main structures limiting inferior subluxation in the dependent position[f]
Negative intra-articular pressure	Limits inferior displacement of the adducted humerus[g]
Inferior glenohumeral ligament	Most effective stabilizer above 45° of abduction[a,d]

Source: Reprinted with permission from E Culham, M Peat, "Functional Anatomy of the Shoulder," *Journal of Orthopaedic and Sports Physical Therapy*, 1993;18(1):345, © 1993, Williams & Wilkins.

Sources: [a]*Journal of Bone and Joint Surgery* (1981;63-A:1208–1217), Copyright © 1981, *The Journal of Bone and Joint Surgery.*

[b]*American Journal of Sports Medicine* (1987;15[2]:144–148), Copyright © 1987, The American Orthopaedic Society for Sports Medicine.

[c]*Acta Orthopedica Scandinavia* (1986;57:324–327), Copyright © 1986.

[d]*American Journal of Sports Medicine* (1990;18[5]:449–456), Copyright © 1990, The American Orthopaedic Society for Sports Medicine.

[e] *Journal of Bone and Joint Surgery* (1985;68-A:724–731), Copyright © 1985, The Journal of Bone and Joint Surgery.

[f]*Clinical Sports Medicine* (1991;10:757–782), Copyright © 1991.

[g]*Journal of Bone and Joint Surgery* (1985;67-B:719–721), Copyright © 1985, The Journal of Bone and Joint Surgery.

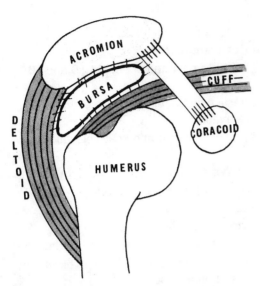

Figure 11–2 Subacromial bursa. The subdeltoid bursa is essentially the inner synovial lining of the deltoid muscle and the undersurface of the acromium. The outer layer of the supraspinatus portion of the cuff is the inner layer of the bursa. In any movement of the arm, the two layers of the bursa glide on each other as the bursa deforms. *Source:* Reprinted with permission from R. Cailliet, *Shoulder Pain*, 3 ed., p. 68, © 1991, F.A. Davis Company.

tendon may also be considered an "unofficial" rotator cuff muscle. Together these five muscles are active during all elevation activities—flexion, abduction, and extension—compressing the humeral head into the glenoid fossa.[5(p373)] The supraspinatus and infraspinatus are also extremely active during internal and external rotation of the humerus, especially when it is in an abducted position.[9(pp81–82)]

Movements of the articular surfaces figure prominently in the understanding of shoulder motion. In the normal GH joint, the humerus is seated slightly inferior to the glenoid. With the initiation of elevation, the humerus actually glides superiorly for about 3 mm and then remains centered in the glenoid throughout arm elevation or rota-tion.[10(pp77–79),11(p193),12(p195)] (This newer biomechanical information is contrary to the conventional belief that the humeral head "depresses" during elevation activities.) Interestingly, if the pathological humerus is initially seated more superiorly than normal, the therapist would have to "inferiorly mobilize" the humerus in order to center it on the glenoid. This may account for the positive results seen with the joint mobilization technique of inferior glide performed on the problem shoulder. (The clinician should stay abreast of the latest research in this controversial area.) The closed-packed position of the GH joint and the shoulder complex is full abduction and external rotation. Any attempt at movement beyond this point of maximal congruency will result in a dislocation of the humeral head.

The most frequently studied motion at the shoulder is scapular plane abduction/elevation (also called "scaption"). The scapular plane is considered to be 30° to 45° in front of the coronal plane (Figure 11–3). During scaption,

- humeral external rotation is not required to prevent GH impingement
- the capsule does not become twisted
- the supraspinatus and deltoid muscles are optimally aligned[13(p252)]

Therefore, scaption places the least passive stresses on the GH joint and is an ideal exercise for initiating a treatment program for an injured GH joint.[10(p68)]

If the scapula is held immobile, the GH joint can attain 120° of elevation passively before the humeral head impinges on the acromial process. If the humerus is held in internal rotation from poor posture or surgery, only 60° of elevation is possible before impingement occurs. Without scapular rotation, active elevation of the humerus is limited to 90° because of deltoid muscle

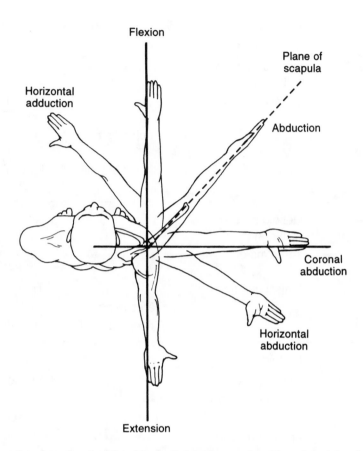

SAGITTAL

Flexion

Plane of
scapula

Horizontal
adduction

Abduction

Coronal
abduction

Horizontal
abduction

Extension

Figure 11–3 Superior view showing the planes of shoulder motion. Note that abduction in the plane of the scapula (dotted line) lies between flexion and abduction. This motion, also termed "scaption," is considered by many authorities to be true abduction. Most functional activities are performed in the scapular plane. *Source:* Adapted with permission from M.J. Kelley, Biomechanics of the Shoulder, in *Orthopedic Therapy of the Shoulder*, M.J. Kelley and W.A. Clark eds., p. 68, © 1995, J.B. Lippincott Company.

shortening and loss of the optimal length-tension relationship in the muscle.[14(p44)] (See Table 11–2 for all muscles and motions.)

Innervation and Blood Supply

The suprascapular, axillary, and lateral pectoral nerves, which are derived from the posterior cord C5-7, innervate the joint capsule. The skin around the shoulder is supplied by the supraclavicular nerves (C-3 and C-4) and by the terminal branches of the sensory component of the axillary nerve.[15(p1861)] Mechanoreceptors have been documented in the inferior aspect of the GH joint capsule.[5(p374)] (Specific muscle innervations are listed in Table 11–2.)

The GH joint receives its blood supply from the anterior and posterior circumflex humeral arteries and the suprascapular arteries.[2(p426)] The blood supply to the supraspina-

Table 11–2 Geriatric Shoulder Complex Motions, Muscles, and Innervations

Motions*	Primary Muscles	Secondary Muscles	Innervation
Glenohumeral joint Flexion 0°–165°	Deltoid (anterior fibers)		Axillary: C-5
	Coracobrachialis		Musculocutaneous: C5-7
		Pectoralis major	Lateral and medial pectoral: C5-8, T-1
		Biceps brachii	Musculocutaneous: C5-7
Extension 0°–44°	Deltoid (posterior fibers)		Axillary: C-5
	Teres major		Lower subscapular: C6-7
	Latissimus dorsi		Thoracodorsal: C6-8
		Teres minor	Axillary: C5-6
		Triceps (LH)	Radial: C7-8
Abduction 0°–165°	Deltoid		Axillary: C-5
	Supraspinatus		Subscapular: C4-6
Adduction (neutral)	Pectoralis major		Lateral and medial pectoral: C5-8, T-1
	Latissimus dorsi		Thoracodorsal: C6-8
		Teres major	Lower subscapular: C6-7
Internal rotation 0°–62°	Pectoralis major		Lateral and medial pectoral: C5-8, T-1
	Subscapularis		Upper and lower subscapular: C5-7
	Latissimus dorsi		Thoracodorsal: C6-8
	Teres major		Lower subscapular: C6-7
		Deltoid (anterior)	Axillary: C-5
External rotation 0°–81°	Infraspinatus		Suprascapular: C4-6
	Teres minor		Axillary: C5-6
		Deltoid (posterior)	Axillary: C-5

continues

Table 11–2 continued

Motions*	Primary Muscles	Secondary Muscles	Innervation
AC, SC, ST joints Scapular elevation	Trapezius Levator scapulae		Accessory: C3-4 C3-4
Scapular depression	Serratus anterior Pectoralis minor		Long thoracic: C5-7 Lateral and medial pectoral: C6-8
Scapular protraction	Serratus anterior Pectoralis minor		Long thoracic: C5-7 Lateral and medial pectoral: C6-8
		Latissimus dorsi	Thoracodorsal: C6-8
Scapular retraction	Trapezius Rhomboids		Accessory: C3-4 Dorsal scapular: C4-5
Scapular upward rotation	Trapezius Serratus anterior		Accessory: C3-4 Long thoracic: C5-7
Scapular downward rotation	Trapezius (eccentric lengthening)		Accessory: C3-4
	Serratus anterior (eccentric lengthening) or forcefully by		Long thoracic: C5-7
	Levator scapulae Rhomboids		C3-4 Dorsal scapular: C4-5

Sources: Gray's Anatomy, ed 35 (pp 423–428, 534–542), by R Warwick and PL Williams (eds), Churchill Livingstone Inc, © 1973.

**Physical Therapy* (1984;64[6]:921), Copyright © 1984, American Physical Therapy Association.

tus muscle by the thoracoacromial artery may be cut off in the so-called "critical zone" by the pressure and tension on the tendon as it passes under the coracoacromial ligament.[15(p1860)] This eventually can lead to further degeneration of the tendon and calcific tendinitis.

The Sternoclavicular Joint

The SC joint consists of the sternal end of the clavicle articulating with both the clavicular notch of the sternum and the cartilage of the first rib. Fibrocartilage covers both articular surfaces.[6(p344)] The joint is divided completely by an articular disc, which also strengthens the joint. The joint capsule is thickest anteriorly and posteriorly and is supported by the anterior and posterior SC ligaments, the interclavicular ligament, and the costoclavicular ligament[2(pp421,422)] (Figure 11–4).

Muscles and Motions

The costoclavicular ligament attaches to the inferior surface of the medial clavicle and the first rib. It is the major stabilizer of the SC joint, preventing excessive clavicular elevation and protraction, and acts as the fulcrum for the following clavicular motions of the SC joint[4(p232),6(p344)]

- elevation of 35° to 45°
- depression of 15°
- protraction of 15°
- retraction of 15°
- longitudinal rotation of 30° to 40°.[16(p4)]

These motions of the clavicle correlate directly with identical motions of the scapula because of the connection of the two bones at the AC joint. Interestingly, no muscles actually cross the SC joint itself, but instead act directly on the clavicle or indirectly through the scapula.

Motion at the SC joint contributes to humeral elevation in the following manner: During the first 90° of humeral abduction or flexion, the distal clavicle (and therefore the scapula) elevates approximately 35° while the sternal end glides inferiorly on the intra-articular disc.[6(p344),14(p41)] If a blockage of motion occurs at the SC joint as a result of direct injury or the accumulated effects of a forward-head posture, decreased shoulder elevation will result.[17(p14)]

Innervation and Blood Supply

The SC joint receives its innervation from the anterior supraclavicular (C-3 and C-4) and subclavian (C-5 and C-6) nerves and its circulation from branches of the internal thoracic and suprascapular arteries.[2(p422)]

The Acromioclavicular Joint

The distal end of the clavicle articulates with the acromial process of the scapula to create the planar, synovial AC joint. Both articular surfaces are covered with fibrocartilage and often are separated by an articular disc, which further strengthens the joint. The fibrous joint capsule is weak and relaxed and is supported by the superior and inferior AC ligaments and the coracoclavicular ligament. The coracoclavicular ligament is considered the major stabilizer of the AC joint and consists of the trapezoid and conoid, which are separated by a bursa (Figure 11–1).[2(pp422,423)]

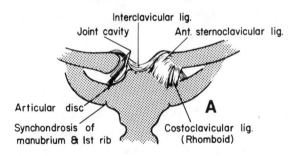

Figure 11–4 Anatomy and ligamentous structures about the sternoclavicular joint. *Source:* Reprinted with permission from *Journal of Bone and Joint Surgery,* Vol. 71A, No. 9, p. 1281, © 1989, The Journal of Bone and Joint Surgery, Inc.

Muscles and Motions

As the scapula rotates to elevate the glenoid fossa, it causes the clavicle to rotate about its longitudinal axis because of the orientation of the trapezoid and conoid. The clavicular rotation is therefore a passive result of tightening of the coracoclavicular ligament. Because of the crank shape of the clavicle, this tightening results in approximately 20° to 25° more scapular elevation with no change in the angle of elevation at the proximal SC joint (Figure 11–5).[14(p42)]

The AC joint also allows the acromion to glide forward and backward, contributing to the motions of protraction and retraction.

Blockage of motion at the AC joint by a screw fixation of the clavicle and coracoid process results in the loss of approximately 20° of humeral elevation.[4(p232)] The scapula can also move about the other two axes of the AC joint in the motions of "scapular winging" and "tilting."[10(p73)] Muscular control of the AC joint is directed mostly by the scapular muscles.

Innervation and Blood Supply

The AC joint receives its innervation from the suprascapular and lateral pectoral nerves (C-5 and C-6) and its blood supply from the suprascapular and thoracoacromial arteries.[2(p423)]

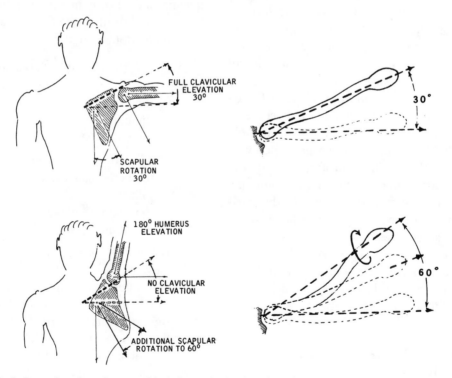

Figure 11–5 Scapular elevation resulting from clavicular elevation and rotation. The upper drawing shows the elevation of the clavicle (without rotation) to 30° that occurs primarily at the sternoclavicular joint. The remaining 30° of scapular rotation, which is imperative in full scapulohumeral range, occurs by rotation of the crank-shaped clavicle about its long axis at the acromioclavicular joint. *Source:* Adapted with permission from R. Cailliet, *Shoulder Pain*, p. 42, © 1991, F.A. Davis Company.

The Scapulothoracic Joint

Although it is not a true joint, the ST joint is considered to be the "articulation" of the scapula with the rib cage. It is convenient to refer to the ST joint to describe the complex motions of the shoulder girdle commonly designated as scapulohumeral rhythm.

Muscles and Motions

The upward scapular rotation that occurs with humeral elevation is controlled by the synergistic actions of the muscles surrounding the scapula. These are the same muscles that cause motion to occur indirectly at the SC and AC joints. During humeral flexion and abduction, the scapula rotates upward through the force-couple action of the upper and lower trapezius along with the serratus anterior. This upward rotation helps to maintain the glenoid's orientation with the humerus to prevent downward dislocation of the humeral head. It also maintains the length-tension relationship of the GH muscles. Of the 180° of available shoulder elevation, the scapula contributes approximately 60°.[18(p153)] The other motions associated with the scapula—such as protraction (abduction), retraction (adduction), elevation, and depression—are also products of the intricate interactions of the scapula muscles, which sometimes act as agonists, antagonists, or stabilizers. These scapular motions correlate directly with similar motions of the clavicle. (See Table 11–2 for specific muscles, motions, and innervations.)

MOTION OF THE SHOULDER COMPLEX

To explain how motion occurs at the shoulder complex as a whole, it is necessary to simplify greatly the actual occurrences. The reader must never lose appreciation for the true complexity of even the most basic shoulder movements.

From the previous discussions, shoulder abduction (in the scapular plane) appears to consist of the following individual joint motions:

- 120° at GH joint
- 35° (elevation) at SC joint
- 40° (rotation) at SC and AC joints
- 25° at AC joint
- 60° at ST joint

This total amounts to 280° of shoulder abduction, where only 180° of motion exists. This is clearly incorrect. Although controversy exists as to the order in which these motions occur, the following simplified sequential model of humeral abduction (scaption) is used to illustrate the interactions of the shoulder joints (Figure 11–5):

1. During the first 30° of abduction
   - the humerus elevates 15° at the GH joint
   - the clavicle elevates 15° at the SC joint

2. Moving toward 90° of abduction
   - the humerus elevates 55° at the GH joint
   - the clavicle elevates full range to 35° at the SC joint

3. Beyond 90° of motion, the clavicle has elevated to its fullest, but the scapula continues to rotate upwardly. This causes the coracoclavicular ligament to tighten, which longitudinally rotates the clavicle passively (40°). Because of the crank shape of the clavicle, the distal end of the clavicle in fact "elevates" 25° at the AC joint.

4. To achieve full abduction of 180°
   - the humerus elevates 120° at the GH joint

- the scapula elevates 60° (35° of clavicular elevation at SC joint and 25° of clavicular elevation at AC joint)

To review, the above sequence is the scapulohumeral rhythm. For every 2° of GH elevation, the scapula rotates approximately 1°; however, the ratio of GH to scapular motion does not maintain a simple 2:1 constant, but varies with the plane and arc of elevation, the amount of load on the arm, and the anatomical variations among individuals.[4(p234)] The clavicular motions at the AC and SC joints are the passive results of the scapula moving on the thorax. They are essentially accessory motions. They allow motion of the shoulder to occur, but they do not cause the motion.

In addition, the posture of the entire spine plays an important role in shoulder range of motion (ROM). In some individuals, forward-head posture results in elevated scapulae, anteriorly rotated clavicles, and sternal depression. This sequence limits the ability to achieve full shoulder flexion.[17(p14)] Kyphotic posture with rounded shoulders can cause the humerus to rotate internally with the resultant loss of 20° to 30° of shoulder abduction due to early acromial impingement. Loss of lumbar lordosis also can prevent full shoulder flexion, as the low back laterally bends or arches during terminal shoulder flexion to help achieve full range.[4(p235)]

Functional Considerations of the Shoulder Complex

The shoulder joint's main function is to move the hand to any desired position in space. The shoulder must provide a stable platform for the hand to perform skilled activities such as reaching, throwing, and eating in an open-kinetic chain and also be able to assume a weight-bearing role during activities such as dusting, writing, and vacuuming in a closed-kinetic chain.

Although it is extremely difficult to calculate the forces acting around the shoulder complex, estimated GH joint reaction forces approach 90% of body weight during elevation activities with the elbow kept extended. (Flexing the elbow reduces the GH joint reaction force by 50%.)[4(pp242–244)] The shoulder is therefore considered to be a weight-bearing joint, even when it is functioning in an open-kinetic chain.

Functional ROM has been defined as 100° of flexion, 90° of abduction, 30° of external rotation, and 70° of internal rotation[19(p1890)]; however, assigning functional ROM norms for the shoulder is difficult because of the large compensatory motions available at the spine, wrist, and elbow. For example, even if the entire shoulder complex were kept completely immobile, the patient would still be able to feed himself or herself independently. More important perhaps than the actual degrees of motion available at the shoulder is the method of achieving that ROM and the ability to be functional. Therapists consider it necessary for the patient to be able to reach above shoulder height, get dressed, and cleanse under the axilla. Consequently, much of the rehabilitation of the elderly shoulder concerns flexion and abduction activities; however, one of the most important functions of the upper extremity is the ability to wipe one's buttocks after a bowel movement. This action requires a combination of shoulder extension, adduction, and internal rotation along with trunk rotation.

Because the upper extremities are involved mostly in skilled activities, functional ROM of the shoulder will be different for each individual. In order to return the patient to functional levels, the therapist must understand the patient's needs as well as the complex interactions of the four shoulder joints and the spine.

SUMMARY

- The shoulder complex comprises four joints: the GH, the SC, the AC, and the ST.
- Together these joints act in concert to allow the shoulder unparalleled mobility in all planes.

- The functional ROM of the GH joint is considered to be 100° of flexion, 90° of abduction, 30° of external rotation, 70° of internal rotation, and approximately 35° of extension.
- Joint reaction forces approach body weight at the GH joint during elevation activities.

REFERENCES

1. Warren RF, O'Brien SJ. Shoulder pain in the geriatric patient, part 1: evaluation and pathophysiology. *Orthop Rev.* January 1989;18:129–135.

2. Warwick R, Williams PL, eds. *Gray's Anatomy.* 35th ed. Edinburgh, Scotland: Churchill Livingstone; 1973.

3. Cooper DE, Anroczky SP, O'Brien SJ, Warren RF, DiCarlo E, Allen AA. Anatomy, histology, and vascularity of the glenoid labrum. *J Bone Joint Surg.* 1992;74-A(1):46–52.

4. Zuckerman J, Matsen FA. Biomechanics of the shoulder. In: *Basic Biomechanics of the Skeletal System.* 2nd ed. Philadelphia: Lea & Febiger; 1989.

5. Wilk KE, Arrigo CA, Andrews JR. Current concepts: the stabilizing structures of the glenohumeral joint. *J Orthop Sports Phys Ther.* 1997;25(6):364–379.

6. Culham E, Peat M. Functional anatomy of the shoulder complex. *J Orthop Sports Phys Ther.* 1993; 18(1):342–350.

7. Cooper DE, O'Brien SJ, Warren RF. Supporting layers of the glenohumeral joint. An anatomic study. *Clin Orthop.* 1993;289:144–155.

8. Clark WA. Anatomy. In: Kelley MJ, Clark WA, eds. *Orthopedic Therapy of the Shoulder.* Philadelphia: JB Lippincott Company; 1994.

9. Hughes RE, An KN. Force analysis of rotator cuff muscles. *Clin Orthop.* 1996;330:75–83.

10. Kelley MJ. Biomechanics of the shoulder. In: Kelley MJ, Clark WA, eds. *Orthopedic Therapy of the Shoulder.* Philadelphia: JB Lippincott Company; 1994.

11. Wuelker N, Schmotzer H, Thren K, Korell M. Translation of the glenohumeral joint with simulated active elevation. *Clin Orthop.* 1994;309:193–200.

12. Poppen NH, Walker PS. Normal and abnormal motion of the shoulder. *J Bone Joint Surg.* 1976;58-A: 195–201.

13. Johnston TB. The movements of the shoulder joint: a plea for the use of the "plane of the scapula" as the plane of reference for movements occurring at the humero-scapular joint. *Br J Surg.* 1937;25:252–260.

14. Cailliet R. *Shoulder Pain.* 3rd ed. Philadelphia: FA Davis Co; 1991.

15. Peat M. Functional anatomy of the shoulder complex. *Phys Ther.* 1986;66(12):1855–1865.

16. Falkel JE, Murphy TC. Shoulder injuries. *Sports Inj Management.* June 1988;1:4–12.

17. Engle R. The shoulder. *Orthop Phys Ther Pract.* 1989;1:12–18.

18. Boissonnault WG, Janos SC. Dysfunction, evaluation, and treatment of the shoulder. In: Donatelli R, Wooden MJ, eds. *Orthopaedic Physical Therapy.* New York: Churchill Livingstone Inc; 1989.

19. Griffin JW. Hemiplegic shoulder pain. *Phys Ther.* 1986;66(12):1884–1893.

12

Treatment of Common Problems of the Shoulder Complex

The shoulder complex is a common site of pain and dysfunction in the elderly population. Because complaints of shoulder pain can be vague, the clinician first must determine whether the pain is being referred from another region, such as the neck or the viscera. Any process stimulating the phrenic nerve can cause pain in the shoulder region, including

- coronary ischemia
- pulmonary embolism
- cholecystitis
- pneumonia
- neoplasm
- splenic injury
- intra-abdominal abscess

The therapist must attempt to distinguish intrinsic from extrinsic causes of pain. Pain originating from the shoulder itself usually is characterized by worsening at night, by motion, and by lying on it.[1(p130)] If the therapist has any doubt as to the origin of pain, immediate referral to the physician is imperative because the shoulder pain could be a symptom of a life-threatening problem.

HUMERAL FRACTURES

Fractures of the humerus can cause severe disability in the elderly population. Often the accompanying injury to the surrounding soft tissue structures can be more damaging than the fracture itself.[2(p310)] In the elderly, the fracture is usually the result of a fall onto an outstretched arm.

Proximal Humeral Fractures

Proximal humeral fractures are about half as common as hip fractures, and the highest incidence occurs between 70 and 85 years of age. Approximately 85% of proximal humeral fractures are of the undisplaced, or group I, category and rarely require surgical fixation.[3(p203),4(p88)] Displaced two- and three-part fractures of the surgical neck (group II or III) require surgery to stabilize them properly. The orthopaedic surgeon may choose one of the following internal fixation devices:

- Rush pins (may damage rotator cuff)
- Kirschner wire (K-wire)
- cancellous lag screws (may cause impingement or migrate)
- interosseous suture
- percutaneous 2.5 mm pins
- wire-loops
- T-plates
- semitubular blade plates
- tension-band wire
- clover-leaf plate[2(p327),5(ppl07–116),6(p508),7(p244),8(p21)]

There is no presently accepted "fixation of choice" for this type of fracture. Each fixation has positive attributes and undesired complications. Complications can include avascular necrosis of the humeral head, subacromial impingement, nerve lesions, and vascular damage.[8(pp22,23)] Depending on the severity of the fracture, displacement of fragments, and available bone stock, the physician selects the most appropriate device.

More severe fractures consisting of three- and four-part fractures and fracture dislocations (groups V and VI) are relatively uncommon and difficult to manage. They can easily disrupt the blood supply (derived from the axillary artery) to the humeral head, causing avascular necrosis. Surgical reconstruction with a clover-leaf plate has been relatively successful in younger patients, but humeral hemiarthroplasty is generally used in the older, osteoporotic patient. Neither fixation allows for good functional return.[5(p120),7(p250)]

Treatment of Proximal Humeral Fractures

The most important goal of the management of the proximal humeral fracture is bony union. The muscular forces are difficult to control at the humerus and tend to pull the fracture fragments apart. Most patients are immobilized for three weeks to allow for callus formation; however, some orthopaedic surgeons may opt to place the patient in a sling for six weeks to allow for complete healing, even though this will result in a stiff shoulder.[2(pp312,329)] Excellent communication between physician and therapist is required to provide optimal management of this condition for each patient.

Postfracture Weeks 1 to 2. The patient is generally in excruciating pain despite potent analgesic medications. The arm is usually placed in a sling and swathe (a wide elastic bandage that is wrapped around the humerus and trunk) to immobilize it. The therapist may recommend that the patient sleep in a semi-upright position (i.e., in a lounge chair or with pillows stacked up in bed).[2(p316)] Ice can be used to decrease pain and swelling. If the fracture is nondisplaced, the therapist should encourage gentle range of motion (ROM) exercises for the elbow, wrist, and hand. The patient generally requires assistance with basic activities of daily living (ADL), especially if the dominant arm is involved. Balance and gait training may be needed as well.

Postfracture Weeks 3 to 6. The exercise prescription is dependent on the stability of the fracture fragments and varies greatly from patient to patient. If the fracture is stable, the patient removes the sling three to five times a day for gentle ROM exercises, such as pendulum exercises and active-assisted elevation activities.[9(p122)] Some physicians discontinue the use of the sling at this time. Active scapular motions such as shoulder shrugging, shoulder circles, and protraction/retraction should be started, and elbow, wrist, and hand motions should be continued. With physician approval, the patient may begin active glenohumeral motions in a very restricted range, concentrating on the quality of the motion and allowing no muscle substitution to occur. Passive ROM and stretching are contraindicated at this time. Ambulation activities should be improving rapidly, but ADL continue to be extremely limited.

Postfracture Weeks 6 to 12. At 6 weeks, the fracture is almost healed. Active ROM exercises progress in the pain-free range to the patient's tolerance. The therapist must ensure that proper scapulohumeral rhythm (SHR) is being reeducated and that muscle substitution is not occurring. A mirror can be a very helpful adjunct in the retraining of SHR. The patient also begins resisted isometric exercise for strengthening purposes (Figure 12–1).

When the humerus is completely healed (at about 8 weeks), therapy becomes more aggressive. Joint mobilization and passive ROM now can be used safely to stretch out soft tissue structures. Supervised pulley work can be helpful in regaining terminal shoulder elevation, but care should be taken to ensure proper SHR. Proprioceptive work with a wobbleboard, BodyBlade, or play ball should be initiated (Figure 12–2). The patient progresses to full-spectrum exercising (resisted isotonics, isometrics, and isokinetics) in the pain-free range. Proprioceptive neuromuscular facilitation (PNF) techniques work well in returning the shoulder to function. Weight-bearing or closed-chain exercises, such as wall push-ups and arm-chair push-ups, should be included in the program. All exercises should also be performed both for power and speed. Overhand ball throwing (with a Nerf-type ball) will enhance coordination and function. If desired, sport activities now can be specifically retrained (see "The Shoulder in Sports" later in this chapter).

Depending on the severity of the fracture and the need for internal fixation, the patient should be independent in most basic ADL, but lifting heavy items (more than 10 lbs), grocery shopping, and reaching overhead may still be difficult.[3(pp203–207)]

Humeral Shaft Fractures

Fractures of the shaft of the humerus are usually the result of a fall on the outstretched arm, but may be due to metastatic disease in the elderly.[9(p124)] The fracture may be repaired surgically with plates and screws or intramedullary nails, but the most frequently

used technique is the conservative method of functional bracing. A plastic cuff (i.e., a Sarmiento orthosis) is placed around the humeral shaft, compressing the soft tissues. The brace allows for gravity-induced traction as well as controlled movement.[10(p97)] In many studies comparing the functional brace to open-reduction internal fixation, this reliable and cost-effective method has resulted in superior strength, ROM, and functional outcomes.[11(p1132),12(p283)]

Treatment of Humeral Shaft Fractures

Treatment of humeral shaft fractures is similar to proximal humeral fractures, but glenohumeral joint motion is not overly emphasized because the joint surfaces are not involved in this injury. Due to the high incidence of radial nerve injury associated with this type of fracture, the therapist should check light touch sensation on the radial aspect of the forearm and hand and the motor ability to dorsiflex the wrist. The fracture needs to be stabilized for at least 6 weeks for bony union to occur. The brace may need to be worn for up to 4 months before the fracture site can withstand the stresses of daily living.[2(pp318–320)] Aggressive therapy is not performed until sufficient healing is confirmed by radiograph.

Summary of Treatment of Humeral Fractures

- Know the type of fracture, the fixation (if any), the stability of the fracture fragments, and any weight-bearing restrictions.

- During the immobilization phase,
  1. use ice to decrease pain
  2. begin ROM exercises for elbow, wrist, and hand
  3. train balance and gait

1. Shoulder flexion
   Loop a sturdy belt around the bottom of your foot. With elbow straight, pull up on belt. Hold for 5 seconds, then relax.

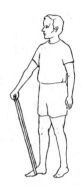

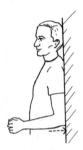

2. Shoulder extension
   Stand with back to wall. Bend your elbow and place it against the wall. Press the point of your elbow into the wall as hard as you can for 5 seconds, then relax.

3. Shoulder abduction
   Stand sideways next to a wall. With your elbow bent, place it against the wall. Push outward against the wall as hard as you can for 5 seconds, then relax.

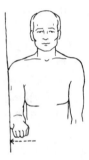

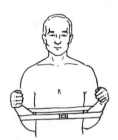

4. Shoulder external rotation
   Fasten a belt into a circle. With elbows bent and held by your side, place both of your wrists inside the belt. Keeping your elbows close by your ribs, push your wrists apart against the belt and hold for 5 seconds, then relax.

5. Shoulder internal rotation
   Stand inside a door frame facing the doorjamb. With your arm by your side with the elbow bent, place your forearm against the doorjamb and press into it as hard as you can for 5 seconds, then relax. (By placing your arm on the opposite side and pressing out, you can strengthen your external rotators.)

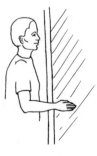

Figure 12–1 Isometric exercises for the shoulder

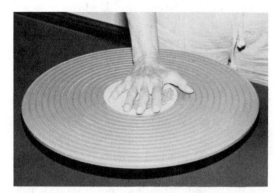
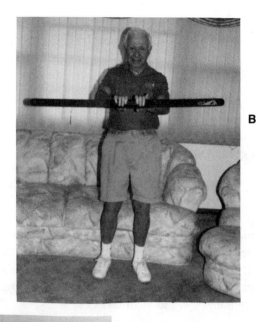
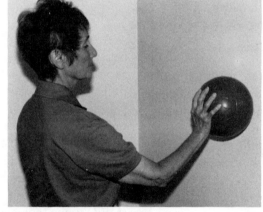

Figure 12–2 Exercises to restore proprioception and control to the shoulder complex. (**A**) The hand and wrist move the wobbleboard in multidirections with weight bearing through the entire upper extremity, (**B**) the BodyBlade™ oscillates during open-chain activities, and (**C**) the patient moves the playball along the wall in an elevation activity in the closed chain.

---

4. do not use affected arm for ADL

- As the fracture stabilizes
  1. discontinue the sling immobilization (proximal humeral fracture only) on physician order
  2. begin active scapular exercises
  3. begin active-assisted shoulder exercises

4. begin using arm for daily activities to tolerance.

- As the fracture heals
  1. discontinue the functional brace (humeral shaft fracture only) on physician order
  2. begin joint mobilization and passive stretching

3. retrain proper SHR and coordination
4. use full spectrum exercises to restore strength and ROM
5. use weight-bearing activities to restore proprioception
6. emphasize functional activities

OSTEOARTHRITIS

Although osteoarthritis (OA) of the glenohumeral (GH) and acromioclavicular (AC) joints is considered to be a very common problem in elderly patients,[1(p130)] little appears in the literature on the best therapeutic approach to these conditions. The patient usually presents with some of the following signs and symptoms of GH OA:

- constant ache in the shoulder region
- difficulty in sleeping on the affected side
- joint crepitance
- capsular pattern: ROM with so much limitation of abduction, more limitation of external rotation (ER), less limitation of internal rotation (IR)[13(p203)]
- point tenderness of the posterior GH joint line[2(p263)]
- hard end-feel
- weakness/disuse atrophy
- osteophyte formation
- narrowing of the joint space
- functional loss

OA of the AC joint commonly goes undiagnosed. The signs and symptoms of this disorder include:

- tenderness at the joint line
- enlarged joint
- joint crepitance[14(p1514)]
- loss of glenohumeral IR[14(p1514)]
- pain when sleeping on affected side[2(p249)]
- pain when arm adducted across chest[2(p249)]
- pain on overhead reaching

- pain with military press and bench weightlifting[2(p249)]

Treatment of Osteoarthritis of the Shoulder

The therapist must design a program that minimizes pain while restoring ROM, strength, coordination, muscle balance, and function to osteoarthritic joints. The physician may prescribe analgesic or anti-inflammatory agents to control the symptoms. Since OA at the GH and AC joints can be caused from overuse, the therapist should carefully look for dysfunctional posture, muscle imbalance, and activities that may contribute to the problem.

Exercise Program

At the beginning of therapy, it is often beneficial to use heat modalities (hydrocolator pack or ultrasound) to reduce pain and to prepare the soft tissues. Since many of the painful symptoms of OA are due to capsular tightness,[2(p279)] joint mobilization to the GH and AC joints can be extremely helpful in decreasing pain and improving motion. Prolonged passive stretching to shortened muscle groups, as well as myofascial release (MFR) to the thoracic inlet, also helps to regain ROM (Figure 12–3). In the extremely painful shoulder, gentle pendulum exercises help initiate motion without compressing the GH joint. Progressive elevation exercises can be performed as the capsule becomes more distensible. Internal and external humeral rotation may cause more grinding and pain than elevation activities and should be monitored carefully.[2(p280)] The therapist also must remember to stretch the GH joint into hyperextension or the patient will have difficulty with basic dressing and toileting activities. Active isometric or isotonic exercise in the

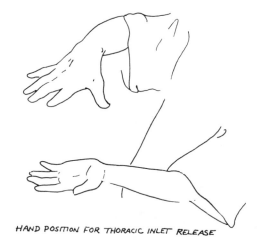

HAND POSITION FOR THORACIC INLET RELEASE

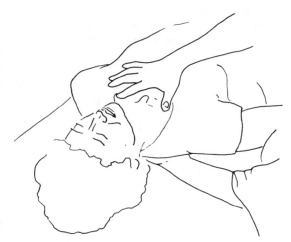

Figure 12–3 Hand placement for thoracic inlet release. *Source:* Reprinted with permission from *Craniosacral Therapy I Study Guide,* © 1987, Upledger Institute Publishing.

newly gained range must follow these techniques to maintain it. The therapist should instruct the patient in gentle self-stretching techniques using a towel or a dowel (Figure 12–4).

Strengthening can be achieved through full-spectrum exercising in the pain-free range with emphasis on proper SHR. The use of PNF D1 and D2 diagonals helps to return the shoulder to function. Weight-bearing exercises, such as wall push-ups, rocking on forearms, and using a wobbleboard (Figure 12–2), may be better tolerated than elevation activities. The patient should progress to light weight-bearing activities that emphasize function, such as vacuuming, washing windows/walls, and dusting. If the patient has access to a therapeutic pool, resistive exercise against the water with hand paddles can provide desired strength levels in a fun manner. As strength improves, the patient begins exercising for speed as well as power.

Activities of Daily Living Program

The therapist should observe the patient perform ADL tasks and offer corrections or alternatives. If reaching and lifting activities can be completed without pain or muscle substitution, they should be encouraged as a functional means of maintaining or improving ROM and strength. Modifications of some activities may be needed to alleviate unnecessary stresses at the joints. For example, carrying heavy purses (or camera bags or suitcases) with shoulder straps that tend to cross over the AC joint causes many AC joint symptoms. In addition, heavy-chested women may compress the AC joint by using bras with narrow straps. By simply "removing the kitchen sink" from a purse or by using a fanny pack or suitcase on wheels, many AC symptoms will disappear. The patient can be discharged from therapy when all functional goals are achieved and the patient understands and can perform the home program independently.

Summary of Treatment of Osteoarthritis of the Shoulder

* Use heat modalities to decrease symptoms.
* Restore functional ROM by using joint mobilization, passive stretch, and MFR.

1. Hyperextension
   While holding a stick or a cane in both hands behind your back, use the unaffected arm to help bring your operated arm into hyperextension.

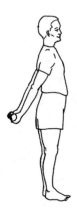

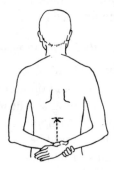

2. Internal rotation
   Behind your back, grasp your operated wrist with your unaffected hand. Slowly pull your hands up your back.

3. Internal rotation (alternate)
   Hold a towel or a stick as shown in the picture, with your unaffected hand grasping it from above and the operated arm from below. Slowly pull the stick or the towel up so that your operated arm moves into internal rotation

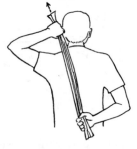

Figure 12–4 Active-assistive exercises in standing position

- Initiate motion exercises with pendulum exercises. Progress to light weight-bearing exercises. Progress to elevation activities.
- Do not emphasize humeral rotations, especially IR, as this motion tends to increase grinding at both the GH and AC joints.
- Strengthen the shoulder complex musculature with full-spectrum exercise within the pain-free range.

- Modify activities to alleviate unnecessary stresses on the GH or AC joints.
- Achieve independent ADL status.

RHEUMATOID ARTHRITIS

Approximately 60% of patients with diagnosed rheumatoid arthritis (RA) complain of some degree of shoulder pain; however, more than half of those patients possibly could attribute their symptoms to a cause other than

RA.[15(p1922)] It therefore behooves the therapist to make a careful assessment of the patient with RA who complains of shoulder pain and not merely assume that the pain is a manifestation of this systemic disease.

The patient often complains of constant pain, swelling, and severe stiffness. On evaluation the therapist usually discovers

- a hot, edematous joint
- tenderness to palpation
- moderate to severe loss of strength in the rotator cuff muscles
- a capsular pattern
- systemic involvement: fatigue, hand or foot deformities

Treatment of Rheumatoid Arthritis of the Shoulder

As discussed in Chapter 6, the goals of the conservative treatment of the rheumatoid arthritic shoulder are more modest than are those for other conditions of a more "curable" nature.

During an acute flare-up, the primary goals of therapy are to reduce inflammation and pain while preventing major losses in shoulder strength and ROM. Anti-inflammatory medications; transcutaneous electrical nerve stimulation (TENS); and cold, wet towels can provide pain relief. Antigravity elevation activities should be avoided at this time, as they greatly increase GH joint reaction forces (see Chapter 11). The patient should perform short-duration isometrics in neutral with emphasis on the weakest muscle groups: the shoulder flexors, abductors, and external rotators.[15(p1926)] Rest is very important during this stage. As the symptoms subside, activity levels can be increased gradually.

During the chronic stages, the patient must learn about joint protection, energy conser-

vation, and work simplification while exercising to increase aerobic capacity and to maximize strength, endurance, and function. The therapist can institute a full-spectrum exercise program within a pain-free range to the patient's tolerance. Care should be taken to prescribe an exercise regimen that does not further aggravate the hands and wrists. Theraband™ looped around the forearm, therefore, is superior to resistive exercise involving dumbbells. Rest sessions must be scheduled into the program as well.

When conservative measures fail, surgical intervention can offer varying degrees of successful pain reduction and subsequent return to function. For uncontrolled synovitis, a synovectomy can provide up to 5 years of pain relief. For impingement syndrome, an acromioplasty (resection of the AC joint) can relieve the pressure on swollen tissues. Rehabilitation after this procedure calls for the protection of the deltoid insertion for up to 2 months postoperatively. Full recovery takes from 4 to 6 months.[16(p107)] For destruction of the joint surfaces, prosthetic replacement (arthroplasty) can restore partial joint function. Arthroplasty is discussed in more detail later in this chapter.

Summary of Treatment for Rheumatoid Arthritis of the Shoulder

- During the acute stage, prevent major losses of strength and ROM through short-duration isometrics to the shoulder flexors, abductors, and external rotators.
- During the chronic stage, maximize strength, endurance, ROM, and function through pain-free exercise.
- Schedule sufficient rest sessions throughout treatment.
- Avoid exercises that aggravate the wrist and hand.

- Teach the patient about the concepts of work simplification, energy conservation, and joint protection.

TOTAL SHOULDER ARTHROPLASTY

Approximately 10,000 total shoulder arthroplasties (TSAs) are performed in the United States annually.[17(p47)] TSA is indicated primarily in the elderly population for patients with OA, RA, or avascular necrosis with destruction of both the humeral head and glenoid surfaces. Prosthetic replacement of only the humeral head is indicated in severe (four-part) fractures of the proximal humerus and in less severe fractures of an osteoporotic humeral head. Contraindications for shoulder arthroplasty include active infection and paralysis of the anterior deltoid and rotator cuff muscles.[18(p3)]

Prosthetic Hardware

Since 1951 a number of different types of TSAs have evolved. The humeral component consists of Mediloy and articulates with a high-density polyethylene glenoid (some components are backed with metal for support). Components usually are cemented in place with polymethyl methacrylate. (See Chapter 4 for more information on acrylic cement.) In general, there are three basic designs:

1. nonconstrained (Neer, Bechtol, O'Leary-Walker models)
2. semiconstrained (Fenlin, UCLA, MacNab-English models)
3. fully constrained (Post, Gristina, Buechel, Zippel, Kessel models)

By far the most popular type of TSA has been the nonconstrained implant (Figure 12–5), which duplicates the anatomical design of the GH joint. This type of prosthesis

relies on soft tissue structures both to stabilize and to move the implant. If the rotator cuff is torn, as is the case in 38% of the population with RA, it must be repaired for this surgery to be successful. In at least half the cases of rotator cuff repair in patients with RA, the rotator cuff fails to function normally postsurgically.[19(p128)] As more constraint is built into a prosthesis, there is less need for a functioning rotator cuff; however, these constrained implants generate higher translational forces and frictional torque than

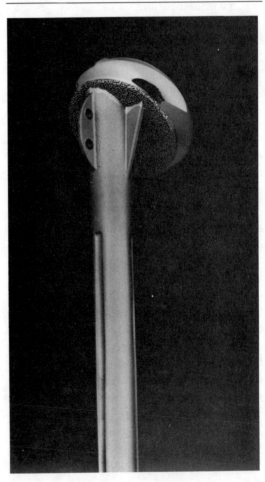

Figure 12–5 Humeral component of the Cofield Shoulder. Courtesy of Richards Medical Co. Inc., Memphis, Tennessee.

the unconstrained implants, and they have a higher rate of loosening and failure.[20(p155), 21(p151)]

Surgical Approach

The shoulder usually is opened anteriorly in a deltopectoral approach (Figure 12–6). The deltoid origin and insertion usually are maintained and only the subscapularis is divided transversely. If the subscapularis is excessively contracted, it may be necessary to lengthen the tendon using a step-cut (Z-plasty) technique.[22(pp198,199)] After dislocating the humeral head anteriorly, a small amount of bone is reamed off the humerus. Any associated pathological condition of the rotator cuff and AC joint is corrected; the subscapularis tendon and the deltoid are repaired carefully.[23(p853),24(pp261,262)] The glenoid fossa is prepared with reamers. The humeral and glenoid components are seated and ce-

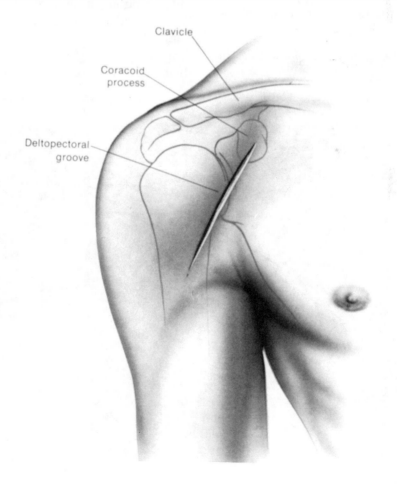

Figure 12–6 Deltopectoral approach. *Source:* Reprinted with permission from S. Hoppenfeld and P. deBoer, *Surgical Exposures in Orthopaedics: The Anatomic Approach,* 2nd Ed., p. 4, © J.B. Lippincott Company.

mented into place. If the humeral component is placed too high, impingement and poor rotator cuff function will occur. If it is placed too low, poor deltoid function will occur. [25(p24)] (See Figure 12–7.) The subscapularis and rotator interval is closed with heavy nonabsorbable sutures.

Complications of Shoulder Arthroplasty

Although good to excellent results occur in over 90% of TSAs, complications inevitably occur. The incidence of complications is approximately 14% and includes:

- instability (related to problems in humeral alignment)

- rotator cuff tear
- ectopic ossification
- glenoid loosening
- intraoperative fracture (due to excessive reaming or impaction)
- axillary nerve injury
- humeral loosening
- infection (0.5% incidence).[17(pp49–65)]

The rate of complication from TSA is considerably higher than for total hip or total knee arthroplasty. There is 9.6% probability of failure in only 5 years and only 75% of TSAs are expected to function 10 years.[17(p66)] In spite of this, shoulder arthroplasty is becoming increasingly popular. Much more research is needed in tech-

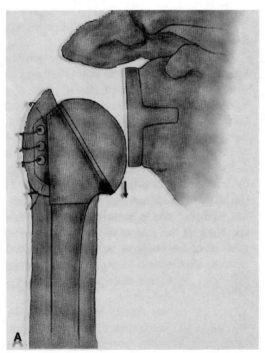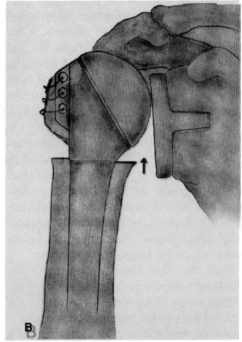

Figure 12–7 (**A**) Prosthesis seated too low causing laxity of deltoid and poor abduction fixation. (**B**) Prosthesis seated too proud causing superior instability and impingement. *Source:* Reprinted with permission from D.M. Dines and R.F. Warren, "Modular Shoulder Hemiarthroplasty," *Clinical Orthopaedics and Related Research*, No. 307, p. 21, © 1994, J.B. Lippincott Company.

nique, design, and materials before TSA approaches the results for other total joint replacements.

Treatment of the Patient with Total Shoulder Arthroplasty

The goals of TSA surgery are to relieve shoulder pain and to improve functional ROM. According to Dr. John Brems, the main goals of TSA rehabilitation should be to restore joint mobility and muscle strength—in that order.[26(p70)] The therapist must know the pathological process preceding the surgery to best treat the patient. Patients with OA usually progress more quickly than do their counterparts with RA, who may have poorer bone stock, muscle myopathy, and systemic involvement. Individually, the postoperative (PO) care depends on the condition of the repair of the rotator cuff, the subscapularis tendon, the insertion of the deltoid, and the general stability of the joint.[27(p1291)] As always, good communication with the orthopaedic surgeon greatly assists the rehabilitative process.

Brems/Holpit Total Shoulder Arthroplasty Protocol[26(pp76–85),28(pp98–108)]

Phase 0 (Preoperative Instruction). As in all elective surgery, the therapist has the luxury of instructing the patient about the rehabilitation program and PO precautions before the surgical insult, answering common questions, and allaying fears of pain and therapy. In addition, the therapist can teach the patient deep breathing and coughing to prevent respiratory problems postoperatively.

The PO precautions should be followed for 2 weeks and consist of:

- no more than 90° of active, painless, gentle shoulder flexion or scaption
- no lifting (with exception of light ob-

jects such as a pen, toothbrush, or fork)
- no weight bearing on arm
- no spray deodorant or perfume (to prevent infection of unhealed incision)
- wearing an immobilizer when a passenger in a car, when sleeping, or in a crowd

Phase I—Stretching (PO Days 1 to 10). Goals: ROM 140° elevation/scaption, 40° external rotation.

Immediately after surgery the arm is immobilized in a sling and swathe. Analgesics are given and moist heat is applied 30 minutes before therapy to decrease pain and stiffness. The program is initially begun in the hospital and then becomes part of the home program. It is done three to five times daily for short duration (5 minutes) with emphasis on quality, not quantity. On PO Day 1 or 2, the patient begins

- *Active elbow, forearm, wrist, and hand motion* for 5 to 10 repetitions.
- *Passive pendulum exercise.* Exercise time: 30 to 60 seconds.
- *Assisted supine elevation/scaption* without a pillow under head, with the therapist applying gentle traction. Exercise time: 15 to 30 seconds.
- *Assisted supine external rotation* with wand and with the arm abducted 4 to 6″ from side of body. Do not exceed 40° ER or rotator cuff repair could be jeopardized. Usually painful. Exercise time: 30 to 45 seconds (Figure 12–8).
- *Assisted elevation with pulley* with pulley placed directly above patient's head or slightly behind the patient. Do not allow motion to be substituted by trunk. Caution if rotator cuff has been repaired. Exercise time: 60 to 90 seconds.
- *Assisted supine abduction* without a pillow under head. Exercise time: 30 to 60 seconds (Figure 12–9).

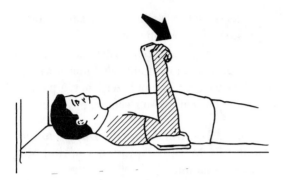

Figure 12–8 Supine passive or active-assisted shoulder external rotation using a wand. The elbow should be placed on a folded towel and be placed 4–6″ from the side of the body. Keep the elbow of the surgical shoulder at 90° through the range of motion to ensure true shoulder external rotation. *Source:* Adapted with permission from L.A. Holpit, "Preoperative and Postoperative Physical Therapy for the Total Shoulder, Hip, and Knee Replacement Patient," *Orthopaedic Physical Therapy Clinics of North America*, Vol. 2, No. 1, p. 101, © 1993, W.B. Saunders Company.

Phase II—Stretching (Begin PO Days 10 to 14). Goals: 160° elevation/scaption and 60° external rotation.

After removal of sutures, begin assisted IR and extension exercises in standing (Figure 12–4). Progress assisted elevation and ER exercises (Figure 12–10). The new exercises are performed after the Phase I stretches and should take approximately 3 to 4 minutes more to accomplish.

Phase III—Stretching (Begin approximately PO Weeks 3 to 6 depending on progress). Goals: 180° elevation/scaption and 80° external rotation.

The last stretching program is designed to help the patient achieve the last 20° of all shoulder motions. It is performed twice daily.

- *Assisted elevation while standing in a corner.* The patient leans into the ele-

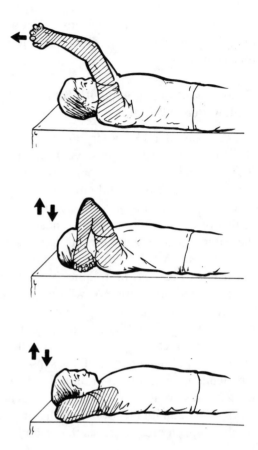

Figure 12–9 Assisted abduction. The patient is positioned supine and uses the uninvolved arm to stretch the involved shoulder overhead. The fingers are intertwined and placed behind the head, and the elbow is gently lowered to the side. *Source:* Reprinted with permission of J.J. Brems, "Rehabilitation Following Total Shoulder Arthroplasty," *Clinical Orthopaedics and Related Research,* Vol. 307, p. 77, © 1994, Lippincott-Raven Publishers.

vated arm pressing the axilla, extended elbow, and hand into the corner.

- *Assisted external rotation* through a doorjamb or in a corner. The patient leans through the opening in the doorjamb, stretching the anterior capsule (and pectoralis major).

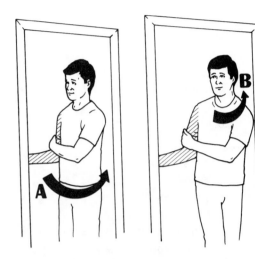

Figure 12–10 Assisted external rotation. The patient stands holding the elbow of the involved arm tight up against his side (**A**). While keeping the forearm held on the doorjamb and turning the body in place (**B**), the arm is pulled into increasing external rotation. *Source:* Reprinted with permission of J.J. Brems, "Rehabilitation Following Total Shoulder Arthroplasty," *Clinical Orthopaedics and Related Research,* Vol. 307, p. 78, © 1994, Lippincott-Raven Publishers.

- *Assisted internal rotation using a table top.*
- *Assisted horizontal adduction/posterior capsule stretch.*

Phase I—Strengthening eccentrically with gravity assist (Begin PO Week 2).

Goals: increase strength of anterior deltoid and supraspinatus muscles.

This program consists of one exercise: active supine elevation with emphasis on eccentrically lowering the surgical arm to the plinth. The elbow is kept flexed. When able to complete 10 repetitions, a 1/2 lb weight is used. This is repeated, progressing by 1/2 lb increments, until 5 lbs can be lifted and lowered for 10 repetitions.

Phase II—Strengthening eccentrically against gravity.

Goals: increase strength of deltoid and rotator cuff muscles.

The patient stands or sits and elevates arm (assisted by uninvolved arm if needed) and then eccentrically lowers arm to side. The elbow is kept flexed. After 10 repetitions can be completed, a 1/2 lb weight is used. This is repeated, progressing by 1/2 lb increments, until 5 lbs can be lifted and lowered for 10 repetitions.

Phase III—Strengthening with Theraband™ tubing.

Goals: increase strength of all shoulder muscles for functional return.

The patient performs isometric and resistive tubing exercises for the anterior and posterior deltoid, the subscapularis (internal rotator), and the infraspinatus (external rotator). These can be performed similarly to the exercises shown in Figure 12–1; however, the shoulder should not be elevated above 45°. The exercises are performed twice daily for about 3 months. The resistance level of the Theraband™ can be increased as well. After 3 months, strengthening of the scapular muscles (trapezius, rhomboids, latissimus dorsi, and pectoralis major) should begin. Coordination of the scapulohumeral muscles is imperative for functional return.

Home Program after Discharge from Formal Therapy

Although the patient has usually been discharged from formal therapy after 3 months, he or she should continue with the home program for up to 2 years for optimal results. What can this patient expect from TSA surgery? The average increase in active forward elevation is 38° (to an average of 124°) and active ER increased by 29° (to 46°). Strength increases by one full grade on a manual muscle test to 4/5.[29(p79)] Three studies have shown that between 82% and 94% of patients with a TSA have no appreciable pain and 75% have no significant functional limitation, although patients with RA did not show as great a functional gain compared to patients with OA.[27(pp1289,1294),29(pp78,79),30(p494)]

Summary of Treatment of the Patient with a Total Shoulder Arthroplasty

- Know the type of TSA, the surgical approach, and the condition of the rotator cuff.
- Preoperatively, orient the patient to the rehabilitation process, answer questions, and instruct in deep breathing and coughing.
- The goals are to restore motion first, then strength.
- During PO Days 1 to 14
  1. begin active elbow, wrist, and hand exercises
  2. begin active-assistive shoulder elevation (scaption) and rotations in supine position
  3. begin passive pendulum exercises
  4. with doctors orders, begin assisted abduction (depends on rotator cuff repair)
- Beginning PO Week 2 (after suture removal)
  1. add assisted IR and extension exercises in standing
  2. progress intensity of stretch in assisted elevation and ER
  3. begin strengthening: active supine elevation with emphasis on eccentric lowering
- Beginning PO Weeks 3 to 6 (depending on progress)
  1. progress stretches of elevation and rotations, add posterior capsule stretch

  2. progress strengthening to active standing elevation with emphasis on eccentric lowering
  3. progress rotator cuff and deltoid strengthening to isometrics and resisted isotonics with Theraband™
  4. begin light ADL only
- Beginning PO Month 3
  1. begin strengthening of large scapular muscles
  2. ensure coordination of scapulohumeral muscles
  3. continue program twice daily for 2 years for optimal results

POSTURAL FAULTS AND MUSCLE IMBALANCES

Postural faults and accompanying muscle imbalances are common in the shoulder region. Kendall and colleagues theorize that persistent postural faults give rise to discomfort, pain, and disability.[31(p3)] It is presently unclear why some obvious postural faults produce no symptoms, whereas some minor postural defects appear to cause severe pain. It is a commonly held belief in physical therapy that the resting position of the scapula is altered in persons with malalignment of the cervicothoracic spine.[32(p343)] In women more than 50 years of age or with an increased thoracic kyphosis, the scapula tilts more forward (in the sagittal plane) by 46%; however, there does not appear to be an increase in the distance from the scapula to the vertebral column (excessively abducted scapulae) or a tendency to downwardly rotate the scapula with increasing age or thoracic kyphosis.[32(p343)]

Although posture is an exceedingly difficult entity to measure reliably,[33(p353)] it has been associated with common muscle imbalances in the shoulder girdle. Forward head and round-shouldered postures are associated with the following short and tight muscles:

- cervical spine extensors
- upper trapezius
- levator scapula
- serratus anterior
- pectoralis minor

In addition, this posture is also associated with lengthened cervical spine flexors, middle trapezius, and lower trapezius muscles.[31(p106),34(p82)] In spite of the fact that the relationship of the many postural variables is presently unknown, significant forward head posture is seen in patients with overuse (impingement-type) injuries of the shoulder.[35(p294)]

Treatment of Postural Faults and Muscle Imbalances in the Shoulder Complex

It is perhaps understandable that therapists are reluctant to engage in a postural retraining program for elderly patients who may have fixed kyphotic or forward head deformities of many years standing. The therapist should know that the goals for treatment are modest (decrease pain and increase function) and do not include the unrealistic expectation of regaining "normal" postural alignment. The program may include:

1. MFR thoracic inlet technique to release anterior structures (Figure 12–3)
2. gentle mobilization of the spine by lying supine on a folded towel or foam roller (Figure 12–11)
3. heat modalities, massage, and stretching to tight muscles
4. inhibitory taping of the upper trapezius muscle[36(p34)] (Figure 12–12)
5. strengthening of middle and lower trapezius muscles (Figure 12–13)
6. proprioception retraining (Figure 12–2)
7. motor retraining of scapulohumeral rhythm
8. functional retraining

IMPINGEMENT SYNDROME

Impingement syndrome is an umbrella term encompassing any disorder to the soft tissue structures in the region of the subacromial arch, such as rotator cuff tendinitis or

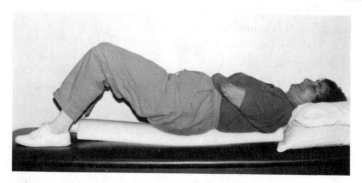

Figure 12–11 Self-mobilization of the thoracic spine with a foam roller. A pillow under the head may be used if necessary. For some patients with thoracic kyphosis, the foam surface is too uncomfortable to lie on. A large towel may be rolled up and used instead. The patient lies on the roller from 20 seconds to 3 minutes. Care must be taken in getting on and off the roller.

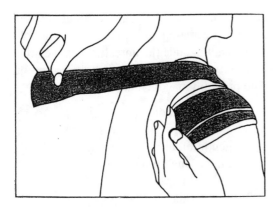

Figure 12–12 Inhibitory taping for the upper trapezius muscle. As taught by J. McConnell, the tape is firmly placed perpendicular to the muscle fibers to inhibit upper trapezius activity and allow easier recruitment of the lower trapezius muscle. The tape is commenced just proximal to the clavicle and firmly pulled over the upper trapezius muscle belly. The tape is anchored toward the thoracic spine. *Caution:* The skin of many elderly patients is too brittle to tolerate the tape used in this technique. *Source:* Adapted with permission from J. McConnell, *Course Notes: The McConnell Approach to the Problem Shoulder*, p. 34, © 1994 McConnell Institute.

subacromial bursitis. It is relatively common in the elderly population. By the fifth decade, many rotator cuffs are pulling away from their insertions. There is thinning of the tendons and erosion of the humeral tubercles.[37(p33)] Classic impingement occurs when the acromion, the coracoacromial ligament, or the undersurface of the acromioclavicular joint abrade the anterior border of the rotator cuff or the long head of the biceps tendon.[2(p112),38(p10),39(pp97,98)] The mechanism of impingement in older patients is often from osteophyte formation on the underside of the acromial surface narrowing the subacromial space. This differs from impingement in younger persons that often arises from a hook-shaped acromion, GH joint instability,

Standing Lower Trapezius Exercise (Facing Wall)

Purpose: To strengthen and shorten the lower trapezius, the muscle that turns the shoulder blade upward.
Position: Standing facing a wall with the arms overhead and slightly out to the side. The thumbs should point away from the wall.
Method: With the arms overhead, pull the shoulder blades back or together.
    Hold for count of _____.
    Repeat _____ times.
    Option: _____ Bring the arms down and relax before repeating the exercise.

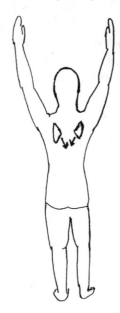

Figure 12–13 Standing lower trapezius exercise facing the wall. *Source:* Reprinted with permission from S. Sahrmann, *Course Notes: Exercises for Correction of Muscle Imbalances.* © 1990.

a tight posterior GH joint capsule, or muscle weakness.[9(p108),40(p355),41(p184),42(p605),43(p194)] Because the rotator cuff stabilizes the GH joint during most shoulder motions[44(p143)] (Table 12–1), repetitive everyday ADL can cause an "overuse" injury, if some of the above-mentioned etiological factors are present. In addition, the loss of vascularity, tendon

Table 12–1 Major Muscle Function of the Shoulder Joint during Eccentric Movements

Movements	Eccentric Working Muscles	Stabilizers
Extension (from flexed position)	Deltoideus anterior Deltoideus medius	Supraspinatus Infraspinatus
Flexion (from extended position)	Deltoideus medius Deltoideus posterior	Subscapularis Supraspinatus
Adduction (from abducted position)	Deltoideus anterior Deltoideus medius Supraspinatus	Infraspinatus
Internal rotation (from external rotated position)	Supraspinatus Infraspinatus	Subscapularis
External rotation (from internal rotated position)	Subscapularis Pectoralis major	Supraspinatus Subscapularis

Note: Kronberg and Brostrom found the rotator cuff muscles stabilize the GH joint during eccentric work of the primary muscle movers. In patients with joint laxity and anterior instability, they found decreased activity of the infraspinatus muscle and increased activity in the supraspinatus and subscapularis muscles. This muscle imbalance may contribute to impingement syndrome.

Source: Adapted with permission from M. Kronberg and L.A. Brostrom, "Electromyographic Recordings in Shoulder Muscles During Eccentric Movements," *Clinical Orthopaedics and Related Research*, Vol. 314, p. 150, © 1995, Lippincott-Raven Publishers.

cellularity, and fiber organization limits the ability of the tendons of the rotator cuff to adapt to stresses and to heal.[45(p164)]

Stage I

Neer has described three progressive phases of shoulder impingement based on the correlation of patient symptoms with the pathological findings he observed in surgery.[44(p70)] According to Neer, the first stage is reversible and generally involves people younger than 25 years of age. Signs and symptoms include:

- tenderness at the greater tuberosity and anterior acromion
- painful arc between 60° and 120° of abduction
- shoulder pain during activity
- possible tenderness at supraspinatus and long head of biceps tendons

Treatment

Initially, the physician usually prescribes an oral anti-inflammatory medication and "active" rest. The Stage 1 impingement syndrome (i.e., rotator cuff tendinitis or subacromial bursitis) responds well to conservative physical therapy modalities, such as ice packs and ultrasound. In addition, the program should include a posterior capsule stretch[46(p215)] (Figure 12–14) and progressive pain-free strengthening exercises for the rotator cuff. Rotator cuff retraining emphasizes endurance work and consists of very low resistance (0 to 3 lbs or yellow Theraband™)

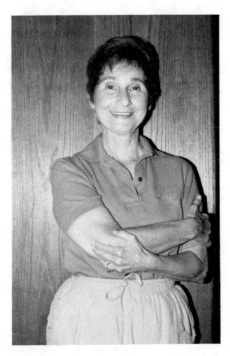

Figure 12–14 Posterior capsule stretch. The patient passively adducts the arm across the body and feels the stretch on the posterior aspect of the GH joint. If pain is felt at the front of the shoulder during this maneuver, the therapist should evaluate the AC joint for dysfunction.

for high repetitions. The exercises include scapular plane elevation in ER (scaption), IR, and standing extension (Figure 12–15). Emphasis is on the concentric phase to prevent further injury.[2(p144)] The stabilizer function of the rotator cuff must also be retrained. This can be accomplished by manually resisting forearm pronation and supination, as well as through open-chain rhythmic stabilization with Theraband™ (Figure 12–16). Because the scapulothoracic musculature works in harmony with the rotator cuff muscles, it is also important to strengthen them. Weight-bearing exercises such as rhythmic stabilization, push-ups, and dips are necessary to restore proximal stability. These exer-

cises can be easily modified for the frailer elderly (Figure 12–17). The mechanism of injury should be determined (e.g., kyphotic or round-shouldered postures, improper tennis service) and corrective measures taken to prevent recurrence.

Stage II

The patient with Stage II impingement syndrome is usually under 40 years of age and presents with some of the following signs and symptoms:

- night pain
- constant shoulder aching and discomfort
- pain with overhead activity
- point tenderness at the coracoacromial ligament
- catching sensation
- impingement sign (full passive flexion, test positive if pain is produced in the last 10° to 15° of elevation)
- decreased ROM[47(pp186–190)]

Treatment

The rehabilitation program is very similar to that in the Stage I program. Treatment for the first 2 weeks consists of rest, application of ice, ultrasound, and gentle stretching. At 2 to 4 weeks, the patient begins progressive strengthening exercises to the rotator cuff (Figure 12–15) and especially to the scapular musculature; however, forward flexion past 90° and abduction are avoided. In addition, it is imperative to concentrate on the concentric contractions and allow the eccentric recovery phase to be done quickly and smoothly in order to prevent further injury.[2(pp143,144)] Scapular taping may be used to help correctly align the GH joint and prevent painful impingement.[48(p803)] After 4 weeks, full ROM is permitted with return to modi-

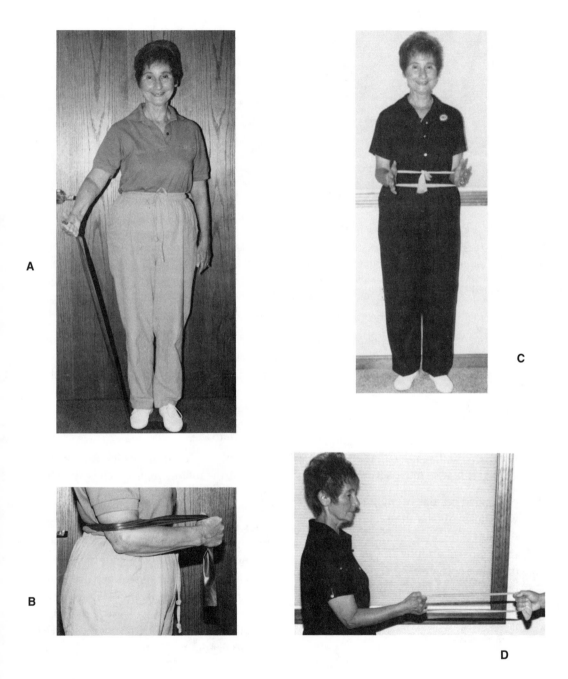

Figure 12–15 Rotator cuff endurance training. Very low resistance is used to prevent the larger surrounding musculature from being recruited. (**A**) Scapular plane elevation in external rotation (scaption), (**B**) internal rotation, (**C**) external rotation, and (**D**) extension from a flexed position. By beginning the exercises in these positions, anterior capsule stress is reduced.

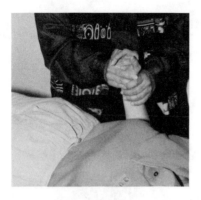
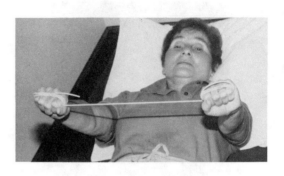

A   **B**

Figure 12–16 Improving rotator cuff stabilizer function. (**A**) Manual resistance to forearm pronation and supination in increasing amounts of elevation causes the rotator cuff to act as a GH joint stabilizer. (**B**) The patient keeps both arms elevated to about 90°. The uninvolved arm rhythmically oscillates the Theratubing™, forcing the rotator cuff muscles on the involved side to stabilize the GH joint.

fied activities.[24(p249)] Surgical decompression may be necessary if conservative measures fail.[1(p134)]

Stage III

The patient with Stage III impingement syndrome is usually older than 40 years of age and presents with more severe symptoms:

- prolonged periods of night pain
- weakness of shoulder abduction and flexion
- infraspinatus atrophy
- partial or complete rotator cuff tears
- bony changes of the acromion or greater tuberosity
- decreased shoulder ROM: active worse than passive[47(p190)]

If the conservative measures indicated fail to resolve the problem, surgical decompression consisting of AC joint resection and excision of the coracoacromial ligament is performed. If torn, the rotator cuff is repaired, with special care taken to protect the suprascapular nerve (which supplies the rotator

cuff).[49(p36)] Surgery is indicated only for elderly patients who understand and will comply with the extensive postsurgical rehabilitation program, which can take up to 1 year.[24(pp249–252)]

Treatment

If only an acromioplasty has been performed, the treatment program is very similar to that in the TSA regimen. Active abduction is avoided initially, and deltoid strengthening does not commence until 6 weeks into the program. Protecting the deltoid is a key part to the rehabilitation program.

When the rotator cuff is repaired, the patient may be placed in an abduction brace or sling for up to 6 weeks. Passive motion is allowed in the brace beginning on PO Day 1. Active pendulum exercises, as well as active elbow, wrist, and hand exercises can also be started immediately. Many patients can use the involved arm to assist in eating and grooming activities. At PO Week 6, the patient begins active strengthening exercises and gradually progresses to resistive exercise with light weights or tubing. Heavier resis-

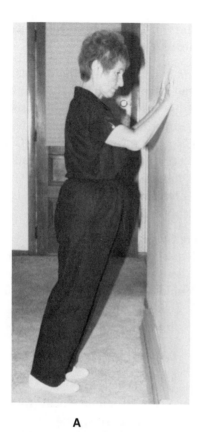

A

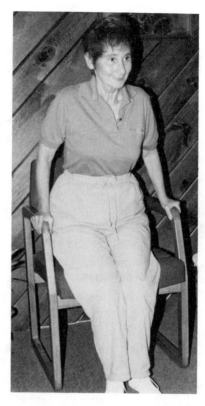

B

Figure 12–17 Modified scapular stabilization exercises in the closed-chain. (**A**) Wall or table push-ups and (**B**) chair push-ups promote proximal stability in the shoulder complex.

tance can begin at PO Weeks 10 to 12. The progression of the rehabilitation program is dependent on the exact procedure used by the surgeon, and close communication is necessary between the therapist and doctor to ensure optimal treatment.[2(p156),24(p258),50(pp155,156)]

Calcific Tendinitis of the Rotator Cuff

Calcium hydroxyapatite crystals may form in the tendons of the rotator cuff, causing an inflammatory disease called calcific tendinitis. The pathogenesis is presently not known, but may have a vascular, mechanical, or metabolic origin.[2(p342)] It occurs most frequently in women over 50 years of age.

Severity of symptoms is unrelated to the size of the calcium deposits.[51(p232)] During the asymptomatic chronic phase, calcium salts are deposited in the tendon. Symptoms begin to occur as the deposits enlarge and cause impingement. During the acute phase, the body reabsorbs the calcium. The pain, although lasting only 3 or 4 days, can be excruciating.[9(p114)]

Treatment

For patients with severe pain, the orthopaedic surgeon can pierce the calcium deposit with a large-bore (18 to 25 gauge) hypodermic needle in a treatment called barbotage or simply "needling." The calcium is sucked up and the area bathed with a local anesthetic and steroid.[2(p343)] Despite the local anesthetic, the pain of this procedure is quite severe and can cause nausea.[51(p234)] At this juncture, some doctors order complete rest in a sling for a week and high-dose anti-inflammatories and ice applications before initiating therapy,[2(p343)] whereas others recommend immediate active ROM exercises to be performed hourly.[51(p234)] Obviously close communication with the surgeon is required for proper treatment. When allowed, the therapist may use moist heat and prolonged, low-load stretches as well as joint mobilization techniques to restore ROM. The patient is instructed in self-stretching techniques. Isometrics are followed by resisted isotonics for strengthening purposes. Scapular exercises, such as push-ups, retractions, and shrugs, are also performed to help restore SHR.

The surgeon can also opt to excise the calcium deposits by splitting the deltoid and removing the white paste-like substance from the tendon. Since this may cause a small rotator cuff tear, the surgeon needs to repair the defect before closing. Although pain relief is immediate with this procedure, strength and function may take up to 6 months to return.[2(pp344,345)] Rotator cuff exercises (Figure 12–15) are usually imperative to restore the commonly atrophied supraspinatus and infraspinatus to adequate strength. These exercises must be progressed into functional activities as discussed previously.

If the pain level is milder and does not require surgical intervention, the patient may be referred to therapy for heat or ice, ultrasound, and ROM and strengthening exercises. The exercises must be performed in a pain-free range to prevent exacerbating the symptoms. More than half the cases respond well to conservative treatment.[2(p344)]

Summary of Treatment of Impingement Syndrome

- For Stage I impingement (rotator cuff tendinitis or subacromial bursitis)
  1. use modalities (ice or pulsed ultrasound) to diminish symptoms
  2. stretch posterior capsule of GH joint
  3. strengthen rotator cuff and scapulothoracic muscles
  4. determine mechanism of injury if possible and correct.

- For Stage II impingement
  1. perform Stage I program at lower intensity
  2. initially avoid elevation past 90°
  3. consider taping scapula to correct alignment (caution for elderly patients)
  4. restore full ROM and functional independence after 4 weeks.

- For Stage III impingement (rotator cuff tendon tear) postsurgical repair
  1. begin passive ROM on PO Day 1 (on doctor's orders)
  2. begin active pendulum exercises only for GH joint
  3. begin active elbow, wrist, and hand exercises
  4. PO Week 6, begin active shoulder exercises and progress
  5. PO Week 10, begin using heavier resistance for strengthening
  6. retrain scapulohumeral rhythm
  7. restore functional independence

- For calcific tendinitis, postsurgical "needling" or excision
  1. begin gentle active-assisted ROM
  2. begin low-load, prolonged stretches and joint mobilization to regain ROM
  3. begin active rotator cuff strengthening, on doctor's orders

4. retrain scapulothoracic musculature
5. restore functional independence

FROZEN SHOULDER

Frozen shoulder (adhesive capsulitis) refers to a lesion of the capsule of spontaneous onset with progressive pain and severe loss of shoulder motion. Although the pathogenesis of this disorder is still unclear, some of the extrinsic factors that may trigger this condition are trauma, immobilization, disease, and faulty body mechanics.[52(p878)] A study by Ozaki et al[53(p1511)] indicates that a contracture of the coracohumeral ligament or rotator interval can also cause this disorder. This condition is generally seen in patients over 40 years of age and is seen more frequently in patients with diabetes and hyperthyroidism. The elderly patient is very susceptible to a faster onset of frozen shoulder, which can develop after only 1 or 2 days of immobilization. Although no precise definition of frozen shoulder exists, the joint capacity can be reduced from a normal volume of 25 ml to 30 ml to a range of 5 ml to 10 ml.[54(p1)] Pathological studies of the capsule and bursal areas show inconsistent findings, possibly due to the studies being done at different phases of the disease. The term "frozen shoulder" therefore, is an "umbrella" diagnosis, with no clear-cut definition or underlying pathology. Clinically, the patient presents with the following symptoms:

- acute pain (initially during both activity and rest, gradually subsiding, and eventually disappearing)
- severely restricted GH motion
- sleep disturbance
- severely restricted function

On evaluation the therapist may also find

- tenderness on the anterior aspect of the joint
- disuse atrophy of deltoid, rotator cuff, biceps, and triceps
- capsular pattern: limitation of abduction, more limitation of ER, less limitation of IR
- capsular end-feel
- limited GH accessory movements (anterior and inferior glides as well as lateral distraction)
- tight internal rotators and adductors
- stretch weakness of the protracted scapular muscles[45(p160)]

Treatment of Frozen Shoulder

Since no precise underlying pathology has been determined for this disorder, it is not surprising that no consensus has yet been reached on the best treatment for frozen shoulder. Although some authorities consider frozen shoulder a self-limiting disease, many patients have continuing impairments up to 10 years later.[55(p738)] In some instances, secondary frozen shoulder may be prevented through patient education on the necessity of continued shoulder motion following an injury to the shoulder complex. For most patients, however, the condition already exists before they seek professional help.

For mild cases of frozen shoulder, conservative treatment including physical therapy begins immediately. In general, the doctor prescribes nonsteroidal anti-inflammatory drugs and analgesics.[54(p2)] In the early stage, physical therapy goals are to decrease pain and inflammation. This can be achieved by

- ice, ultrasound, TENS, or iontophoresis
- gentle active/active-assistive exercises within pain-free ROM, performed frequently throughout the day (one set every 2 hours)

- joint mobilization for pain modulation (small amplitude within available range)
- postural training
- thoracic inlet release (Figure 12–3)
- patient education[45(p161),52(p1881)]

During the later stages of frozen shoulder, therapy becomes aggressive in order to restore glenohumeral ROM. Because any residual loss of motion can reinitiate the frozen shoulder cycle, it is imperative to restore full ROM to the shoulder.[37(p69)] Treatment for frozen shoulder, unlike that for other dysfunctions of the shoulder, often causes pain with the initial attempts to regain motion; however, the pain should not be severe and should not set off an inflammatory response lasting for more than 12 hours. The patient begins full-spectrum exercising. PNF techniques, including rhythmic stabilization in a weight-bearing posture (prone-on-elbows or quadruped), work well in restoring strength, ROM, stability, and coordination. As the patient progresses, the therapist can adjust resistance and timing easily with this therapeutic type of exercise. This intensive program should also include:

- ultrasound
- retraining of SHR
- GH joint mobilization (multidirectional glides)
- thoracic inlet release (Figure 12–3)
- passive stretching and self-stretching (Figures 12–4, 12–8, 12–9, 12–18, and 12–19)
- prolonged stretch (up to 30 minutes) of arm elevated on a sofa armrest
- proprioception and motor control exercises (Figure 12–2)
- home program of short duration performed five times daily
- patient education to prevent recurrence

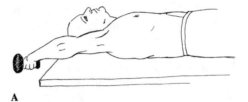

A

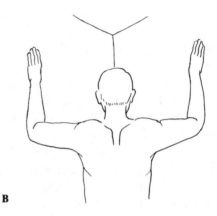

B

Figure 12–18 Passive self-stretching into (**A**) flexion in the supine position with a 1- or 2-lb dumbbell and (**B**) abduction/external rotation with the patient facing a corner.

In a recent study by Mao, Jaw, and Cheng, a 6-week physical therapy program significantly improved ROM and increased joint space in patients with acute frozen shoulder syndrome.[56(p857)]

If conservative measures fail, the orthopaedic surgeon has several options available, none of which has been proven conclusively better than another.

1. Injection of methylprednisolone acetate in GH joint.[54(p2)]
2. Manipulation under anesthesia, with or without arthroscopy.[57(p30)]
3. Hydraulic distension and rupture of the subacromial bursa.[58(p803)]
4. Combination of the above three treatments.[59(p105)]

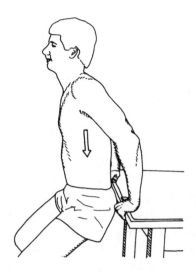

Figure 12–19 Self-stretch to increase shoulder extension and internal rotation. By placing the hand more toward the center of the back (not shown), greater internal rotation will be achieved. *Source:* Adapted with permission from C. Kisner and L.A. Colby, *Therapeutic Exercise: Foundations and Techniques*, 3 ed, p. 316, © 1996, F.A. Davis Company.

There are no clear guidelines as to the progression of a physical therapy program after any of the above procedures. The doctor must communicate clearly to the therapist any contraindications present and the intensity of the rehabilitation program desired.

HEMIPLEGIC SHOULDER PAIN

A fine line is crossed by labeling hemiplegic shoulder pain—essentially a neurological problem—an orthopaedic injury; however, the line is in our minds only, as surely the body does not differentiate between neurological and orthopaedic insults. In any event, soft tissue injuries result as a consequence of the neurological lesion and must be addressed.

After a cerebrovascular accident (CVA), a patient may present with some of the following symptoms:

- severe paralysis
- pain at the shoulder (may extend to the elbow or hand) that is present at rest but worsens with passive motion, dependent position, and at night
- localized tenderness over biceps and supraspinatus
- GH joint subluxation
- edema of the wrist and hand[60(p1884)]

Although hemiplegic shoulder pain is not completely understood, many of the causes of pain and the resultant disability are correctable and preventable.[61(p52)] With an understanding of normal shoulder function and biomechanics, the therapist in coordination with the entire rehabilitation team can prevent some of the soft tissue injuries.

Pathomechanics

During the flaccid stage, the trunk tends to lean or shorten toward the hemiparetic side, which causes the scapula to descend from its normal horizontal level. The trapezius and serratus anterior also become flaccid, causing the scapula to rotate downwardly. Without normal tone, the rotator cuff can no longer maintain the integrity of the GH joint. These conditions contribute to a subluxating GH joint with a stretched and weakened joint capsule. Passive ROM at this stage can cause further subluxation, capsular stretch, and rotator cuff tears.[37(pp201,202),61(p54)]

During the spastic stage, the pectoralis major and minor, rhomboids, levator scapulae, and latissimus dorsi can become hypertonic, further rotating the scapula downward. The subscapularis also can be a site of increased tone and can cause the humerus to be in a state of internal rotation, which can lead to impingement syndrome or frozen shoulder.[37(p203),61(pp55,56)]

The above discussion on the pathomechanics of the flaccid and spastic stages after a CVA presupposes that the paralysis is the cause of the shoulder dysfunction. It is of course entirely possible that a degree of shoulder impingement or arthritis existed prior to the CVA and that the paralysis merely exacerbated an underlying condition. No clear-cut explanation yet exists for hemiplegic shoulder pain; but left untreated (or in some cases because of treatment) the condition can develop into frozen shoulder, brachial plexus or peripheral nerve injuries, shoulder-hand syndrome, or thalamic pain.[60(pp1885–1888)]

Treatment of the Hemiplegic Shoulder

The soft tissue management of the hemiplegic shoulder, not the neurological facilitation required to promote "return," is addressed here.

Clearly, the most obvious treatment for the flaccid or spastic shoulder is the most difficult to accomplish—proper positioning of the arm and trunk. To prevent both subluxation and spasticity from occurring or worsening, adequate support for the arm is essential. If the patient is ambulating, the affected arm must be supported manually by the therapist in the antispasticity position of ER or, if necessary, with a sling. Taping the GH joint to maintain correct alignment is proving beneficial during the first three weeks after the stroke. Functional electrical stimulation over the supraspinatus has also been helpful in maintaining GH joint integrity.[62(p73)] When the patient is seated, the arm can be supported on a table, on a lapboard, by an overhead sling, or on pillows. The difficulty in maintaining proper positioning generally

comes from the inability of the rest of the rehabilitation team and family members to follow through with proper positioning. Well-meaning staff, friends, and family can inadvertently "yank" on the affected extremity while trying to help the patient.

Another cause of shoulder pain results from improperly administered passive exercise leading to an impingement syndrome.[60(p1888)] Simply bringing the arm through full range without regard for scapular position is destined to tear an already stretched and weakened rotator cuff. SHR must be maintained passively during ROM activities. For this reason, using pulleys on a flaccid upper extremity is absolutely contraindicated. Although untrained staff or family should not perform passive ROM, the patient can easily be taught to range the affected shoulder independently and safely.

If the prophylactic measures above do not prevent the onset of hemiplegic shoulder pain, the following conservative treatment program may be helpful:

- modalities: heat, cold, TENS
- active exercise to GH and ST joints, including weight-bearing exercise
- gentle stretching of the internal rotators if tight
- manual compression of the humerus into the glenoid
- aggressive management of hand edema [60(p1890)]

THE SHOULDER IN SPORTS

The geriatric athlete needs additional sport-specific training in order to prevent soft tissue injury upon return to sport. Two sports favored by the geriatric population, swimming and golf, involve extensive use of the upper extremities.

Swimming

Swimmers often complain of shoulder pain that is usually due to impingement syndrome. Primary impingement in the suprahumeral space occurs during the recovery phase of the free-style stroke (when the arm is out of the water). It is usually caused by fatigue of the external rotators and scapular stabilizers. The external rotators should have at least 50% of the endurance of the internal rotators. If the endurance falls below 50%, the patient is much more prone to impingement syndrome. Mechanical impingement due to positioning of the GH joint in adduction and IR occurs mostly during the mid pull-through phase of the free-style stroke (when the hand is in the water)[63(p311)]; therefore, biceps training is also important to the swimmer, as the long head is one of the prime movers during this phase.[64(pp115–121)] A prophylactic program for the geriatric swimmer includes:

- out-of-water strength and endurance training for the entire rotator cuff (Figure 12–15) and scapular stabilizers (Figures 12–13 and 12–17) with low weights and high repetitions
- stretching of the posterior capsule (Figure 12–14)
- stretching of the pectoralis major and minor, upper trapezius, levator scapulae, biceps, and triceps muscles

- proprioception retraining (Figure 12–2)
- SHR retraining including combined movement patterns
- functional retraining, including stroke simulation[63(pp315,316),65(p220)]

Golf

Golf is one of the few sports that involve bilateral low-level deltoid activity and high-level rotator cuff activity. Also, unlike most sports, golf does not require the shoulder to have full ROM in order to play. With the exception of the follow-through phase, after the ball has been hit, the shoulder need not elevate beyond 90°, which is probably why so many older persons are able to enjoy it. Postural alignment is also an important aspect of the proper golf swing. The conditioning program therefore concentrates on resisted rotator cuff exercises within the limited ROM needed for the sport, postural awareness, trunk rotation exercises, and a gradual return to golfing.[66(p1911),67(pp44,45)]

With healthier aging, many elders are continuing to enjoy a variety of sports into their eighth and ninth decades. These more-informed consumers of health care will no longer be satisfied with "giving up" the activities they love (and that keep them "young"). More will be seeking out physical therapy to return them to function following a sport-related injury.

DOCUMENTATION TIPS: DEMONSTRATING SKILL

Therapists are constantly asked (by third-party payers) to demonstrate that they are providing a skilled service to their patients. Many denials of payment are based on the lack of skilled treatment perceived by the insurance reviewer. Documenting skilled care does not involve long, copious notes, which no one wants to write (or read for that matter). To illustrate, a sample objective portion of a progress note written for a

continues

DOCUMENTATION TIPS: continued

patient with impingement syndrome is shown below. The words shown in italics are the brief descriptors that need to be added to the progress note in order to demonstrate skilled care. (They do not have to be included in every progress note written, but should be included at least once a week.) The assessment portion should briefly recap the patient's progress and deliver the therapist's professional opinion as to the efficacy of the treatment plan.

S- "My arm is hurting less, especially when I put on my sweater. But I still can't do what I want. Even driving hurts."

O- Alternating isometrics at 90° with yellow Theraband™ *for GH proprioception*
Modified push-ups and rowing exercises *to enhance proximal stability*
Patient instructed in independent posterior capsule stretch
Begin Sahrmann lower trap exercise *to promote muscle balancing*
Visual feedback needed in mirror *for control of scapulohumeral rhythm* as patient continues to be upper trap dominant
5 min ice massage *to control pain and inflammation*
Patient given (enclosed) home program

A- Patient showing steady improvement with decreased shoulder pain, but ADL still painful. More work needed in motor control to restore SHR, before strengthening can be truly effective.

P- Continue independent home program. Progress program next week.

The note written above is not by any means "the perfect progress note," but it is a good note that conveys skilled care and can realistically be written under prevailing time constraints. In addition to the small descriptors mentioned, the note should also include short-term treatment goals. This is covered in the Documentation Tips section at the end of Chapter 10.

REFERENCES

1. Warren RF, O'Brien SJ. Shoulder pain in the geriatric patient, part 1: evaluation and pathophysiology. *Orthop Rev.* January 1989;18:129–135.

2. Haig SV. *Shoulder Pathophysiology: Rehabilitation and Treatment.* Gaithersburg, MD: Aspen Publishers, Inc; 1996.

3. Koval KJ, Gallagher MA, Mariscano JG, et al. Functional outcome after minimally displaced fractures of the proximal part of the humerus. *J Bone Joint Surg.* 1997;79-A:203–207.

4. Cornell CN, Schneider K. Proximal humerus. In: Koval KJ, Zuckerman JD, eds. *Fractures in the Elderly.* Philadelphia: Lippincott-Raven Publishers; 1998.

5. Wallace WA, Bunker TD. Management of proximal humeral fractures. In: Bunker TD, Colton CL, Webb JK, eds. *Frontiers in Fracture Management.* Gaithersburg, MD: Aspen Publishers, Inc; 1989: 107–120.

6. Jaaberg H, Warner JJP, Jakob RP. Percutaneous stabilization of unstable fractures of the humerus. *J Bone Joint Surg.* 1992;74-A(4):508–515.

7. Esser RD. Open reduction and internal fixation of three and four part fractures of the proximal humerus. *Clin Orthop.* 1994;299:244–251.

8. Szyskowitz R, Seggl W, Schleifer P, Cundy PJ. Proximal humeral fractures: management techniques and expected results. *Clin Orthop.* 1993;292: 13–25.

9. Malone TR, Richmond GW, Frick JL. Shoulder pathology. In: Kelley MJ, Clark WA, eds. *Orthopedic Therapy of the Shoulder.* Philadelphia: Lippincott-Raven Publishers; 1995.

10. Georgiadis GM, Behrens FF. Humeral shaft. In: Koval KJ, Zuckerman JD, eds. *Fractures in the Elderly.* Philadelphia: Lippincott-Raven Publishers; 1998.

11. Klestil T, Rangger C, Kathrein A, Brenner E, Beck E. Conservative and surgical treatment of humeral shaft fractures. *Chirurg.* 1997;68(11):1132–1136.

12. Wallny T, Westermann K, Sagebiel C, Reimer M, Wagner UA. Functional treatment of humeral shaft fractures—indications and results. *J Orthop Trauma.* 1997;11(4):283–287.

13. Cyriax J. *Textbook of Orthopaedic Medicine. Diagnosis of Soft Tissue Lesions.* 7th ed. London: Bailliere Tindall: 1978.

14. Cibulka MT, Hunter HC. Acromioclavicular joint arthritis treated by mobilizing the glenohumeral joint. *Phys Ther.* October 1985;65:1514–1516.

15. Gibson KR. Rheumatoid arthritis of the shoulder. *Phys Ther.* December 1986;66:1920–1929.

16. Sculco TP, ed. *Orthopaedic Care of the Geriatric Patient.* St Louis: CV Mosby Co; 1985.

17. Wirth MA, Rockwood CA. Complications of shoulder arthoplasty. *Clin Orthop.* 1994;307:47–69.

18. Craig EV. Shoulder arthroplasty. In: Scott WN, Stillwell WT, eds. *Arthroplasty: An Atlas of Surgical Technique.* Gaithersburg, MD: Aspen Publishers, Inc; 1987:1–28.

19. Thomas BJ, Amstutz HC, Cracchiolo A. Shoulder arthroplasty for rheumatoid arthritis. *Clin Orthop.* 1991;265:125–128.

20. Brostrom LA, Wallensten R, Olsson E, Anderson D. The Kessel prosthesis in total shoulder arthroplasty. *Clin Orthop.* 1992;277:155–160.

21. Severt R, Thomas BJ, Tsenter MJ, Amstutz HC, Kabo JM. The influence of conformity and constraint on translational forces and frictional torque in total shoulder arthroplasty. *Clin Orthop.* 1993;292:151–158.

22. Watson KC. Total Shoulder replacement. In: Paulos LE, Tibone JE, eds. *Operative Techniques in Shoulder Surgery.* Gaithersburg, MD: Aspen Publishers, Inc; 1991.

23. Hughes M, Neer C II. Glenohumeral joint replacement and postoperative rehabilitation. *Phys Ther.* August 1975;55:850–858.

24. Warren RF, O'Brien SJ. Shoulder pain in the geriatric patient, part II: treatment options. *Orthop Rev.* February 1989;18:248–263.

25. Dines DM, Warren RF. Modular shoulder hemi-arthoplasty for acute fractures. *Clin Orthop.* 1994;307:18–26.

26. Brems JJ. Rehabilitation following total shoulder arthroplasty. *Clin Orthop.* 1994;307:70–85.

27. Brenner BC, Ferlic DC, Clayton ML, Dennis DA. Survivorship of unconstrained total shoulder arthroplasty. *J Bone Joint Surg Am.* October 1989; 71-A:1289–1296.

28. Holpit LA. Preoperative and postoperative physical therapy for the total shoulder, hip, and knee replacement patient. *Orthop Phys Ther Clin N Am.* 1993;2(1):97–118.

29. Norris BL, Lachiewicz. Modern cement technique and survivorship of total shoulder arthroplasty. *Clin Orthop.* 1996;328:76–85.

30. Friedman RJ, Thornhill TS, Thomas WH, Sledge CB. Non-constrained total shoulder replacement in patients who have rheumatoid arthritis and class-IV function. *J Bone Joint Surg Am.* April 1989;71-A:491–496.

31. Kendall FP, McCreary EK, Provance PG. *Muscles: Testing and Function.* 4th ed. Baltimore: Williams & Wilkins; 1993.

32. Culham E, Peat M. Functional anatomy of the shoulder complex. *J Orthop Sports Phys Ther.* 1993; 18(1):342–350.

33. Harrison AL, Barry-Greb T, Wojtowicz G. Clinical measurement of head and shoulder posture variables. *J Orthop Sports Phys Ther.* 1996;23(6): 353–361.

34. Cantu RI, Grodin AJ. *Myofascial Manipulation. Theory and Clinical Application.* Gaithersburg, MD: Aspen Publishers, Inc; 1992.

35. Greenfield B, Catlin PA, Coats PW, Green E, et al. Posture in patients with shoulder overuse injuries and healthy individuals. *J Orthop Sports Phys Ther.* 1995;21(5):287–295.

36. McConnell J. The McConnell Approach to the Problem Shoulder. Course Notes. Marina Del Rey, California: McConnell Institute; 1994.

37. Cailliet R. *Shoulder Pain.* 3rd ed. Philadelphia: FA Davis Co; 1991.

38. Soslowsky LJ, An CH, Johnston SP, Carpenter JE. Geometric and mechanical properties of the coracoacromial ligament and the relationship to rotator cuff disease. *Clin Orthop.* 1994;304:10–17.

39. Burns WC, Whipple TL. Anatomic relationships in the shoulder impingement syndrome. *Clin Orthop.* 1993;294:96–102.

40. Oxner KG. Magnetic resonance imaging of the musculoskeletal system. Part 6—the shoulder. *Clin Orthop.* 1997;334:354–373.

41. Corso G. Impingement relief test: an adjunctive procedure to traditional assessment of shoulder impingement syndrome. *J Orthop Sports Phys Ther.* 1995;22(5):183–192.

42. Frieman BG, Albert TJ, Fenlin JM. Rotator cuff disease: a review of diagnosis, pathophysiology, and current trends in treatment. *Arch Phys Med Rehabil.* 1994;75(5):604–609.

43. Warner JJ, Micheli LJ, Arslanian LE, Kennedy J, Kennedy R. Scapulothoracic motion in normal shoulders and shoulders with glenohumeral instability and impingement syndrome. *Clin Orthop.* 1992;285:191–199.

44. Neer CS. Impingement lesions. *Clin Orthop.* 1983;173:70–77.

45. Boissonnault WG, Janos SC. Dysfunctions, evaluation and treatment of the shoulder. In: Donatelli R, Wooden MJ, eds. *Orthopaedic Physical Therapy.* New York: Churchill Livingstone Inc; 1989:151–172.

46. Kamkar A, Irrgang JJ, Whitney SL. Nonoperative management of secondary shoulder impingement syndrome. *J Orthop Sports Phys Ther.* 1993; 17(5):212–224.

47. Thein LA. Impingement syndrome and its conservative management. *J Orthop Sports Phys Ther.* November 1989;11:183–191.

48. Host HH. Scapular taping in the treatment of anterior shoulder impingement. *Phys Ther.* 1995;75(9): 803–812.

49. Warner JJ, Krushell RJ, Masquelet A, Gerber C. Anatomy and relationships of the suprascapular nerve: anatomical constraints to mobilization of the supraspinatus and infraspinatus muscles in the management of massive rotator cuff tears. *J Bone Joint Surg.* 1992;74-A(1):36–45.

50. Kracht JJ. Rehabilitation of the postoperative shoulder. A basis for early mobilization. *Orthop Phys Ther Clin N Am.* 1993;2(2):149–159.

51. Wainner RS. Management of acute calcific tendinitis of the shoulder. *J Orthop Sports Phys Ther.* 1998;27(3):231–237.

52. Wadsworth CT. Frozen shoulder. *Phys Ther.* December 1986;66:1878–1883.

53. Ozaki J, Nakagawa Y, Sakurai G, Tamai S. Recalcitrant chronic adhesive capsulitis of the shoulder. *J Bone Joint Surg Am.* December 1989;71-A: 1511–1515.

54. Biundo JJ. Frozen shoulder. *Bull Rheum Dis.* 1994;43(8):1–3.

55. Shaffer B, Tibone JE, Kerlan RK. Frozen shoulder. A long-term follow-up. *J Bone Joint Surg.* 1992; 74-A(5):738–746.

56. Mao CY, Jaw WC, Cheng HC. Frozen shoulder: correlation between the response to physical therapy and follow-up shoulder arthrography. *Arch Phys Med Rehabil.* 1997;78:857–859.

57. Pollock RG, Duralde XA, Flatow EL, Bigliani LU. The use of arthroscopy in the treatment of resistant frozen shoulder. *Clin Orthop.* 1994;304:30–36.

58. Rixk TE, Gavant ML, Pinals RS. Treatment of adhesive capsulitis (frozen shoulder) with arthrographic capsular distension and rupture. *Arch Phys Med Rehabil.* 1994;75(7):803–807.

59. Ekelund AL, Rydell N. Combination treatment for adhesive capsulitis of the shoulder. *Clin Orthop.* 1992;282:105–109.

60. Griffen JW. Hemiplegic shoulder pain. *Phys Ther.* December 1986;66:1884–1893.

61. Cailliet R. The painful shoulder in hemiplegia. *Top Geriatr Rehabil.* July 1987;2:52–58.

62. Faghri PD, Rodger MM, Glaser RM, et al. The effects of functional electrical stimulation on shoulder subluxation, arm function recovery, and shoulder pain in hemiplegic stroke patients. *Arch Phys Med Rehabil.* 1994;75(1):73–79.

63. Allegrucci M, Whitney SL, Irrgang JJ. Clinical implications of secondary impingement of the shoulder in freestyle swimmers. *J Orthop Sports Phys Ther.* 1994;20(6):307–318.

64. Falkel JE, Murphy TC. Shoulder injuries. *Sports Inj Management.* June 1988;1:109–125.

65. Allegrucci M, Whitney SL, Lephart SM, Irrgang JJ, Fu FH. Shoulder kinesthesia in healthy unilateral athletes participating in upper extremity sports. *J Orthop Sports Phys Ther.* 1995;21(4):220–226.

66. Moynes DR, Perry J, Antonelli DJ, Jobe FW. Electromyography and motion analysis of the upper extremity in sports. *Phys Ther.* December 1986;66: 1905–1911.

67. Sobel J. The shoulder in the older athlete. *Top Geriatr Rehabil.* 1991;6(4):34–46.

SUGGESTED READING

Cyriax J. *Textbook of Orthopaedic Medicine.* Diagnosis of Soft Tissue Lesions. 7th ed. London: Bailliere Tindall; 1978;1.

13

The Elbow Joint

The elbow helps to place the hand in position for skilled activities, as well as provide stability to allow forceful movements of the hand. It is extremely resilient to the effects of time, with very little change occurring with age.

ANATOMY OF THE ELBOW JOINT

The elbow complex, also called the cubital articulation, is made up of three distinct joints: the humeroulnar, the humeroradial, and the superior radioulnar joints. All three joints create a compound synovial joint with 2 degrees of freedom, allowing the motions of flexion/extension and rotation to occur.[1(p247)]

The humeroulnar joint consists of the trochlear surface of the humerus and the trochlear notch of the ulna (Figure 13-1). Both the trochlea and the trochlear notch are angulated 45° anteriorly, resulting in an increased ability to flex the elbow.[2(p200)] Because the articulating surfaces are not completely congruent, they form a modified hinge joint that primarily provides flexion and extension, as well as tiny amounts of conjunct rotation at the extremes of range.[3(p429)] As a whole, the humeroulnar joint is one of the most stable joints in the body, with the olecranon process of the ulna locking into the olecranon fossa of the humerus during extension and the coronoid process of the ulna mating with the coronoid fossa of the humerus during flexion.[4(p280)]

The humeroradial joint is the articulation of the capitulum of the humerus and the head of the radius (Figure 13-1). It is a uniaxial joint that acts both as a hinge, during flexion and extension with the humeroulnar joint; and as a pivot, during longitudinal rotations of the forearm.[3(p429),4(p280)]

The superior radioulnar joint is comprised of the medial rim of the radial head and the concave radial notch of the ulna (Figure 13-1). It is a uniaxial joint that produces the rotations of pronation and supination in conjunction with the inferior radioulnar joint. Most of the motion occurs at the radius, with the ulna remaining relatively stationary.[4(p281)]

Ligaments

The entire cubital articulation is encased by one joint capsule. It is broad and thin anteriorly and thin posteriorly where it blends with the tendons of the triceps and anconeus.[3(p429)] Like all hinge joints, the elbow complex is stabilized by two strong collateral ligaments.

The ulnar collateral ligament (UCL) is on the medial side of the joint and consists of

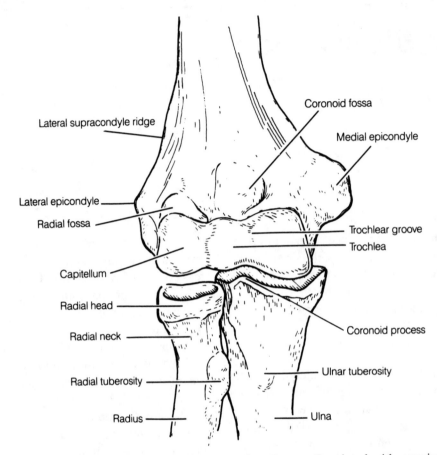

Lateral supracondyle ridge

Lateral epicondyle

Radial fossa

Capitellum

Radial head

Radial neck

Radial tuberosity

Radius

Coronoid fossa

Medial epicondyle

Trochlear groove

Trochlea

Coronoid process

Ulnar tuberosity

Ulna

Figure 13–1 The osseous anatomy of the elbow complex. *Source:* Reprinted with permission from M. Stroyan, K.E. Wilk, "The Functional Anatomy of the Elbow Complex," *Journal of Orthopaedic and Sports Physical Therapy*, Vol. 17, No. 6, p. 280, © 1993, Williams & Wilkins.

three parts: the anterior bundle, the posterior bundle, and the transverse ligament[3(p430)] (Figure 13–2). The anterior bundle is the strongest ligament at the elbow and controls the entire range of motion (ROM).[5(p170)] It is also the primary constraint to valgus stress. Damage to this structure leads to a major instability of the elbow joint.[6(p187),7(p67)] The posterior bundle of the UCL is taut in flexion.[5(p170)] The transverse ligament is not well developed.[2(p202)]

The radial collateral ligament, on the lateral aspect of the joint, blends with the origins of the supinator and extensor carpi radialis brevis muscles.[3(p430)] It extends from the lateral epicondyle to the annular ligament. It is taut throughout range, but is much weaker than the anterior bundle of the UCL.

The annular ligament encircles the head of the radius, keeping it in contact with the radial notch. On its internal surface is a thin layer of cartilage, where it meets the radial head. The ligament maintains the stability of the superior radioulnar joint during pronation and supination.[3(p432)]

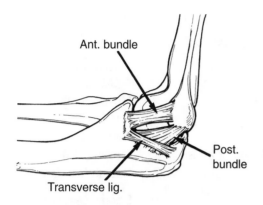

Ant. bundle

Post. bundle

Transverse lig.

Figure 13–2 Drawing of the medial view of the right elbow, showing the ulnar collateral-ligament complex. *Source:* Reprinted with permission from J.E. Conway, et al., "Medial Instability of the Elbow in Throwing Athletes," *Journal of Bone and Joint Surgery,* Vol. 74-A, No. 1, p. 67, © 1992, The Journal of Bone and Joint Surgery, Inc.

Muscles and Motion

Both the humeroulnar and humeroradial joints allow approximately 0 to 140° of extension to flexion at the elbow complex.[8(p251)] With the elbow full extended and the forearm fully supinated, a valgus angulation of 10 to 17° occurs between the humerus and the ulna. This "carrying angle" prevents the arm from contacting the thigh and is generally greater in women than in men. The valgus angulation is caused by the medial edge of the trochlear projecting 6 mm below the lateral edge and the obliquity of the superior articulating surface of the coronoid process in relation to the ulna.[3(p430)]

Pronation and supination occur primarily at the humeroradial and superior radioulnar joints. The axis of rotation does not remain stationary and is dependent on the actual curvature of the radial head. In general, the average amount of pronation available is 70° and the average amount of supination is 85°.[8(p252)]

To perform activities of daily living (ADL), only 70% of normal ROM is required at the elbow complex, assuming surrounding joints have normal motion. Most functional activities can be performed with 30 to 130° of flexion and 50° of both pronation and supination.[9(pp873,874)] If this motion is unavailable, the shoulder, wrist, and spine can usually provide compensatory motion to complete most functional tasks.

Depending on elbow and forearm positions, different muscles alternate as the primary versus secondary movers and stabilizers. During flexion, the brachialis muscle acts regardless of forearm position, whereas the biceps fires primarily when the forearm is supinated or in neutral position. In addition, the brachioradialis is most effective in midpronation and is recruited for speed work.[3(p431),8(p254)] During extension, the middle head of the triceps is the prime mover, with the lateral and long heads recruited for extra power.[10(p37)] The anconeus muscle also assists in extension and is a major elbow stabilizer during hand and wrist motions.[8(p255)] During pronation, the pronator quadratus is the primary mover, regardless of elbow or forearm position. The pronator teres assists in rapid movements or against resistance. Slow, unresisted supination is provided by the supinator. The biceps is recruited during fast movements or against resistance.[8(pp256,434)] (See Table 13–1 for muscle actions and innervations.)

Innervation and Blood Supply

The elbow complex is innervated mostly by the musculocutaneous, median, and radial nerves. (See Table 13–1 for muscle actions and innervations.) Compression of these nerves can cause both sensory and motor impairments. The musculocutaneus nerve arises from the lateral cord of the

Table 13–1 Motions, Muscles, and Innervations of the Cubital Articulation

Motion*	Primary Muscles	Secondary Muscles	Innervation
Elbow Flexion 0°–140°	Brachialis		Musculocutaneus: C-5, C-6
	Biceps brachii		Musculocutaneus: C-5, C-6
	Brachioradialis		Radial: C-5, C-6
		Pronator teres	Median: C-6, C-7
		Flexor carpi radialis	Radial: C-6, C-7
Elbow Extension 0°	Triceps		Radial: C-7, C-8
		Anconeus	Radial: C-7, C-8
Forearm Supination 0°–85°	Supinator		Radial: C-6
	Biceps brachii		Musculocutaneus: C-5, C-6
Forearm Pronation 0°–70°	Pronator quadratus		Anterior interosseous branch of median: C-8, T-1
	Pronator teres		Median: C-6, C-7

Sources: Gray's Anatomy, ed 35 (pp 431–434) by R Warwick and PL Williams (eds), Churchill Livingstone Inc, © 1973; *Basic Biomechanics of the Musculoskeletal System, 2nd ed (pp 251–252), M Nordin, V Frankel (eds), Lea & Febiger, © 1989.

brachial plexus and can become entrapped between the biceps tendon and the brachialis fascia when the elbow is extended and pronated. The median nerve originates from the lateral and medial cords of the brachial plexus and can be compressed between the heads of the pronator teres with highly repetitive pronation movements. The radial nerve comes off the posterior cord of the brachial plexus and can become entrapped with repetitive pronation and supination (e.g., during racquet sports).[4(pp283,284)]

The brachial artery is the continuation of the axillary artery and is easily palpated at the medial humerus. It divides into the radial and ulnar arteries one centimeter below the elbow joint. Its many branches (arteria profunda brachii, main nutrient artery, superior and inferior ulnar collateral, and muscular branches) supply nutrients to the elbow and forearm complex.[3(pp649,650)]

KINETICS OF THE ELBOW COMPLEX

Until recently, the elbow complex has been considered a non-weight bearing joint; however, simply flexing the elbow causes a compression force to occur at the elbow. Holding a 1-kg weight in the hand while flexing the elbow increases that joint reaction force by 2.5 times.[8(p258)] The closer the weight is held to the elbow joint, the less compressive forces. For example, carrying a purse at the crook of the elbow rather than at the wrist reduces the joint reaction force by two-thirds and decreases the work done by the biceps muscle by one-half. This is in keeping with the principle of joint protection to place any load as close as possible to the affected joint.[11(pp135,136)]

During dressing and eating activities, the joint reaction forces at the elbow are approximately one-half the body weight. Activities, such as getting out of a chair by pushing up with one's arms, can generate joint reaction forces of more than double the body weight.[8(p258)] The therapist must keep these forces in mind when designing an exercise or functional program for patients with injured elbow joints.

SUMMARY

- The elbow complex or cubital articulation is made up of three joints:
  1. the humeroulnar joint
  2. the humeroradial joint
  3. the superior radioulnar joint.

- Elbow flexion and extension of 0 to 140° occurs at the humeroulnar and humeroradial joints.

- Forearm supination of 85° and pronation of 70° occurs at the humeroradial and superior radioulnar joints (in conjunction with the inferior radioulnar joint).

- Functional ROM at the elbow complex consists of 30 to 130° of flexion/extension and 50° of both pronation and supination.

- The anterior bundle of the UCL is the strongest ligament at the elbow and helps control valgus stress throughout range.

- The elbow complex is innervated mostly by the musculocutaneous, median, and radial nerves.

- Large compression forces of more than double the body weight occur at the elbow joint during many ADL.

REFERENCES

1. Magee DJ. *Orthopaedic Physical Assessment.* 3rd ed. Philadelphia: WB Saunders Company; 1997.

2. Winkel D. *Diagnosis and Treatment of the Upper Extremities.* Gaithersburg, MD: Aspen Publishers, Inc; 1997.

3. Warwick R, Williams PL, eds. *Gray's Anatomy.* 35th ed. Edinburgh, Scotland: Churchill Livingstone; 1973.

4. Stroyan M, Wilk KE. The functional anatomy of the elbow complex. *J Orthop Sports Phys Ther.* 1993; 17(6):279–288.

5. Regan WD, Korinek SL, Morrey BF, An KN. Biomechanical study of ligaments around the elbow joint. *Clin Orthop.* 1991;271:170–179.

6. Morrey BF, Tanaka S, An KN. Valgus stability of the elbow: a definition of primary and secondary constraints. *Clin Orthop.* 1991;265: 187–195.

7. Conway JE, Jobe FW, Glousman RE, Pink M. Medial instability of the elbow in throwing athletes. *J Bone Joint Surg.* 1992;74-A(1):67–83.

8. Zuckerman JD, Matsen FA. Biomechanics of the elbow. In: Nordin M, Frankel VH, eds. *Basic Biomechanics of the Musculoskeletal System.* 2nd ed. Philadelphia: Lea & Febiger; 1989.

9. Morrey BF, Askew L, An KN, Chao EY. A biomechanical study of normal functional elbow motion. *J Bone Joint Surg.* 1981;63-A:872–877.

10. Netter FH. The CIBA Collection of Medical Illustrations. Vol. 8, Musculoskeletal System. *Part I: Anatomy, Physiology, and Metabolic Disorders.* Summit, NJ: CIBA-GEIGY Corporation; 1987.

11. Roberts SL, Falkenburg SA. *Biomechanics: Problem Solving for Functional Activity.* St Louis: Mosby-Year Book; 1992.

14

Treatment of Common Problems of the Elbow

The elbow complex serves two purposes. It helps to position the hand and assists in carrying loads.[1(p107)] Normal function of this joint is taken for granted throughout the thousands of upper extremity tasks performed daily. When the elbow is injured, however, even the simplest activities, such as lifting a glass of water, become excruciatingly painful or impossible to perform.

ELBOW FRACTURES

Most elbow fractures in the elderly occur from low-energy falls. The incidence of this type of fracture actually decreases with increasing age.[1(p108)] The complication rate following elbow fracture is higher than with most other joints. The primary complication in adults is loss of motion and stiffness. Other common complications include heterotopic ossification and neurovascular compromise.[2(pp40,44)]

Distal Humeral Fracture

Fractures of the distal humerus account for about 1 to 2% of all fractures.[3(p26)] In the elderly population, there is increasing evidence that this injury is osteoporotic in nature. Epidemiological trends indicate that this fracture is increasing at an alarming rate, doubling in the past 25 years.[4(p159)] There are three common types of distal humeral fractures in adults:

1. supracondylar
2. intercondylar
3. articular[5(p2309)]

Depending on the location and stability of the fracture segments, the surgeon can opt for conservative or surgical correction. Supracondylar fractures, which are transverse fractures of the distal one-third of the humerus, are usually treated with a hanging cast or coaptation splint. Neurovascular injuries from this type of fracture include laceration of the brachial artery (which can lead to compartment syndrome), or damage to the radial or median nerves.[5(p2309)]

Intercondylar fractures in the elderly are often highly comminuted with many free-floating articular fragments[1(p118)]; therefore, this injury is extremely difficult to stabilize surgically. Open reduction with rigid fixation (Figure 14–1) has been relatively successful.[3(pp29–31),5(p2312)] Closed reduction using the "bag of bones" technique is used most often in the elderly with good results. This method involves immobilizing the elbow in 90° or more of flexion in a sling for 2 to 3 weeks,

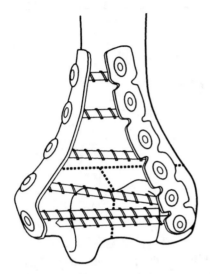

Figure 14–1 One-third tubular plate and reconstruction plate fixation for an intercondylar fracture of the distal humerus. (Fracture site represented by dotted line.) *Source:* Adapted with permission from D.L. Helfert and G.J. Schmeling, "Bicondylar Intraarticular Fractures of the Distal Humerus in Adults," *Clinical Orthopaedics and Related Research,* Vol. 292, p. 31, © 1993, Lippincott-Raven Publishers.

allowing gravity to assist in reducing the fracture fragments.[1(p118),6(p278)]

The most common articular fracture is a shear fracture of the capitellum, which is caused by a fall on the outstretched arm. Because closed reduction is rarely successful, surgery is performed to either remove the fractured fragments or internally stabilize them.[1(p122),5(p2320)]

Treatment of Distal Humeral Fractures

If medical treatment is conservative, the fracture site is immobilized and active range of motion (ROM) exercises usually are allowed at the shoulder, wrist, and hand. After bony union is confirmed, gentle active ROM is allowed at the elbow. Passive stretching, joint mobilization, and resisted motion are

all contraindicated at this time, as they result in periarticular hemorrhage and fibrosis and risk of joint ankylosis.[5(p2317),6(p278)]

After closed reduction, active-assisted ROM to the elbow can begin on Postoperative (PO) Day 5 on doctor's orders.[7(p551)] A splint or sling keeps the fracture site protected between exercise periods during the first 3 weeks after surgery. Once again, although early motion is highly desirable, aggressive physical therapy is contraindicated during early elbow rehabilitation.[5(p2317)] Five years postfracture, Manueddu et al found the average elbow extension/flexion after distal humeral fracture to be 29 to 127°, forearm pronation 68°, and forearm supination 85°. Patients mobilized before PO Day 5 showed significantly greater flexion than those mobilized PO Day 5 or later. They also found a major loss of elbow strength, with extension more adversely affected than flexion.[7(p551)]

Olecranon Fractures

Olecranon fractures are common injuries in adults and are usually the result of a fall with a direct impact on the point of the elbow.[1(p113)] Nondisplaced fractures may be immobilized for 2 to 3 weeks in a splint.[2(p45)] Displaced fractures require open reduction and internal fixation, because the biceps and triceps muscle action pulls the fracture site apart (Figure 14–2). Fixation with tension band wiring (Figure 14–3) counters the muscular traction forces, while allowing early mobilization of the elbow joint.[8(p238),9(p55)] Depending on the severity of the fracture, screw or plate fixation may also be used.[9(p55),10(p229)]

Treatment of Olecranon Fractures

For nondisplaced fractures or severely comminuted fractures in the elderly, nonoperative management and gentle, active exer-

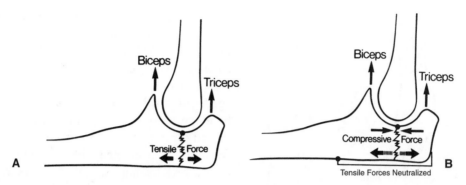

Figure 14–2 (**A**) The forces of an olecranon fracture. (**B**) The forces of an olecranon fracture after adding a tension band wire. *Source:* Reprinted from G. Horne, "Olecranon Fractures: Classification and Techniques of Internal Fixation," *Techniques in Orthopaedics*, Vol. 1, No. 1, p. 56, © 1986, Aspen Publishers, Inc.

cise initiated within 10 days of fracture, have proven a successful combination[1(p113)]; however, full elbow extension and strength do not generally occur.

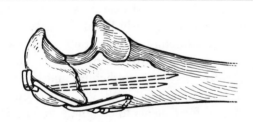

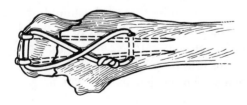

Figure 14–3 Tension band wiring of an olecranon fracture. *Source:* Adapted with permission of S.A. Rowland and S.S. Burkhart, "Tension Band Wiring of Olecranon Fractures," *Clinical Orthopaedics and Related Research*, Vol. 277, p. 238, © 1992, Lippincott-Raven Publishers.

The key to a good result following olecranon fractures is early stabilization (i.e., within 72 hours of injury)[11(p46)] and early mobilization within one week of surgery.[8(p238)] The arm is usually placed in a posterior splint with the elbow maintained at 90°.[5(p2325)] On PO Days 5 to 7, the splint is removed for exercise and gentle active flexion and extension begins. Emphasis should be on regaining extension, which is often lost after an olecranon fracture.[9(pp57,58)] Pronation and supination are rarely limited. The splint can be removed approximately 1 month after surgery. Functional return is usually predicated on the amount of articular involvement. Strengthening exercises can begin around PO Week 8. Optimal ROM, strength, and function occur approximately 6 to 12 months following surgery.[5(p2326)]

Radial Head Fractures

Radial head fractures are almost always the result of a fall onto an outstretched hand. There are three types of radial head fracture (Figure 14–4) according to the Mason classification:

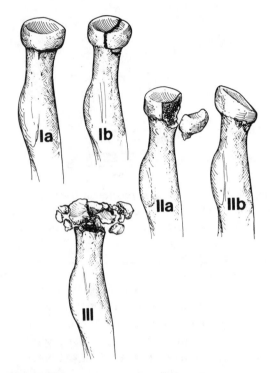

Figure 14–4 Patterns of radial head fracture: I, nondisplaced fractures; Ia, radial neck fracture with minimal angulation or impaction; Ib, vertical shear fracture with less than 2 mm of incongruity; II, displaced/impacted fractures; IIa, vertical shear fracture with greater than 2 mm displacement; IIb, radial neck fracture with marked angulation or impaction; III, comminuted fracture. *Source:* Reprinted with permission from P.A. Davidson et al., "Radial Head Fracture," *Clinical Orthopaedics and Related Research*, Vol. 297, p. 227, © 1993, Lippincott-Raven Publishers.

1. nondisplaced
2. two-part displaced
3. comminuted[11(p226)]

Nondisplaced fractures are stable, but displaced fractures are associated with medial collateral ligament tears and valgus instability. Other soft tissue injuries may include tears of the interosseous membrane and damage to the triangular fibrocartilage complex.[12(pp224,230)] This fracture can also result in a change in the "carrying angle."

Nondisplaced fractures are usually managed with a splint for 5 to 7 days. An elastic bandage secures the splint and can be removed for icing to control edema. Displaced fractures can be treated with internal fixation (screw or Kirschner wire)[13(p48)] or by resection of the radial head.

Treatment of Radial Head Fractures

For all types of radial head fracture, controlling edema is important. Because the elbow joint has a small volume capacity, any fluid can greatly limit motion and cause pain.[2(p49)] During early rehabilitation, the affected area should be iced and elevated four to five times a day. After surgery, the posterior splint is usually removed after 1 week and replaced with a sling. Early active and active-assisted ROM exercises can then be started. Although early ROM decreases the risk of contracture, the program progresses gradually. Aggressive therapy, including mobilization, is contraindicated until bony union is confirmed.[5(p2331),13(p935)] It is quite common for patients to complain of pain at the wrist as well, because of the inferior radioulnar articulation. Strengthening and ROM exercises to uninvolved joints, as well as a conditioning program, should be prescribed as needed. Although ROM, strength, and functional gains continue for up to 6 months following injury, many patients never regain full pronation and supination.

Summary of Treatment of Elbow Fractures

- Early mobilization is associated with better ROM and function.

- Aggressive therapy is associated with decreased ROM and contractures.
- Edema control is important because of the small volume capacity of the elbow joint.
- Strengthening exercises can begin after bony union is confirmed.
- Strength, ROM, and functional gains continue up to 1 year postinjury.

ARTHRITIS

Degenerative arthritis at the elbow is rare and is usually the result of a previous injury, such as an intra-articular fracture. Passive flexion is more limited than passive extension (i.e., capsular pattern) and forearm rotations tend to be normal. A bony end-feel may be present. The joint space narrows and osteophytes may form. The patient usually complains of a general ache around the elbow. The treatment may consist of a cortisone shot, followed by a week of rest with gradual return to functional activities.[14(pp234–235)] Depending on the severity of symptoms, other treatment options include "no treatment" and total elbow arthroplasty (TEA).

Rheumatoid arthritis at the elbow can cause a painful synovitis, which forces the patient to maintain a flexed elbow posture. In the early stages of the disease, the patient can achieve good pain relief with synovectomy and radial head excision[15(p95)]; however, long-term results are poor, with many patients requiring revision surgery.[16(p918)] As the disease progresses, synovitis, ligamentous instability, loss of ROM, ulnar neuropathy, and joint destruction can occur. Physical therapy consisting of modalities, gentle stretching, strengthening, motor retraining, and functional training provides some pain relief and functional gains. If the pain continues to be unbearable, the surgeon may opt for TEA.

TOTAL ELBOW ARTHROPLASTY

The TEA has been evolving over the past 10 years. In general, TEAs are indicated for patients with rheumatoid arthritis, traumatic arthritis, and for elderly patients with distal humeral fractures.[17(p826)] Initial results from totally constrained arthroplasties in the late 1970s were poor, with high rates of loosening and failure.[18(p177)] Resurfacing devices lessen the rate of loosening, but have problems with instability. Semiconstrained implants are designed to allow for some varus and valgus motion, provide inherent stability, and decrease the rate of loosening.[19(p479)] Morrey and Adams report good to excellent long-term results with their semiconstrained Coonrad TEA. Patients had good pain relief and an average ROM of 20 to 129° of extension to flexion and 77° of both supination and pronation; however, 10% of the patients required additional operations.[19(p479)] Nonconstrained prostheses rely on soft tissues for stability. As a result, they have a lower rate of loosening, but higher rates of dislocation, infection, and ulnar nerve problems.[18(p177)] In general, TEAs provide good satisfaction, but still have unacceptably high rates of complications.

Treatment of Patients with Total Elbow Arthroplasty

The therapist should communicate carefully with the physician regarding the rehabilitation process and any contraindications, as few treatment protocols exist for TEA. In general, the elbow is splinted after surgery. Gentle active ROM for the elbow and forearm begins PO Days 3 to 4. The exercises should be performed every 1 to 2 hours, with the elbow kept in a splint when not exercising. Passive ROM and strengthening exercises can be initiated on doctor's orders, 3 to 8 weeks postoperatively.

EPICONDYLITIS

Overuse injuries at the elbow can occur from repetitive use or misuse of the elbow, forearm, or wrist; however, the actual etiology of the tendinitis that can occur at the medial or lateral epicondyle remains unknown. Some researchers believe that degenerative changes contribute to epicondylitis, but the decreasing incidence in the elderly of this inflammatory process counters that theory.[14(p246),20(p78)] Other proposed causes include radiohumeral bursitis, microtendinous tears, myofasciitis, calcification, radial nerve entrapment, cervical radiculopathy, and inflammation of the annular ligament.[21(p135)]

Lateral Epicondylitis (Tennis Elbow)

Lateral epicondylitis, or tennis elbow, is a lesion of the wrist extensors and the common extensor tendon. The incidence in the general population varies from 1 to 3%, with an exceptionally high incidence of up to 39% in recreational tennis players.[20(p73)] Repetitive use of the wrist extensors while the hand is grasping an object (such as a screwdriver, hammer, or racquet) may cause this injury. There are five types of tennis elbow (Figure 14–5), with injury to the extensor carpi radialis brevis or the extensor digitorum occurring most frequently.[14(pp246,247)]

The signs and symptoms associated with lateral epicondylitis are:

- palpable pain at the lateral epicondyle
- pain on active or resisted wrist extension
- pain with passive wrist flexion with the elbow extended
- pain with grasping

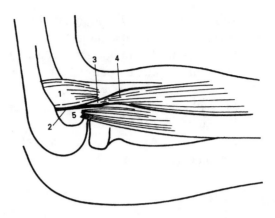

Figure 14–5 The five types of tennis elbow. 1, Origin of the extensor carpi radialis longus; 2, origin of the extensor carpi radialis brevis; 3, tendon of the extensor carpi radialis brevis; 4, muscle belly/musculotendinous junction of the extensor carpi radialis brevis; 5, origin of the extensor digitorum. *Source:* Reprinted from D. Winkel, "Pathology of the Elbow," in *Diagnosis and Treatment of the Upper Extremities*, p. 248, © 1997, Aspen Publishers, Inc.

- pain with activities of daily living (opening a doorknob, brushing teeth, or picking up a cup)
- decreased strength of the wrist extensors[6(p270),14(p249),22(p61),23(p387),24(p64)]

Treatment of Lateral Epicondylitis

The physician may prescribe nonsteroidal anti-inflammatory drugs (NSAIDs) with "active" rest, inject the area with cortisone, order physical therapy, or as a last resort, surgically excise the pathological tissue and repair adjacent tissues. Cortisone injection and surgical intervention remain controversial.[20(p79),22(p62),24(p67),25(p99)]

Physical therapy goals for lateral epicondylitis include:

- decrease pain and inflammation
- identify and correct causal factors

- restore strength and flexibility to wrist extensors
- return patient to function or sport [23(pp387, 388),26(p78)]

The therapist can augment healing by applying modalities to the lateral epicondylar region. In the acute stage, ice, phonophoresis, or iontophoresis help to lessen inflammation and pain. As the pain subsides, heat, ultrasound, and transverse friction massage can increase local circulation, minimize scar formation, and eliminate metabolic waste products. [14(p249),23(p388),27(p23)] Counterforce bracing with a tennis elbow strap diminishes pressure on the injured elbow by creating a "new" origin for the extensor carpi radialis brevis. This "new" muscle origin not only alters the magnitude and direction of the muscle force, but it also effectively bypasses the injured muscle fibers, allowing them to heal. [28(p71)]

The therapist must determine for each patient the underlying factors that increase the risk of tennis elbow. For many patients, decreased strength or flexibility of the wrist extensors predisposes them to develop tennis elbow. Loss of motion at the elbow joint is not compensated for by shoulder or wrist motions, causing excessive stress to be placed at the elbow. [29(p89)] A progressive stretching and strengthening program, as shown in Figure 14–6, must be implemented to restore pain-free function to the patient. Both concentric and eccentric muscle contractions need to be strengthened and low-level endurance needs to be retrained.

Use of poor technique or improperly fitting equipment contributes to this syndrome when playing tennis. If the racquet grip is too large or too small, both the finger flexors and wrist extensors may be overused. If the strings on the racquet are too taut, the vibration transmitted to the elbow and wrist on ball impact may be too great for the soft tissue to absorb. [14(p249),23(p388)] Overpronation during the forehand stroke of an overhead serve may cramp the lateral compartment of the elbow joint. In most instances, correction of these causal factors eliminates the need for more invasive treatment. [30(p182)]

As the symptoms subside, the patient should gradually return to sporting or other functional activities. The above exercise and modification program should be maintained and performed to prevent recurrence. In general, the patient may complain of intermittent symptoms (e.g., painful twinges) when performing various activities, such as opening a jar or lifting an object. These painful reminders tend to last up to one year from original injury.

Medial Epicondylitis

Medial epicondylitis is a lesion of the common tendon of the wrist flexors (flexor carpi radialis and ulnaris) or the pronator teres tendon where they originate on the medial epicondyle. The incidence of medial epicondylitis is much less than lateral epicondylitis, but the symptoms tend to be more acute. Repetitive wrist flexion from sports or vocational activities tends to cause this condition. [14(p245),24(p64)]

The signs and symptoms associated with medial epicondylitis are:

- pain at medial epicondyle, radiating down volar aspect of forearm
- pain on active or resisted wrist flexion (with elbow extended)
- pain on resisted pronation
- pain on passive wrist extension. [6(p271), 14(p246),24(p64)]

Treatment of Medial Epicondylitis

The medical and rehabilitative goals and treatment of medial epicondylitis are very

Elbow Exercise Program

1. Deep Friction Massage:
   Deep transverse friction across area of elbow that is sore. 5 minutes, several times daily. (Not shown)
2. Grip:
   Grip apparatus, putty, small rubber ball, etc. Use as continuously as possible all day long. (Not shown)
3. Stretch Flexors:
   Straighten elbow completely. With palm facing up, grasp the middle of the hand and thumb. Pull wrist down as far as possible. Hold for 10 counts. Release and repeat 5–10 times before and after each exercise session.

4. Stretch Extensors:
   Straighten elbow completely. With palm facing down, grasp the back of the hand and pull wrist down as far as possible. Hold for a 10 count. Release and repeat 5–10 times, before and after each exercise session.

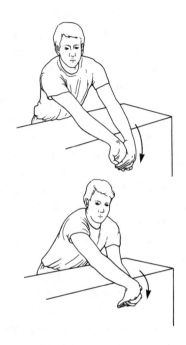

Progressive Resistive Exercises (PRE)
Begin each PRE with 1 set of 10 repetitions without weight, progressing to 5 sets of 10 repetitions as tolerable. When you are able to easily perform 5 sets of 10 repetitions, you may begin adding weight. Begin each PRE with 1 set of 10 repetitions with 1 lb. progressing to 5 sets of 10 as tolerable. When you are able to easily perform 5 sets of 10 repetitions with 1 lb., you may begin to progress your weight in the same manner.

In a preventive maintenance program (excluding specific rotator cuff exercises) it is permissible to advance weight as tolerable with strengthening exercises, taking care to emphasize proper lifting technique.

Figure 14–6 Elbow exercise program. *Source:* Reprinted with permission from Elbow Exercise Program in *Preventive & Rehabilitative Exercises for the Shoulder & Elbow,* © 1997, American Sports Medicine Institute.

continues

Figure 14–6 continued

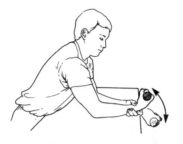

5. Wrist Curls:
   The forearm should be supported on a table with hand off edge; palm should face upward. Using a weight or hammer, lower that hand as far as possible and then curl it up as high as possible. Hold for a 2 count.

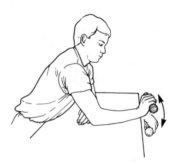

6. Wrist Reverse Curls:
   The forearm should be supported on a table with hand off edge; palm should face downward. Using a weight or hammer, lower the hand as far as possible and then curl wrist up as high as possible. Hold for a 2 count.

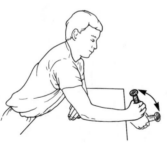

7. Neutral Wrist Curls:
   The forearm should be supported on table with wrist in neutral position and hand off table. Using a weight or hammer held in a normal hammering position, lower wrist into ulnar deviation as far as possible. Then bring into radial deviation as far as possible. Hold for a 2 count. Relax.

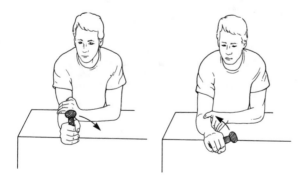

8. Pronation:
   The forearm should be supported on a table with wrist in neutral position. Using a weight or hammer held in a normal hammering position, roll wrist and bring hammer into pronation as far as possible. Hold for a 2 count. Raise back to starting position.

continues

Figure 14–6 continued

9. Supination:
   The forearm should be supported on the table with the wrist in neutral position. Using a weight or hammer held in a normal hammering position, roll wrist bringing hammer into full supination. Hold for a 2 count. Raise back to the starting position.

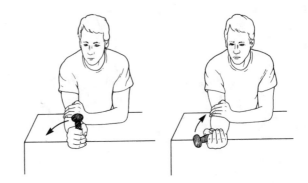

10. Broomstick Curl Up:
    Use 1–2 foot broom handle with a 4–5 foot cord attached in the middle with a 1–5 lb. weight tied in the center.
    A. Extensors:
       Grip the stick on either side of the rope with the palms down. Curl cord up by turning stick toward you (cord is on side of stick away from you). Once the weight is pulled to the top, lower the weight by unwinding the stick, rotating it away from you. Repeat 3–5 times.
    B. Flexors:
       Same as above exercise (Extensors), but have palms facing upward.

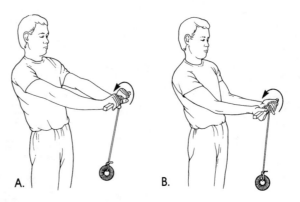

A.   B.

11. Bicep Curl:
    Support arm on opposite hand. Bend elbow to full flexion, then straighten arm completely.

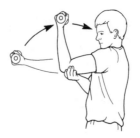

continues

Figure 14–6 continued

12. French Curl:
    Raise arm overhead. Take opposite hand and give support at elbow. Straighten elbow over head, hold for a 2 count.

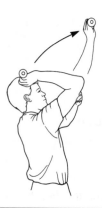

similar to lateral epicondylitis. Oral anti-inflammatories (NSAIDs), rest, and modalities can be used to decrease pain and inflammation. Counterforce bracing can be helpful by creating a "new" muscle origin for the wrist flexors and pronators. (Counterforce bracing will not help if medial epicondylar pain occurs due to valgus instability or ulnar nerve entrapment and can, in fact, worsen these conditions.[28(p78)])

Determining and correcting the cause of the overuse syndrome remain the key to proper treatment. Five sporting activities tend to increase the risk of medial epicondylitis:

1. pitching a baseball: especially throwing a curve ball or screw ball
2. driving a golf ball using an improper technique

DOCUMENTATION TIPS: BUZZWORDS

Sometimes documentation of patient care seems like a pinball game played between the pinball wizard (a.k.a. the therapist) and an inhuman machine (a.k.a. the insurance company.) If the therapist chooses the wrong terminology and writes the "wrong" words, such as "maintained" or "independent," the pinball machine tilts, the patient's benefits expire, and the game ends. So how does the therapist lengthen the game and maybe even get a "free ball?" The answer is through documentation that demonstrates a skilled level of care. (See Documentation Tips in Chapter 12.) Some words are clearly better to use when documenting than others. These

"buzzwords" are supposed to magically convey patient progress to third-party payers and guarantee continued patient benefits. Although this is not necessarily true, a few "buzzwords" and "buzz phrases," as well as "don't use" words and phrases, are presented in Table 14–1.

Buzzwords and phrases should be used to document patient care and patient progress accurately. In and of themselves, they are not a panacea for getting more patient visits (the free ball in pinball) and they are certainly not a substitute for providing skilled care; however, when used properly, they can facilitate reimbursement.

Table 14–1 Buzzwords and Taboo Words for Documenting Skilled Patient Care and Progress

Buzzwords and Buzz Phrases	Taboo Words and Phrases
Strength deficit[†]	Generalized weakness[*]
Acute[*]	Chronic[*]
Evaluated[†]	Monitored[*] or observed[†]
Attention span deficit[†]	Confused[†]
Gait disturbance or deviation[†]	Poor gait[†]
Verbal (or tactile) cues[†]	Reminders[†]
Bed-confined[*]	Stays in bed[*]
Continues to progress[*]	Has progressed[*]
Measurable amount[*] (ie, 20°, 12 sec, etc.)	Scant, little, much, great, etc.[*]
Instructed[†]	Practiced[†]
Balance deficits	Wobbly
Motor control deficits or uncoordination	
Proprioception deficits	
Reddened area[*]	Slightly red[*]
	Independent
	Maintain or maintenance
	No problem[*]
	Within normal limits[*]
Retro-walking	Walking backwards
Agility training	
Open- or closed-chain exercises	

Sources:

*Data from L Phillippi, "The ABCs of Medicare Part A and Part B for Clinicians," p. 9, © MJ Therapy & Associates, Inc, 1991.

†Data from A Baeten, "Documentation Tips," *GeriNotes* (1995;2(3):4), © Section on Geriatrics, American Physical Therapy Association, 1995.

---

3. backstroking in swimming using an improper technique
4. playing excessive racquetball
5. serving in tennis[22(p63),23(p389)]

Each of the above activities increases the use of the wrist flexors or pronators. Patients may need to seek out a specialized coach or professional athlete to correct the improper technique contributing to the injury.

Other causes of medial epicondylitis are decreased strength and flexibility of the wrist flexors. A progressive stretching and strengthening program, as shown in Figure 14–6, must be implemented. As with lateral epicondylitis, emphasis is on a pain-free program with both concentric and eccentric work occurring. Implementation of the conservative program is imperative, because cortisone injections have not been efficacious in treating this problem.[31(p1648)]

Summary of Treatment of Epicondylitis

- use modalities, rest, and counterforce bracing to decrease pain and inflammation

- determine and correct causal factors contributing to epicondylitis
- restore strength and flexibility to the elbow and wrist joints
- return to functional activities gradually

REFERENCES

1. Weirich S, Jupiter J. Elbow. In: Koval K, Zuckerman JD, eds. *Fractures in the Elderly.* Philadelphia: Lippincott-Raven Publishers; 1998.

2. Shapiro MS, Wang JC. Elbow fractures: treating to avoid complications. *Phys Sportsmed.* 1995;23(4):39–50.

3. Helfet DL, Schmeling GJ. Bicondylar intraarticular fractures of the distal humerus in adults. *Clin Orthop.* 1993;292:26–36.

4. Palvanen M, Kannus P, Niemi S, Parkkari J. Secular trends in the osteoporotic fractures of the distal humerus in elderly women. *Eur J Epidem.* 1998; 14(2):159–164.

5. Crenshaw AH. Fractures of the shoulder girdle, arm, and forearm. In: Canale ST, ed. *Campbell's Operative Orthopaedics,* 9th ed., Vol. 3. St Louis: Mosby-Year Book; 1998.

6. Shankman GA. *Fundamental Orthopaedic Management for the Physical Therapist Assistant.* St Louis: Mosby-Year Book; 1997.

7. Manueddu CA, Hoffmeyer P, Haluzicky M, Blanc Y, Borst F. Distal humeral fracture in adult: functional evaluation in 30 patients. *Rev Chirurg Orthop Reparat.* 1997;83(6):551–560.

8. Rowland SA, Burkhart SS. Tension band wiring of olecranon fractures. *Clin Orthop.* 1992;277:238–242.

9. Horne G. Olecranon fractures: classification and techniques of internal fixation. *Techniques Orthopaed.* 1986;1(1):54–58.

10. Hume MC, Wiss DA. Olecranon fractures. A clinical and radiographic comparison of tension band wiring and plate fixation. *Clin Orthop.* 1992;285:229–235.

11. Teasdall R, Savoie F, Hughes JL. Comminuted fractures of the proximal radius and ulna. *Clin Orthop.* 1993;292:37–47.

12. Davidson PA, Mosely B, Tullos HS. Radial head fracture. A potentially complex injury. *Clin Orthop.* 1993;297:224–230.

13. Bradley JB. Elbow injuries. In: Fu FH, Stone DA, eds. *Sports Injuries: Mechanisms, Prevention, Treatment.* Baltimore: Williams & Wilkins; 1994.

14. Winkel D. *Diagnosis and Treatment of the Upper Extremities.* Gaithersburg, MD: Aspen Publishers, Inc; 1997.

15. Ruth JT, Wilde AH. Capitellocondylar total elbow replacement. *J Bone Joint Surg.* 1992;74-A(1):95–100.

16. Gendi NST, Axon JMC, Carr AJ, et al. Synovectomy of the elbow and radial head excision in rheumatoid arthritis: predictive factors and long term outcome. *J Bone Joint Surg.* 1997;79-B(6):918–923.

17. Cobb TK, Morrey BF. Total elbow arthroplasty as primary treatment for distal humeral fractures in elderly patients. *J Bone Joint Surg.* 1997;79-A(6):826–832.

18. Kasten MD, Skinner HB. Total elbow arthroplasty. An 18-year experience. *Clin Orthop.* 1993;290:177–188.

19. Morrey BF, Adams RA. Semiconstrained arthroplasty for the treatment of rheumatoid arthritis of the elbow. *J Bone Joint Surg.* 1992;74-A(4):479–490.

20. Wittenberg RH, Schaal S, Muhr G. Surgical treatment of persistent elbow epicondylitis. *Clin Orthop.* 1992;278:73–79.

21. Lee DG. "Tennis elbow": a manual therapist's perspective. *J Orthop Sports Phys Ther.* 1986;8(3):134–142.

22. Fox GM, Jebson PJL, Orwin JF. Overuse injuries of the elbow. *Phys Sportsmed.* 1995;23(8):58–66.

23. Massie DL, Sager J, Spiker JC. Rehabilitation of the injured elbow. *Orthop Phys Ther Clin N Am.* 1994;3(3):385–401.

24. Hannafin JA, Schelkun PH. How I manage tennis and golfer's elbow. *Phys Sportsmed.* 1996;24(2):63–68.

25. Solveborn SA, Buch F, Mallmin H, Adalberth G. Cortisone injection with anesthetic additives for radial epicondylagia (tennis elbow). *Clin Orthop.* 1995;316:99–105.

26. Andrews JR, Wilk KE, Groh D. Elbow rehabilitation. In: Brotzman SB, ed. *Handbook of Orthopaedic Rehabilitation.* St Louis: Mosby-Year Book; 1996.

27. Demirtas RN, Oner C. The treatment of lateral epicondylitis by iontophoresis of sodium salicylate and sodium diclofenac. *Clin Rehabil.* 1998;12(1):23–29.

28. Harding WG. Use and misuse of the tennis elbow strap. *Phys Sportsmed.* 1992;20(8):65–74.

29. O'Neill OR, Morrey BF, Tanaka S, An KN. Compensatory motion in the upper extremity after elbow arthrodesis. *Clin Orthop.* 1992;281:89–96.

30. Ilfeld FW. Can stroke modification relieve tennis elbow? *Clin Orthop.* 1992;276:182–186.

31. Stahl S, Kaufman T. The efficacy of an injection of steroids for medial epicondylitis. A prospective study of 60 elbows. *J Bone Joint Surg.* 1997;79-A(11): 1648–1652.

15

The Wrist and Hand

The human wrist and hand are so complex that anatomists and researchers are still unclear as to how they interrelate and function. Massive texts have focused on the detailed anatomy and intricate interactions of the 27 bones, overlapping ligaments, intrinsic and extrinsic musculature, and the sensory and motor nerves. A brief and basic review of the wrist and hand anatomy is presented here. The reader is referred to the many hand texts available for more in-depth information.

ANATOMY OF THE WRIST AND HAND

From the forearm to the fingertips lie seven levels of joints:

1. inferior radioulnar joint
2. radiocarpal or wrist joint
3. midcarpal or intracarpal joint
4. carpometacarpal (CMC) joints
5. metacarpophalangeal (MCP) joints
6. proximal interphalangeal (PIP) joints
7. distal interphalangeal (DIP) joints.

The inferior radioulnar joint is the articulation between the head of the ulna and the ulnar notch of the distal radius. A triangular-shaped fibrocartilaginous disc and the ulnocarpal ligament (Figure 15–1) form the trian-gular fibrocartilage complex (TFCC) that binds the distal radius and ulna together.[1(p432),2(p438)] Together with the superior radioulnar joint (see Chapter 13), the motions of pronation and supination occur.

The radiocarpal or wrist joint is the articulation between the concave surface of the radius and the ulnar fibrocartilaginous disc with the convex proximal row of carpal bones: the scaphoid, lunate, and triquetrum (Figure 15–2). Both the distal radius and ulna are mainly comprised of cancellous bone, but the radius has a very thin cortex, which makes it susceptible to fracture. The ulnar articular disc bears 40% of the load and the distal radius bears 60% of the load.[3(p153)] There are five ligaments (Figure 15–1) about this joint:[1(pp435,436),4(p209)]

1. volar radiocarpal ligament
2. volar ulnocarpal ligament
3. dorsal radiocarpal ligament
4. ulnar collateral ligament
5. radial collateral ligament.

The volar (or palmar) ligaments are thick and more highly developed than the dorsal and collateral ligaments. In addition to stabilizing the wrist, these ligaments also induce bony displacement and transmit loads.[5(p262)]

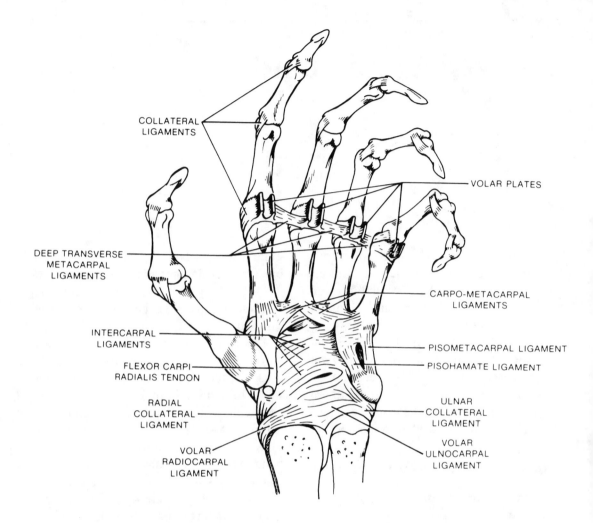

Figure 15–1 Ligaments of the wrist and hand. *Source:* Reprinted with permission from C.T. Wadsworth, "Clinical Anatomy and Mechanics of the Wrist and Hand," *The Journal of Orthopaedic and Sports Physical Therapy*, Vol. 4, No. 4, p. 209, © 1983, Williams & Wilkins.

This joint has two axes of rotation allowing wrist flexion and extension, as well as ulnar and radial deviations to occur.

The midcarpal or intracarpal joint is the articulation between the proximal and distal rows (trapezium, trapezoid, capitate, and hamate) of carpal bones. Short, irregular ligaments connect the two rows on the dorsal, palmar, radial, and ulnar surfaces. This "compound articulation" also contributes to both flexion/extension and ulnar/radial deviations at the wrist.[1(p437)]

The CMC joints of metacarpals 2 through 5 are the articulations between the proximal carpal bones and the metacarpals, forming the base of the "finger rays" of the hand.

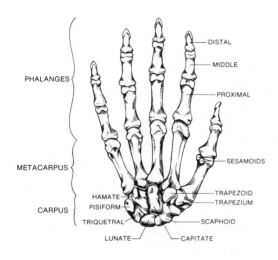

PHALANGES
DISTAL
MIDDLE
PROXIMAL

METACARPUS
SESAMOIDS

HAMATE
PISIFORM
TRAPEZOID
TRAPEZIUM
CARPUS
TRIQUETRAL
SCAPHOID
LUNATE
CAPITATE

Figure 15–2 Hand skeleton. *Source:* Reprinted with permission from C.T. Wadsworth, "Clinical Anatomy and Mechanics of the Wrist and Hand," *The Journal of Orthopaedic and Sports Physical Therapy,* Vol. 4, No. 4, p. 207, © 1983, The Orthopaedic and Sports Physical Therapy Sections of The American Physical Therapy Association.

These planar joints are bound by dorsal and palmar and interosseous ligaments, which allow small gliding movements to occur. The CMC joint of the thumb is a sellar (or saddle-shaped) joint, which connects the first metacarpal bone to the trapezium. Lateral, dorsal, and palmar ligaments also support this joint and are important in the thumb movements of flexion, extension, abduction, adduction, and opposition.[1(pp439,440)]

The MCP joints of metacarpals 2 through 5 are triaxial joints connecting the convex metacarpal heads to the concave phalangeal bases. The joint capsules are reinforced by a dorsal hood apparatus (Figure 15–3) and volar plates (Figure 15–1). The cartilaginous volar plates provide additional stability and prevent hyperextension of the MCP joints. Strong, cord-like collateral ligaments support the joints. They are lax in extension and taut in flexion, when they limit joint abduction and adduction. When contractures form in these ligaments, significant loss of MCP flexion can occur. Additionally, the deep transverse metacarpal ligaments, consisting of three short, wide bands, connect the palmar ligaments of these joints, forming the distal transverse arch. Full extensibility of these ligaments is necessary for prehension. MCP motions include flexion, extension, adduction, abduction, circumduction, and some rotation. The first MCP joint is a hinge joint allowing flexion and extension; however, side-to-side movements are greatly restricted.[1(pp440,441),4(pp209,210),6(p116),7(p1008)]

The interphalangeal joints are uniaxial hinge joints surrounded by a fibrous capsule, a palmar ligament, and two collateral ligaments. The collateral ligaments provide stability throughout range, but are most taut at 25° of flexion.[1(p441),4(p210),6(p117)]

Muscles and Motion

The interplay between the extrinsic and intrinsic muscles of the forearm, wrist, and hand is complex and not completely understood. The position of the different joints of the upper extremity has a profound effect on available range of motion (ROM) and muscle recruitment. The basic joint motions and the primary and secondary muscle movers are shown in Table 15–1. It is beyond the scope of this text to describe the muscles or their actions in greater detail.

Wrist Kinematics

As stated previously, the wrist complex moves in two planes and can flex, extend, abduct, adduct, or move in combination. Wrist motions vary widely in individuals with average wrist flexion at 85°, extension (dorsiflexion) at 75°, radial deviation at 15°,

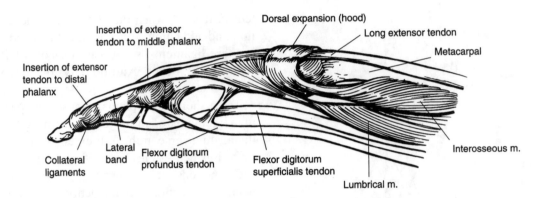

Figure 15–3 Lateral view of joint apparatus of a digit. *Source:* Reprinted from J.A. Sutin, *Tissue and Joint Impairments in Rheumatoid Arthritis* (Chapter 3), in *Rehabilitation of Persons with Rheumatoid Arthritis,* R.W. Chang (ed), p. 20, Copyright © 1996, Aspen Publishers, Inc.

and ulnar deviation at 40°.[5(pp265,266),8(p126)] During flexion and extension, the axis of rotation passes between the lunate and capitate; during radial and ulnar deviations, it passes through the head of the capitate.[8(p130)] During flexion and extension, most of the motion occurs at the radiocarpal joint, but the midcarpal joint also contributes. During ulnar deviation, the proximal carpal row rotates dorsally and radially, with the motion occurring at both the radiocarpal and midcarpal joints. During radial deviation, the proximal carpal row rotates ventrally with most of the motion occurring at the midcarpal joint.[9(p3447)]

Functional ROM values at the wrist also vary considerably. Almost all activities of daily living (ADL) can be performed with 40° of both flexion and extension, and 40° of combined radial and ulnar deviation.[10(p432)] Many activities, such as eating, reading, and dressing, can easily be performed with only 10° of flexion and 35° of extension.[5(pp266–268)] The functional position of the wrist (i.e., the position that provides the greatest efficiency for hand prehension activities) is 20 to 40° of extension and 10 to 15° of ulnar deviation.[8(p144),11(p289)]

Hand Kinematics

The basic motions and muscle actions of the hand are summarized in Table 15–2. In addition, the insertions of the flexor and extensor muscles of the fingers are shown in Figure 15–3. Recent research indicates that individuals employ different motor strategies to accomplish varying types of manual tasks. In other words, one person may use one of the thumb muscles as a prime mover, while another uses it as a stabilizer. This means that there is not one "correct" way to retrain motor control of the hand. In addition, wrist position alters the motor strategies used.[12(p129)]

The thumb, with its unique relation to the rest of the hand, provides the motion of opposition (abduction with rotation at the CMC joint), giving the human hand amazing dexterity and agility. The CMC joints of finger rays two and three fit tightly together, forming the "immobile unit" of the hand. The CMC joints of finger rays four and five permit small amounts of movement, allowing for the motions of "cupping" and "gripping."[13(pp277,278)] This "cupping" or "hollowing" of the hand forms three basic arches[8(p148)]:

1. transverse arch, consisting of the carpal arch continuing into the metacarpal arch
2. longitudinal arch, spanning from the CMC joints to the DIP joints
3. oblique arch, formed during thumb opposition.

The ability to alter the dimensions of these arches (i.e., change the shape of the hand) is necessary for grasping and manipulating objects. The thenar, hypothenar, lumbricals, and interosseous muscles and palmar ligaments maintain and control the arches of the hand.

Table 15–1 Motions, Muscles, and Innervations of the Wrist

Motion[†]	Primary Muscles[††]	Secondary Muscles[¥]	Innervation[††]
Extension 0°–75°	Extensor carpi radialis longus		Radial: C6-7
	Extensor carpi radialis brevis		PIB* Radial: C7-8
	Extensor carpi ulnaris		PIB Radial: C7-8
Flexion 0°–85°	Flexor carpi radialis		Median: C6-7
	Flexor carpi ulnaris		Ulnar: C7-8
	Palmaris longus		Median: C7-8
		Flexor digitorum superficialis	Median: C7-8
Radial deviation 0°–15°	Extensor carpi radialis longus		Radial: C6-7
	Extensor carpi radialis brevis		PIB Radial: C7-8
	Flexor carpi radialis		Median: C6-7
		Abductor pollicis longus	PIB Radial: C7-8
		Extensor pollicis brevis	PIB Radial: C7-8
Ulnar deviation 0°–40°	Extensor carpi ulnaris		PIB Radial: C7-8
	Flexor carpi ulnaris		Ulnar: C7-8

*PIB = Posterior interosseous branch of the radial nerve

Source: [†]*Basic Biomechanics of the Musculoskeletal System,* 2nd ed. (pp 265–266) by M Nordin, VH Frankel (eds), Lea & Febiger, © 1989.

[††]*Gray's Anatomy,* ed 35 (pp 543–550) by R Warwick and PL Williams (eds), Churchill Livingstone Inc, © 1973.

[¥]*The Physiology of the Joints, Vol I—The Upper Limb* (pp 142,143) by IA Kapandji, Churchill Livingstone Inc, © 1970.

Table 15–2 Motions, Muscles, and Innervations of the Hand

Motions[†]	Primary Muscles[††]	Secondary Muscles[¥]	Innervation[††]
Finger extension			
MCP	Extensor digitorum		PIB* Radial: C7-8
0° to +30°		Extensor indicis	PIB Radial: C7-8
		Extensor digiti minimi	PIB Radial: C7-8
PIP 0°	Dorsal and palmar interossei		Ulnar: C8-T1
	Lumbricals: index and middle fingers		Median: C8-T1
	Lumbricals: ring and little fingers		Ulnar: C8-T1
	Extensor digitorum		PIB Radial: C7-8
		Extensor indicis	PIB Radial: C7-8
		Extensor digiti minimi	PIB Radial: C7-8
DIP 0°–15°	Dorsal and palmar interossei		Ulnar: C8-T1
	Lumbricals: index and middle fingers		Median: C8-T1
	Lumbricals: ring and little fingers		Ulnar: C8-T1
Finger flexion			
MCP 0°–90°	Lumbricals: index and middle finger		Median: C8-T1
	Lumbricals: ring and little fingers		Ulnar: C8-T1
	Dorsal and palmar interossei		Ulnar: C8-T1
		Flexor digitorum superficialis	Median: C7-8
		Flexor digitorum profundus	AIB** Median: C8-T1 Ulnar nerve: C8-T1
PIP 0–100° to 110°	Flexor digitorum superficialis		Median: C7-8
		Flexor digitorum profundus	AIB Median: C8-T1 Ulnar nerve: C8-T1

continues

Table 15–2 continued

Motions[†]	Primary Muscles[††]	Secondary Muscles[¥]	Innervation[††]
DIP 0°–90°	Flexor digitorum profundus		AIB Median: C8-T1 Ulnar nerve: C8-T1
Finger abduction 0°–20°	Dorsal interossei Abductor digiti minimi		Ulnar: C8-T1 Ulnar: C8-T1
Finger adduction 0°	Palmar interossei		Ulnar: C8-T1
Opposition of little finger (at MCP joint)	Opponens digiti minimi		Ulnar: C8-T1
Thumb extension			
CMC	Abductor pollicis longus		PIB Radial: C7-8
		Extensores pollicis	PIB Radial: C7-8
MCP 0°	Extensor pollicis brevis	Extensor pollicis longus	PIB Radial: C7-8
IP 0° to +15	Extensor pollicis longus		PIB Radial: C7-8
Thumb flexion			
CMC 0°–45°	Flexor pollicis brevis superficial head deep head		Median: C8-T1 Ulnar: C8-T1
		Abductor pollicis brevis	Median: C8-T1
MCP 0°–50° up to 90°	Flexor pollicis brevis superficial head deep head		Median: C8-T1 Ulnar: C8-T1
	Flexor pollicis longus		AIB median: C8-T1
		Opponens pollicis	Lateral terminal branch of median: C8-T1
		1st palmar interosseous	Ulnar: C8-T1
IP 0°–85°	Flexor pollicis longus		AIB median: C8–T1

continues

Table 15–2 continued

Motions[†]	Primary Muscles[††]	Secondary Muscles[¥]	Innervation[††]
Thumb abduction 0°–60°	Abductor pollicis brevis		Median: C8–T1
	Abductor pollicis longus		PIB Radial: C7–8
Thumb adduction 0°–30°	Adductor pollicis		Ulnar: C8-T1
		1st palmar interosseous	Ulnar: C8-T1
Thumb opposition	Opponens pollicis		Lateral terminal branch of median: C8-T1
		Flexor pollicis brevis superficial head	Median: C8–T1
		deep head	Ulnar: C8–T1

*PIB = Posterior interosseous branch of the radial nerve

**AIB = Anterior interosseous branch of the median nerve

Source: [†]*Basic Biomechanics of the Musculoskeletal System,* 2nd ed. (pp 278–279) by M Nordin, VH Frankel (eds), Lea & Febiger, © 1989.

[††]*Gray's Anatomy,* ed 35 (pp 550–557) by R Warwick and PL Williams (eds), Churchill Livingstone Inc, © 1973.

[¥]*The Physiology of the Joints, Vol I—The Upper Limb* (pp 170–180) by IA Kapandji, Churchill Livingstone Inc, © 1970.

Innervation and Sensation

The hand is the major organ of touch. Sensory feedback is necessary for the precision movements associated with normal hand function. The three major nerves that innervate the wrist and hand are the median nerve, the radial nerve, and the ulnar nerve.

The Median Nerve

The median nerve (Figure 15–4) originates from two roots off the medial and lateral cords of the brachial plexus (C6 through T1) and courses down the inner arm, through the pronator teres at the forearm, and under the flexor retinaculum at the wrist, where it splits into a motor and sensory branch. It supplies the forearm pronators and wrist and finger flexors (see Table 15–1 and Figure 15–4 for more specific muscle innervations). Cutaneous sensation of the hand supplied by the median nerve includes (Figure 15–5):

- part of the palm and thenar surface
- palmar aspect of the thumb, index, middle finger, and half of ring finger
- tips of digits two, three, and four.

Damage to the median nerve (common in carpal tunnel injuries or Colles fractures) results in the inability to perform precision ma-

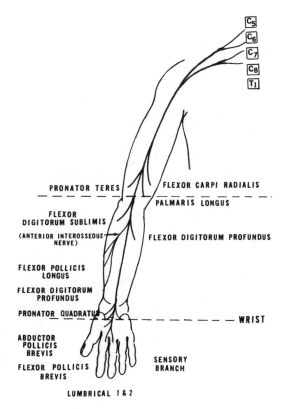

C5
C6
C7
C8
T1

PRONATOR TERES

FLEXOR CARPI RADIALIS

PALMARIS LONGUS

FLEXOR DIGITORUM SUBLIMIS

(ANTERIOR INTEROSSEOUS NERVE)

FLEXOR DIGITORUM PROFUNDUS

FLEXOR POLLICIS LONGUS

FLEXOR DIGITORUM PROFUNDUS

PRONATOR QUADRATUS

WRIST

ABDUCTOR POLLICIS BREVIS

SENSORY BRANCH

FLEXOR POLLICIS BREVIS

LUMBRICAL 1 & 2

Figure 15–4 Median nerve. *Source:* Reprinted with permission from R. Cailliet, Nerve Control of the Hand, *Hand Pain and Impairment*, 4 ed., p. 84, © 1994, F.A. Davis Company.

neuvers due to weakness in thumb flexion and opposition. Loss of power grip may also occur due to the instability of the joints about the thumb.[1(p1041),4(pp214,215),14(pp83–92)]

The Radial Nerve

The radial nerve (Figure 15–6) originates from roots C5 through T1 off the posterior cord of the brachial plexus, winding down the humerus, and entering the forearm between the brachialis and brachioradialis muscles. Its motor supply is confined to the forearm, where it innervates the supinator and wrist and finger extensors (see Table 15–1 and Figure 15–6 for more specific muscle in-

nervations). Cutaneous sensation of the hand supplied by the radial nerve (Figure 15–5) includes most of the dorsum of the hand, thumb, and fingers. Damage to the radial nerve will diminish hand function due to the lack of wrist and MCP extension, and the inability to extend or abduct the thumb.[4(p215),14(pp100,106)]

The Ulnar Nerve

The ulnar nerve (Figure 15–7) originates from roots C8 and T1 off the medial cord of the brachial plexus, courses down the inside of the arm behind the medial epicondyle of the humerus (the funny bone), along the medial side of the forearm, lateral to the pisiform bone at the wrist, and divides past the hamate bone into a superficial and deep terminal branch. It supplies the interossei, lumbricals three and four, and the wrist and deep finger flexors.[1(p1043),14(pp94,95)] See Table 15–1 and Figure 15–7 for more specific muscle innervations. Cutaneous sensation of the hand supplied by the ulnar nerve includes (Figure 15–5):

- the ulnar side of the hand
- the little finger
- the ulnar half of the ring finger.

Damage to the ulnar nerve can produce a weak lateral pinch and power grip, and can result in a claw hand deformity with flattening of the transverse arches.[4(p214)]

Blood Supply

The radial and ulnar arteries are the terminal branches of the brachial artery and supply blood to the wrist and hand. The radial artery begins 1 cm below the bend of the elbow and passes along the radial side of the forearm to the wrist, where the radial pulse can easily be felt. It winds laterally around the dorsum of the wrist and enters the palm between the first and second metacarpal and

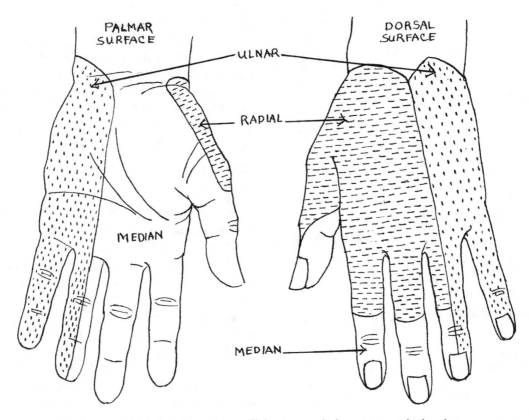

Figure 15–5 Sensory map of median nerve, radial nerve, and ulnar nerve at the hand.

eventually unites with the deep branch of the ulnar artery to form the deep palmar arch.[1(p651)] Near the scaphoid, the radial artery also has a superficial palmar branch that unites with the ulnar branch to form the superficial palmar arch.[4(p215)] The ulnar artery is larger than the radial artery and runs down the forearm medially to the wrist. After crossing the wrist, lateral to the pisiform bone, it gives off a deep branch (which forms the deep palmar arch) and continues across the palm to form the superficial palmar arch.[1(p654)] The deep and superficial palmar arches branch into metacarpal and digital arteries, supplying the fingers.

Venous drainage is important in the prevention of edema at the hand. Both superficial and deep veins, mostly on the dorsum of the hand, drain the hand. The venous plexus becomes the cephalic vein (laterally) and the basilic vein (medially).

KINETICS OF THE WRIST AND HAND

The forces that cross the multiple joints of the fingers and wrist vary depending on the postural alignment of those joints; therefore, although research has been performed in this area, data only exist for activities easily reproduced in a biomechanics laboratory and may not accurately reflect functional conditions.

Prehension: Precision and Power Grip

Everyday function requires the hand to manipulate and handle objects of varying

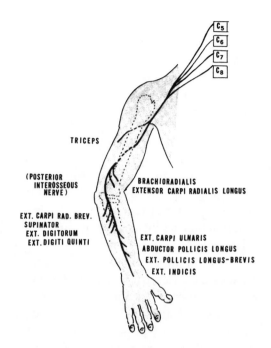

Figure 15–6 Radial nerve. *Source:* Reprinted with permission from R. Cailliet, Nerve Control of the Hand, *Hand Pain and Impairment*, 4 ed., p. 100, © 1994, F.A. Davis Company.

sizes and shapes. Although many classifications have been made, there are two basic patterns of prehension: precision grip and power grip.

The precision grip usually involves the manipulation of small objects between the thumb and palmar aspects of the fingers. The thumb is abducted and opposed. Some of the different types of precision grips are:

- tip pinch (e.g., picking up a needle)
- pad pinch (e.g., picking up a pencil)
- lateral pinch (e.g., putting a key into a keyhole)
- dynamic tripod or chuck grip (e.g., writing with a pen)

In general, greater pinch strength is observed in the dominant hand, males, and in younger persons. During lateral pinch,

women average 10.6 lbs (4.8 kg) and men average 16 lbs (7.3 kg). During pad pinch, women average 7.7 lbs (3.5 kg) and men average 11.2 lbs (5.1 kg).[15(p114),16(pp153,154)] A pinch strength of 5 to 7 lbs is necessary for most ADL.[17(pp292,293)]

The power grip involves the forceful holding of an object between flexed fingers and an adducted thumb. The wrist is usually extended 30 to 40° to facilitate the tension in the flexor tendons.[8(p291)] The power grip is strengthened significantly if the wrist is kept in a neutral position (i.e., not radially or ulnarly deviated).[16(p153)] By altering thumb placement, elements of precision can be attained with the power grip. Gender and age also significantly influence grip strength,

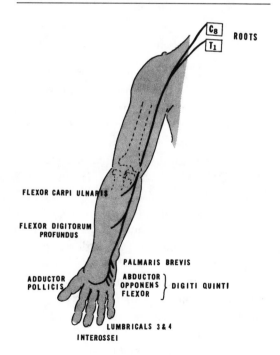

Figure 15–7 Ulnar nerve comprising roots C8 and T1. *Source:* Reprinted with permission from R. Cailliet, Nerve Control of the Hand, *Hand Pain and Impairment*, 4 ed., p. 94, © 1994, F.A. Davis Company.

with men and persons aged 20 to 29 years showing the greatest strengths. For all age groups, women's power grip averages 55 lbs (25 kg) and men's power grip averages 100 lbs (45.5 kg).[10(p432),17(p293)]

Kinetics of the Wrist

One major function of the wrist joint is to transmit forces to and from the forearm and hand. Compressive forces are thought to be directed through the head of the capitate to the scaphoid and lunate and then to the radiocarpal joint and the TFCC. The TFCC seems to act as a cushion, protecting the joint surfaces from degenerative forces.[8(pp270,271)] Uneven or excessive loading of the lunate is thought to cause Kienbock's disease, or avascular necrosis of the lunate.[10(p434)]

Kinetics of the Hand

During precision and power grips, the hand muscles generate large forces. In general, the extrinsic tendon forces are 4 to 5 times the applied external force, and the intrinsic tendon forces are 1.5 to 3 times the applied force. Joint compression forces are the least at the DIP joints, with the PIP and MCP joints having about the same compressive forces. In addition, precision work can result in up to double the forces generated in the muscle tendons than does power grip.[5(pp294,295)]

This information contains significant clinical implications for patients with hand dysfunctions, such as rheumatoid arthritis or carpal tunnel syndrome. Many times these patients switch vocational or avocational activities from "heavy" types of work to "light" types of work. The evidence seems to indicate that this supposedly "light" work requiring precision handling causes more forces to be generated in the hand and could be more damaging than the "heavier" activities.

EFFECTS OF AGING ON HAND FUNCTION

With aging, many changes occur that directly affect hand function. Studies have shown a correlation between diminished hand function and increased use of health care services, as well as need for institutionalization. Some of the changes that affect hand function are included in this section.

The palmar skin is normally thicker and moister than the dorsal skin. The moisture provides increased friction at the fingertips, which allows easier gripping of objects. With aging, loss of some oil glands causes the palmar skin of elderly persons to become drier and smoother. In persons over 80 years of age, this results in more difficulty with precision handling skills. Due to the loss of friction at the fingers, elderly persons have to grip harder and longer to manipulate an object.[18(p450)] After repeated trials, older adults are able to adapt and improve their precision grip force to more optimal levels.[19(p501)]

In a study by Weir et al, the amount of time and timing patterns for prehensile activities were measured for younger and older subjects. When reaching for an object, movement times were comparable between younger and older individuals; however, deceleration and hand enclosing times took longer. In addition, transporting the newly grasped object to a location 30 cm away also took longer for older persons. The greater the precision needed for a task, the longer it took both groups to perform. The relative timing patterns were also similar in both groups.[20(p79)]

As noted previously, grip strength diminishes with age; however, a major loss of grip strength is one of four risk factors that predict dependency—the other three risk factors include age, education, and psychological status.[21(p905)] Increasing grip strength is not an easy goal to accomplish. In another study by Rantanen et al, elderly persons trained hand grip, elbow flexion, and knee extension by performing routine housework, walking, and gardening. Although knee extension improved over 5 years, hand grip and elbow flexion decreased significantly. In people with a high activity level, hand grip remained adequate for independent living.[22(p1439)]

SUMMARY

- The radiocarpal joint and midcarpal joint comprise the wrist complex, allowing the motions of flexion, extension, radial deviation, and ulnar deviation.
- Functional ROM at the wrist consists of 40° of both flexion and extension, and 40° of combined radial and ulnar deviation.

- Stability of the hand occurs through the complex interaction of the many interosseous and collateral ligaments, volar plates, extrinsic muscle tendons, and intrinsic muscles.
- The hand has three arches and an opposable thumb that allows for prehensile activities.
- The three peripheral nerves that supply the hand are the radial, median, and ulnar nerves.
- The radial and ulnar arteries communicate with each other to become the deep and superficial palmar arches, supplying the hand and digits with blood.
- The hand manipulates objects by using a variety of precision and power grips.
- Elderly individuals perform prehensile activities slower and with less efficiency than younger persons, but timing patterns and adaptability remain the same.

REFERENCES

1. Warwick R, Williams PL, eds. *Gray's Anatomy,* 35th Br. ed. Edinburgh, Scotland: Churchill Livingstone; 1973.

2. Bednar MS. Clinical evaluation of the wrist and the hand. In: Nordin M, Andersson GBJ, Pope MH, eds. *Musculoskeletal Disorders in the Workplace: Principles and Practice.* St Louis: Mosby-Year Book; 1997.

3. Palmer AK, Werner FW. The triangular fibrocartilage complex of the wrist: anatomy and function. *J Hand Surg Am.* 1981;6:153–162.

4. Wadsworth CT. Clinical anatomy and mechanics of the wrist and hand. *J Orthop Sports Phys Ther.* 1983;4(4):206–216.

5. Stuchin S. Biomechanics of the wrist. In: Nordin M, Frankel VH, eds. *Basic Biomechanics of the Musculoskeletal System.* 2nd ed. Philadelphia: Lea & Febiger; 1989.

6. Pagonis JF. Imaging for the wrist and hand. *Orthop Phys Ther Clin N Am.* 1995;4(1):95–121.

7. Moran CA. Anatomy of the hand. *Phys Ther.* 1989;69(1):1007–1013.

8. Kapandji IA. *The Physiology of the Joints,* Vol. 1—Upper Limb. Edinburgh, Scotland: Churchill Livingstone; 1970.

9. Wright PE. Wrist. In: Canale ST, ed. *Campbell's Operative Orthopaedics,* 9th ed, Vol. 4. St Louis: Mosby-Year Book; 1998.

10. An KN. Biomechanics of the wrist and hand. In: Nordin M, Andersson GBJ, Pope MH, eds. *Musculoskeletal Disorders in the Workplace: Principles and Practice.* St Louis: Mosby-Year Book; 1997.

11. Magee DJ. *Orthopaedic Physical Assessment.* 3rd ed. Philadelphia: WB Saunders Company; 1997.

12. Johanson ME, Skinner SR, Lamoreux LW. Phasic relationships of the intrinsic and extrinsic thumb musculature. *Clin Orthop.* 1996;322: 120–130.

13. Bejjani FJ, Landsmee JMF. Biomechanics of the hand. In: Nordin M, Frankel VH, eds. *Basic Biomechanics of the Musculoskeletal System.* 2nd ed. Philadelphia: Lea & Febiger; 1989.

14. Cailliet R. *Hand Pain and Impairment.* 4th ed. Philadelphia: FA Davis Company; 1994.

15. Swanson AB, Goran-Hagert C, Swanson G. Evaluation of impairment of hand function. In: Hunter JM, Schneider LH, Mackin EJ, Callahan AD, eds. *Rehabilitation of the Hand.* St Louis: CV Mosby Co; 1990.

16. Lamoreaux L, Hoffer MM. The effect of wrist deviation on grip and pinch strength. *Clin Orthop.* 1995;314:152–155.

17. Phillips C. Management of the patient with rheumatoid arthritis: the role of the hand therapies. *Hand Clin.* 1989;5:291–309.

18. Kinoshita H, Francis PR. A comparison of prehension force control in young and elderly individuals. *Europ J Appl Physiol Occup Physiol.* 1996;74(5):450–460.

19. Weir PL, MacDonald JR, Mallat BJ, Leavitt JL, Roy EA. Age-related differences in prehension—the influence of task goals. *J Motor Behav.* 1998;30(1):79–89.

20. Kawai S, Tsuda H, Kinoshita H, et al. Effects of aging on force adaptation during manipulation of a small object using a precision grip. *Japan J Phys Fitness Sports Med.* 1997;46(5):501–512.

21. Hughes S, Gibbs J, Dunlop D, et al. Predictors of decline in manual performance in older adults. *J Am Geriatr Soc.* 1997:45(8):905–910.

22. Rantanen T, Era P, Heikkinen E. Physical activity and the changes in maximal isometric strength in men and women from the age of 75 to 80 years. *J Am Geriatr Soc.* 1997;45(12):1439–1445.

16

Treatment of Common Problems of the Wrist and Hand

The hand is both an adroit prehensile tool and the major sense organ of touch. The ability of the hand to manipulate the environment is highly interconnected with its sensory function. With age, the accumulated effects of environmental exposure (to pressure, chemicals, toxins, and hot surfaces) and decreased circulation contribute to skin breakdown and the decreased ability to feel. The loss of oil glands makes the palmar surface slippery and less efficient in grasping objects. Decreased coordination affects precision hand movements and is evident in the reduced handwriting speed found in elderly persons over 60 years.[1(pp84,85,233)] The therapist must remember the effects of "normal aging" when designing a rehabilitation program for an elderly patient with dysfunction of the wrist and hand.

FRACTURES OF THE WRIST AND HAND

Fracture of the Distal Radius (Colles' Fracture)

Distal radial fractures are one of the most common fractures in orthopaedics, constituting one-sixth of all fractures that are treated in emergency rooms. The greatest frequency of this type of fracture occurs in children ages 6 to 10 and women over 40 (average age 60 to 69 years).[2(p461),3(p243)] The elderly are at increased risk for fracturing the distal radius due to osteoporosis and increased incidence of falling.[4(p127)] Fractures of the distal radius usually result from a fall onto an outstretched hand. The direction of force dictates the type of fracture.

Types of Fracture of the Distal Radius

Eponyms commonly classify distal radial fractures. A Colles' fracture (Figure 16–1) is a dorsally angulated, displaced fracture of the radius within 1.5 inches of the articular surface. A fracture of the ulnar styloid and avulsion of the triangular fibrocartilage complex often accompany it. The scaphoid and radial head may also fracture.[5(pp107,108)] A Smith's fracture is a volarly angulated, displaced fracture of the radius, and a Bartons' fracture is a fracture of the rim of the distal radius.[4(p130)] There are many other classification systems for distal radial fractures based on mechanism of injury, intra-articular involvement, amount of displacement, and joint involvement[2(pp461,462)]; at present, however, there is no universally accepted classification for this fracture type.

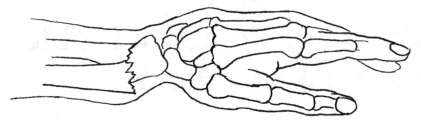

Figure 16–1 Colles' fracture with dorsal displacement of the distal radial fragment. This injury usually occurs from a fall onto the outstretched hand.

Medical Management of Distal Radial Fractures

The fragile bone stock of the elderly makes stabilization of this fracture difficult for the orthopaedic surgeon. Closed fixation with casting increases bone loss due to prolonged immobilization; however, insertion of pins (externally or internally) also increases osteoporosis.[6(pp91,92)] Surgical options are limited because of the small size of the fracture fragments, limited surgical access, and complex soft-tissue structures in the region.[7(pp49,50)] The orthopaedic surgeon can choose from the following types of fixation, depending on bone stock and fracture fragments:

- closed-reduction with plaster casting
- closed-reduction with percutaneous injection of bone cement
- percutaneous pinning
- metal external skeletal-fixation devices
- internal fixation with plate (buttress, T-plate, or cloverleaf) and screws.[2(pp464–466),4(pp134–137),7(pp52–54),8(p110)]

Results from the differing types of fixations are mixed. Although most distal radial fractures are treated with plaster casting, internal and external fixation may result in increased stability and improved function.[7(pp59,60),9(p588),10(p57),11(p212)] In the elderly, plaster casting still remains the most common form of treatment in minimally displaced fractures. It is less invasive, maintains the stability of the fracture fragments, and has good results.[4(p138),12(p46)]

Complications Following Fracture of the Distal Radius

Serious complications to the surrounding soft tissue structures can arise from this type of fracture or the attempt to stabilize the fracture. The complication rate is very high, ranging from 20 to 31%.[13(p144)] Complications can affect the skin, flexor or extensor tendons, the fascia, the vascular structures, or the peripheral nerves.

At the skin, pressure sores can result from incorrect timing of cast application or cast placement. Tendon complications include: stenosing tenosynovitis, adhesive tendinitis, entrapment, rupture, and laceration.[13(pp144,145)] Fascial complications are rare and can involve compartment syndrome or an exacerbation of Dupuytren's disease.[13(p150)] Vascular compromise leading to reflex sympathetic dystrophy (RSD) commonly occurs after a Colles' fracture, but is usually of short duration. Symptoms include pain, tenderness, vascular instability, swelling, and stiffness of the limb.[6(p95)] (See Dupuytren's disease and RSD later in this chapter.)

Injury to any of the peripheral nerves—median, radial, or ulnar—can occur, but the most common complication is secondary median neuropathy due to increased carpal tunnel compression. The pressure in the carpal tunnel changes with wrist position, with the least amount of pressure (~15 mm Hg) occurring with the wrist in neutral and the greatest amount with the wrist in flexion or extension. A Colles' fracture and the edema that follows the injury changes the angulation of the wrist and can cause median nerve compression.[14(p212)] Proper wrist position is critical in the prevention of this secondary injury. Prompt recognition of any of these complications minimizes functional loss and disability.

Treatment

Active finger, elbow, and shoulder range of motion (ROM) exercises begin immediately after stabilization of the fracture fragments and should be performed on an hourly basis. (All splints or casts should end proximal to the metacarpal heads to optimize finger function.) In addition, it is important to instruct the patient in edema control techniques, which include elevation of the hand above heart level and use of Coban® wrapping on the fingers and thumb.

At postfracture 4 to 6 weeks, the cast is removed and the patient is fitted with a removable wrist splint worn between exercising sessions and at night. Wrist and forearm ROM exercises begin at high frequency (hourly) and short duration (5 to 10 minutes). The intensity of the program is dependent on the amount of fracture healing. At approximately 6 to 8 weeks postfracture, the treatment progresses to include resistive exercises for strength and functional activities.[15(p68)] All exercises must be pain free and edema must be controlled to prevent the onset of RSD.

In addition to the obvious treatment of the upper extremity, the therapist may also need to train the patient's balance and gait to prevent further falls.[6(p97)] (See Chapter 17 on Balance Intervention for the Orthopaedic Patient.) Because the distal radial fracture is considered to be "an osteoporotic fracture," closed-chain or weight-bearing exercises for the upper extremity are extremely appropriate to help build bone mass (after complete fracture healing has occurred).

Outcomes following distal radial fractures depend on the complications following the injury or fixation.[16(p200)] Warwick et al report that 85% of patients had a satisfactory functional outcome 10 years after suffering a Colles' type fracture. The major complication associated with negative outcome was RSD.[17(p270)]

Carpal Fractures

The scaphoid is the most frequently fractured carpal bone, with 70% of fractures occurring in the middle or "waist" of the scaphoid.[5(p114)] This fracture mostly occurs as a result of a fall on the outstretched hand. Wrist movements are painful and limited. Palpation of the scaphoid (through the anatomical "snuff box") is tender. Radiographs may be negative.[14(p207)] Scaphoid fractures have varied healing rates. The distal third and middle of the scaphoid are supplied by the dorsal branch of the radial artery and heal relatively quickly in 8 to 12 weeks; however, the proximal pole has a limited blood supply and can take up to 23 weeks to heal.[18(pp4,6)] In some cases, nonunion or avascular necrosis occur in proximal pole fractures. Treatment consists of prolonged immobilization in a cast or splint. (It is difficult to know exactly when the scaphoid is healed, because radiographs do not necessarily show the fracture or the callus formation.) Pain-free active forearm, wrist, and thumb motions begin on an hourly basis when immobilization is discontinued.[15(p61)] Passive stretching and joint mobilization are contraindicated until the fracture is well healed.[19(p290)] Returning to activity prematurely or overly aggressive therapy can jeopardize the recovery from this injury.

Fractures of the hamate bone are common in golf and tennis. In golfers, the fracture usually involves the hook of the hamate on the nondominant hand and is called "golfer's wrist."[20(p27)] Fractures on the dominant hand mostly occur in tennis. Signs and symptoms include palmar pain, decreased grip strength, and painful palpation of the hook of the hamate.[21(p9)] In golf, the injury is usually related to poorly fitted equipment—such as a club that is too short.[20(p27)] Treatment consists of possible splinting for several weeks, followed by ROM and strengthening exercises performed with high frequency and short duration. Often, surgical removal of the hook of the hamate affords the best function, with the patient returning to sport in 6 weeks.[21(p9)]

Summary of Treatment of Wrist and Hand Fractures

- know the type of fracture and fixation (if any) performed
- control edema and pain to prevent RSD
- perform ROM exercises hourly (when mobilization allowed)
- ensure intensity of program is predicated on fracture healing
- retrain balance and gait to prevent recurrence of falls

ARTHRITIS

Rheumatoid Arthritis

Rheumatoid arthritis (RA) is a systemic disease that is two to four times more prevalent in women than in men. The earliest joints affected are usually the small joints of the hand and feet. It generally attacks the body symmetrically, causing inflammation of the synovium of the joints and tendons. The long flexor and extensor tendons are affected most often. Synovial effusion weakens the periarticular tissues and increases the intra-articular pressure that may interfere with cartilage nutrition, contributing to cartilage breakdown.[14(p224),22(pp17,18),23(pp293,294)]

Wrist deformities occur due to ligamentous loosening on the radial aspect, causing ulnar displacement of the proximal carpal row with secondary radial rotation of the distal carpal row and metacarpals. In addition, synovitis at the distal radioulnar joint results in dorsal subluxation of the distal ulnar. This causes pain and decreased ability to extend the wrist. The extensor carpi ulnaris may slip ulnarly and volarly, transforming into a wrist flexor.[22(p22)]

Synovitis at the metacarpophalangeal (MCP) joints and proximal interphalangeal (PIP) joints can erode and sublux the joints, impairing hand function. Flexor tenosynovitis occurs in 38 to 55% of patients with RA and may cause digital stiffness, loss of active finger flexion, or tendon rupture. Flexor tenosynovitis also contributes to the swan-neck deformity of the fingers (flexion of MCP and distal interphalangeal [DIP] joints with hyperextension of PIP joint). The extensor tendons may slip ulnarly between the MCP heads, causing them to deviate in an ulnar direction. The extensor tendons are also prone to rupture, which can cause a Boutonniere deformity (hyperextension of MCP and DIP joints with flexion of PIP joint). Disruption of the MCP collateral ligaments along with the natural pull of the flexor tendons causes ulnar deviation to begin at the MCP joints. As the joints begin to deform, the intrinsic muscles and the force of gravity contribute to the progression of greater hand deformities.[14(pp232–239),22(pp20–23)]

Medical Management of Rheumatoid Arthritis of the Wrist and Hand

The goals of nonsurgical management include:

- decreasing pain
- decreasing inflammation
- preventing deformities
- slowing inevitable joint destruction.[24(p67)]

Since RA is progressive with no cure presently available, the medical treatment consists of pharmacological agents, "active" rest, and therapy. A team approach to treatment is better to manage the multidimensional aspects (physical, psychological, emotional, and social) of this disease.

Surgical Management of Rheumatoid Arthritis of the Wrist and Hand

The goals of surgical intervention include:

- pain relief
- function restoration
- additional deformity prevention
- cosmesis.[24(p68)]

In recent years, surgical correction of minor deformities has been successful in preventing the formation of marked deformities and their associated functional losses. Synovectomy (removal of inflamed synovium and pannus) eliminates pain and delays joint destruction. The procedure lasts about 5 years.

Arthroplasties for the wrist, MCP, and interphalangeal (IP) joints have had varying degrees of success. Total wrist arthroplasty has undergone three generations of design over the past 30 years. Major complications have occurred, including fracture about the prosthesis, bone resorption, and malalignment. As the prostheses' design more approximates the wrist joint's center of rotation, more encouraging results have been observed. At present, the clinical outcomes have not been favorable.[25(p451)] A constrained ball-and-socket arthroplasty for the trapeziometacarpal joint (of the thumb) could not control the forces at this joint and failed in 40% of the cases.[26(p121)] Silicone-rubber implants at the MCP and IP joints have had much greater success. Correction of deformities, improved ROM, functional return, and cosmetic appearance have lasted up to 16 years.[27(p3)] Research continues into the design and implantation of replacement joints for the wrist and hand.

Treatment

Physical or occupational therapy during the acute inflammatory stage of RA consists of modalities (ice or cool towels), rest, and gentle active or active-assisted exercise to reduce the pain and inflammation. Early splinting can reduce pain and swelling, while maintaining proper alignment. Various splints (e.g., wrist futuro or cock-up, thumb spica) can be fabricated depending on the assessed need. The therapist should also assess the patient for assistive devices for activities of daily living (ADL) and educate the patient on joint protection principles.[28(p1094)]

During the subacute stage, gentle active exercises and light ADL can be initiated. Modalities, such as paraffin or whirlpools, can reduce joint pain and muscle splinting. In addition, rest periods should be scheduled into the day to prevent fatigue.[23(p294)]

During the chronic (or inactive inflammation) stage, progressive exercising to increase strength and endurance can be started. (Depending on the level of joint destruction, aggressive therapy may be contraindicated.) Although some strength loss and stiffness is due to myositis and joint destruction, much of the loss of power and flexibility is from immobilization. As in the healthy population, exercise benefits to patients with RA include:

- decreased pain
- decreased swelling
- decreased stiffness
- decreased weakness
- decreased fatigue
- decreased bone loss.[29(p92)]

Strengthening activities for the patient with RA should be of high frequency but short duration. Exercise-induced pain is acceptable only if it lasts 2 hours or less. Aerobic exercises, such as brisk walking, dancing, or Tai Chi, has been found to increase all areas of function. Cross-training is important so that the same muscles or joints are not stressed each exercise session.[29(pp96,97,100)] ADL are emphasized with joint protection principles applied. Joint protection techniques allow performance of ADL with minimal amounts of stress. Some of the basic principles of joint protection and energy conservation are:

- respect pain, but do no fear it
- maintain muscle strength and ROM
- balance work and rest (without guilt when leaving tasks undone!)
- avoid deforming positions (such as prolonged grasp)
- use stronger and larger joints when possible
- avoid one position for prolonged periods of time
- use necessary adaptive equipment
- conserve energy (become organized and efficient)[28(pp1094,1095)]

Postoperative (PO) therapy following joint replacement is dependent on the joint involved and the orthopaedic surgeon. In general, the patient is splinted with a dynamic splint that aligns the joints into desired positions. Gentle, careful exercises for finger

flexion and radial deviation begin around PO Week 6. Progressive strengthening and night splints continue up to PO Month 4.

Osteoarthritis

For reasons still unknown, the articular cartilage of weight-bearing joints undergoes progressive degeneration with increasing age. The cartilage loses its ability to absorb shock, placing more stress on the subchondral bone. The joints in the hand most commonly affected by osteoarthritis (OA) are the finger DIP and thumb carpometacarpal (CMC) joints. Because the thumb contributes so highly to prehensile activities, this "benign" disease can cause major functional loss.

The signs and symptoms of OA include:

- joint stiffness
- grip strength decrease
- joint aching
- edema
- decreased ability to perform ADL due to pain.[23(p291)]

Treatment

Modalities, such as fluidotherapy or whirlpool, can be used to decrease joint stiffness. Grade I and II joint mobilizations can also be helpful in reducing pain. Ultrasound or phonophoresis followed by massage can reduce inflammation. Gentle ROM and stretching exercises, as well as light gripping exercises, can be performed during fluidotherapy or whirlpool or in a tub of warm water at home. An important exercise to perform to prevent loss of ROM is the "hook" exercise or claw fist (Figure 16–2).[23(p291)] The "hook" exercise promotes gliding of the flexor digitorum profundus (FDP) tendon on the bone.[30(p1068)] Acutely painful joints may have to be temporarily immobilized in a

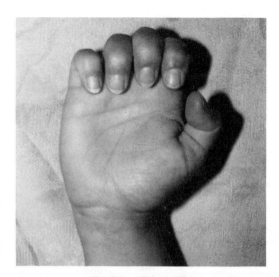

Figure 16–2 "Hook" exercise or claw fist. This exercise (or stretch) involves flexion at the DIP and PIP joints while simultaneously maintaining extension at the MCP joints and promotes gliding of the flexor digitorum profundus tendon.

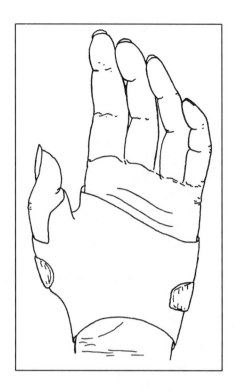

Figure 16–3 Thumb carpometacarpal stability splint. The splint places the first metacarpal in abduction and extends the site of force along the first metacarpal distally beyond the metacarpal joint. The distal aspect of the first metacarpal should be stabilized and the interphalangeal joint should be allowed unrestricted motion. *Source:* Adapted from R.M. Duncan, "Basic Principles of Splinting the Hand," *Physical Therapy,* Alexandria, Virginia, American Physical Therapy Association, 1989, Vol. 69, No. 12, p. 1106, the American Physical Therapy Association.

static extension splint, until the symptoms subside. Small lifestyle modifications should also be introduced to the patient with OA of the thumb CMC joint. A CMC immobilization orthosis (Figure 16–3) should be worn daily until the symptoms subside and then gradually weaned.[23(p293)] Lateral pinch (key pinch) should be avoided as it generates more forces than other grips. (See Chapter 15 for more information on grip and grasp.) Other gripping patterns should be minimized by use of appliances and tools, such as electric can openers and weeders.

Summary of Treatment of Arthritis of the Wrist and Hand

- During the acute stage of RA
  1. use modalities, rest, and gentle active or active-assistive exercise
  2. use splints and assistive devices as needed

  3. educate patient on joint protection and energy conservation principles
- During the subacute stage of RA
  1. begin active exercises and light ADL
  2. use modalities to reduce pain
- During the chronic stage of RA
  1. begin strengthening exercises as tolerated
  2. begin aerobic exercises

3. continue education on joint protection and energy conservation principles

- For patients with OA of the wrist or hand
  1. use modalities to decrease joint stiffness and inflammation
  2. immobilize acutely painful joints in temporary static splints
  3. begin gentle ROM and light strengthening exercises
  4. use appliances and tools to minimize pressure on hand joints

NEUROVASCULAR INJURIES

Carpal Tunnel Syndrome

Carpal tunnel syndrome (CTS) refers to a compression neuropathy of the median nerve as it passes through the carpal tunnel. The carpal tunnel (Figure 16–4) is bounded by the transverse carpal ligament and the carpal bones and contains within it the median nerve and the nine tendons of the flexor pollicis longus and the FDP and flexor digitorum superficialis (FDS). Because space within the tunnel is limited, any condition or injury that increases pressure in the tunnel can cause CTS. The condition is twice as common in women than in men and occurs most often after 55 years of age.[31(p190)] Some of the causes or risk factors for developing CTS include:

- flexor tenosynovitis (from repeated grasping or vibration)
- fracture (Colles' or carpal)
- tumors
- direct trauma
- obesity
- arthritis (OA or RA) at the wrist
- systemic conditions (diabetes or thyroid disease)[23(p296),31(p190),32(p106),33(p166)]

The following signs and symptoms are associated with CTS:

- tingling, burning, and painful paresthesias of the palmar surfaces of the thumb, index finger, middle finger, and radial half of the ring finger that worsen at night
- weakness in grasp and grip with atrophy of the thenar eminence

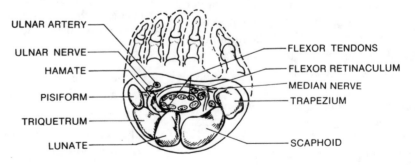

Figure 16–4 Carpal tunnel–space between concave carpus and transverse retinacular ligament, enclosing the median nerve and flexor tendons of the fingers. *Source:* Reprinted from C.T. Wadsworth, "Clinical Anatomy and Mechanics of the Wrist and Hand," *The Journal of Orthopaedic and Sports Physical Therapy,* Vol. 4, No. 4, p. 207, © 1983, Williams & Wilkins.

- positive Tinel's sign (onset of tingling after tapping the volar surface of the wrist)
- positive Phalen's test (onset of tingling after holding wrist in fully flexed position for 60 seconds)[14(p114),23(p297)]

Note: It is imperative for the therapists to rule out the cervical spine as the source of hand symptoms. Cervical arthritis is very common in the elderly patient and can be contributing to apparent CTS.

Treatment

Conservative treatment consists of removing causative factors, splinting the wrist in neutral for 2 weeks (especially at night), and use of oral anti-inflammatory medication or cortisone injection.[14(p115),34(p1244)] The wrist must be splinted in neutral (0°) due to the small amount of compression that occurs in the carpal tunnel at that angle. Even small amounts of extension (as is found in a standard 20° cock-up splint) can be detrimental to the patient.[34(p1243)] Modalities, such as iontophoresis, and soft-tissue mobilizations of the hand and forearm can be used.[23(p297)]

The surgeon can also opt to release the pressure on the median nerve by cutting or lengthening the transverse carpal ligament with or without a synovectomy. Surgery can be performed endoscopically or by open procedure. The wrist is usually immobilized for 2 weeks after surgery. After suture removal, soft tissue massage around the suture line helps to soften the maturing scar. Ice or cold towels can be used to control edema. The patient begins active motions of the digits. To prevent adhesions, gentle selective tendon gliding can be achieved by three exercises:

1. "hook" exercise: isolates FDP (Figure 16–2)
2. sublimis fist or flat-fist: causes FDS to glide on stationary FDP (Figure 16–5)

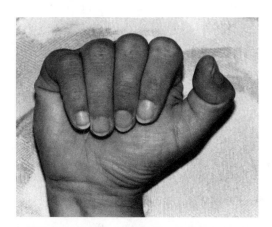

Figure 16–5 Sublimis fist or "flat-fist." This exercise (or stretch) involves flexion at the MCP and PIP joints while simultaneously maintaining extension at the DIP joint and promotes gliding of the flexor digitorum superficialis tendon.

3. full fist: causes gliding of FDP and FDS tendons on each other[30(pp1068,1069)]

Light ADL are allowed around PO Weeks 2 to 3, but no forceful activities or exercises are permitted until PO Weeks 4 to 6.[35(p3691)] Strength returns slowly (over 6 months) and sometimes without reversal of thenar muscle atrophy.

Summary of Treatment of Carpal Tunnel Syndrome

- nonoperative management
  1. identify and eliminate causative factors
  2. splint the wrist in neutral (0°) for 2 weeks
  3. rule out the cervical spine as the source of hand symptoms

- PO management after carpal tunnel release
  1. control edema with ice or cold towels

2. massage around (but not on) suture line
3. begin active finger motion around PO Days 10 to 14
4. ensure tendon gliding to prevent flexor tendon adhesions
5. begin light ADL around PO Weeks 2 to 3
6. begin strengthening exercises after PO Week 6

Reflex Sympathetic Dystrophy

RSD is a term used to indicate a group of clinical conditions occurring in an extremity after a trauma that results from an abnormal or prolonged response of the sympathetic nervous system. The group includes causalgia, Sudeck's atrophy, shoulder-hand syndrome, and Leriche posttraumatic pain syndrome; and has in common the following characteristics:

- excruciating pain (seemingly disproportionate to the injury)
- swelling
- joint stiffness
- skin color changes
- hyperhidrosis (excessive sweating)
- osteoporosis.[36(p1052),37(pp3836,3837)]

Three stages of RSD have been described. In the acute stage (Stage I), the hand is cyanotic, cool to the touch, and hyperhidrotic. Soft and pitted edema are present at the dorsum of the hand and the IP joints, causing joint stiffness. In Stage II, the pain worsens, the edema becomes hard and brawny, the skin becomes red, shiny, and dry, and osteoporosis becomes generalized throughout the hand. In the chronic stage (Stage III), the pain begins to subside, the joints display extreme stiffness, the IP joints are thickened, the skin is pale and dry, and the osteoporosis (demineralization) worsens.[36(p1053)]

Treatment of RSD of the Hand

The goals of treatment are to disrupt the abnormal sympathetic reflex by decreasing pain, and to control the development of edema and joint stiffness.[14(p153),36(pp1053,1054)] No treatment plan has proven completely effective, much to the frustration of the medical community. Physical therapy in conjunction with some type of sympathetic nerve block is the most widely recommended treatment.[37(p3838)]

The therapist can use modalities, such as transcutaneous electrical nerve stimulation and mild heat or cold applications, to relieve the pain. Heat applications should be applied in conjunction with elevation to minimize edema. Resting splints can also be used to calm painful symptoms, but must be removed often to allow for exercise. When the pain lessens, gentle, active exercise can be initiated.[14(p149),36(p1053)] It is imperative to control the development of edema in order to prevent joint deformities. Edema control may include the following interventions:

- elevation (with the hand above the elbow and the elbow above the shoulder)
- exercises to accelerate drainage (Figure 16–6)
- retrograde massage
- compressive dressing (e.g., Isotoner® gloves, Tubigrip gloves, Coban® wrap)[38(pp1062,1063)]

Joint stiffness can be controlled through gentle, active, and passive ROM exercises and with dynamic splinting. Exercise should be directed at all the joints of the upper extremity. Aggressive exercise or painful passive muscle stretching can exacerbate the symptoms and are contraindicated. Dynamic splints can usually be initiated after the pain subsides in Stage III. It is also important to encourage the patient to use the hand for the

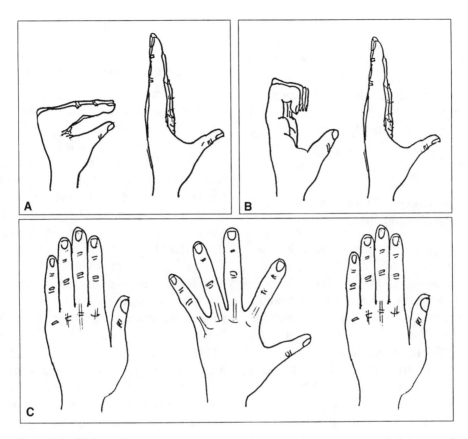

Figure 16–6 Muscle pumping exercises for edema reduction. Modified fist achieved by isolated metacarpophalangeal joint flexion (**A**) and isolated interphalangeal joint flexion (**B**). Digital abduction and adduction to stretch web spaces (**C**). *Source:* Reprinted from J.W. Howell, *Physical Therapy,* Alexandria, Virginia, American Physical Therapy Association, 1989, Vol. 69, No. 12, p. 1081, with permission of the American Physical Therapy Association.

basic ADL of grooming, dressing, and eating. The patient can easily become apprehensive about increasing the severity of the condition and avoid using the hand for normal function.[36(p1054)]

Summary of Treatment of RSD of the Hand

- disrupt the abnormal sympathetic reflex by decreasing pain
- control the development of edema with gentle exercise, massage, and compressive dressings with the hand in an elevated position

- minimize joint stiffness with gentle, active exercise

DUPUYTREN'S CONTRACTURE

Dupuytren's contracture (or disease) is a fibroplasia of the palmar fascia, causing the formation of cords and nodules that can cause progressive flexion contractures of the fingers. This painless disease progresses over several years, occurring most commonly in men over 50 years of age.[39(p3675)] As the fascia becomes fibrotic, it contracts and causes the skin to "dimple." Further progression of the disease compromises the circulation, leading to atrophy of the skin.[14(p181)] Although the etiology is unknown, genetics is known to influence the development of the contracture. In addition, Travell and Simons have consistently found multiple trigger points in the palmaris longus muscle belly.[40(p526)]

Medical and Surgical Treatment of Dupuytren's Contracture

Many medical and therapeutic techniques (including ultrasound and splinting) have been tried unsuccessfully to delay the progression of the disease. Travell and Simons recommend vapocoolant "spray-and-stretch" or injection of the active trigger points with 0.5% procaine solution, but the long-term effects of these procedures on Dupuytren's contracture are not yet known.[40(p528)]

Surgical intervention is the most successful treatment available and is performed easier in the early stages of the disease. Partial fasciectomy is the most common procedure done and involves removal of the mature, deformed tissues. In older persons, a subcutaneous fasciotomy (cutting of the fascial cords) can be performed percutaneously under local anesthetic. The results are less cosmetic and may not last long, but this procedure still provides benefits for persons in poor health.[9(p3678),24(p64)]

Postsurgical Treatment of Dupuytren's Contracture

After a partial fasciectomy, the hand is kept elevated for at least 2 days. The patient should gently exercise the PIP joints actively and often. The therapist must monitor the wound and be aware of excessive pain in the hand (with fever) that may indicate the undesired development of a hematoma. On PO Days 3 to 5, the first dressing is changed and the patient begins ROM exercises. The patient is warned not to allow the limb to hang in a dependent position. The patient should also wear a resting pan splint at night, with fingers maintained in full extension. At PO Week 2, the sutures are removed and active ROM exercises can continue in warm (not hot) water. Passive stretching is contraindicated. After PO Week 3, the patient can use the hand for more functional activities with physician approval. Strengthening exercises with therapeutic putty can augment the program. Depending on physician preference, the pan splint is worn at night up to PO Months 3 to 6.[39(pp3681,3682)]

If the less invasive fasciotomy is performed, only a pressure dressing is required over the area for 24 hours. Therapy consists of active exercise for the fingers, hand, and wrist.

DOCUMENTATION TIPS: THE LEGAL RECORD

It perhaps cannot be overstated in our litigious society, how important documentation is in providing evidence during a legal action. The therapist's evaluation, opinions, and notes (along with the notes of the other members of the health care community) reflects both the patient's condition and the quality of the care provided. There is nothing extraordinary about a note that can "stand up in court" versus a standard progress note that documents patient progress. They should both

continues

DOCUMENTATION TIPS: continued

contain the same information. In other words, a good progress note *will* stand up in court. That being said, a few additional documentation tips are still in order.

(*Author's Note:* In a society where my coffee cup now has giant, red letters warning me that the contents are "hot," it is important to point out that providing good quality care and documenting that care judiciously is still no guarantee against legal action. To cover myself legally, therefore, I should like to add that the list below is not 100% comprehensive and does not cover every contingency of note writing. For the therapist in need of more information on this topic, complete texts are available. Also consider liability insurance.)

1. ***Notes should be written professionally:*** They should be legible and comprehensible and should contain correct spelling and standard abbreviations. All notes should be dated and signed.

2. ***Notes should be written in a timely fashion:*** Occasionally, a therapist will "get behind" on note writing. This can be problematic for two reasons:
   a. The therapist may actually forget all the details of the treatment session when the note is written hours, days, perhaps even weeks, after the treatment was given and may be unable to render an actual account of the session.
   b. Records, with incomplete notes, can be sealed and locked up for protection against "tampering with the evidence," not allowing

the therapist to ever document what happened.

3. ***Corrections:*** All notes should be written in ink. If a mistake in writing occurs, the therapist should place one strike through the word or sentence with ERR and therapist's initials written above the corrected text. The words being corrected *must be readable*. The therapist must not "white out" the text! (Writing ERR shows that the therapist made an honest documentation error and is not trying to hide anything.)

4. ***Notes must be factual and accurate:*** The therapist can write only what he or she did, observed, felt, smelled, heard, or experienced. The notes must never *editorialize* or *judge* a situation, patient, or family member.

5. ***Incidences must be documented immediately:*** Many facilities have "incident reports" that need to be filled out (in triplicate). Although unpleasant to write, they generally ascertain the necessary facts needed for legal purposes. If the facility does not have an incident report, the therapist still must document in detail what happened, the patient's condition, and any actions taken.

6. ***Identification:*** Notes should include the patient's full name, as well as the full names and relationships of family members or friends who attend therapy.

continues

DOCUMENTATION TIPS: continued

7. Confidentiality: The therapist and office workers must make sure that the patient's privacy is protected when sending facsimile (fax) transmissions to insurance providers, lawyers, and doctors, or when mailing progress notes.

8. Keep originals in the medical record: Only the originals of evaluations, notes, home programs, prescriptions, and correspondence are kept in the medical record. Xeroxed copies can be hiding alterations and are therefore unacceptable.

REFERENCES

1. Spirduso WW. *Physical Dimensions of Aging.* Champaign, IL: Human Kinetics; 1995.

2. Jupiter JB. Current concepts review: fractures of the distal end of the radius. *J Bone Joint Surg.* 1991;73-A(3):461–469.

3. Singer BR, McLaughlan GJ, Robinson CM, Christie J. Epidemiology of fractures in 15,000 adults—the influence of age and gender. *J Bone Joint Surg.* 1998;80-B(2):243–248.

4. Dinowitz MI, Koval KJ, Meadows S. Distal radius. In: *Fractures in the Elderly,* Koval KJ, Zuckerman JD, eds. Philadelphia: Lippincott-Raven Publishers; 1998.

5. Pagonis JF. Imaging for the wrist and hand. *Orthop Phys Ther Clin N Amer.* 1995;4(1):95–121.

6. O'Connor LJ. Females and fractures. *Orthop Phys Ther Clin N Am.* 1996;5(1):85–117.

7. Jupiter JB, Lipton H. The operative treatment of intraarticular fractures of the distal radius. *Clin Orthop.* 1993;292:48–61.

8. Jupiter JB, Winters S, Sigman S, Lowe C, Pappas C, et al. Repair of 5 distal radius fractures with an investigational cancellous bone cement—a preliminary report. *J Orthop Trauma.* 1997;11(2):110–116.

9. Rikli DA, Regazzoni P. Fractures of the distal end of the radius treated by internal fixation and early function: a preliminary report of 20 cases. *J Bone Joint Surg.* 1996;78-B:588–592.

10. Van Dijk JP, Laudy FGJ. Dynamic external fixation versus non-operative treatment of severe distal radial fractures. *Injury.* 1996;27:57–61.

11. Rodriguezmerchan EC. Plaster cast versus percutaneous pin fixation for comminuted fractures of the distal radius in patients between 46 and 65 years of age. *J Orthop Trauma.* 1997;11(3):212–217.

12. Zmurko MG, Eglseder WA, Belkoff SM. Biomechanical evaluation of distal radius fracture stability. *J Orthop Trauma.* 1998;12(1):46–50.

13. Kozin SH, Wood MB. Early soft-tissue complications after fractures of the distal part of the radius. *J Bone Joint Surg.* 1993;75-A(1):144–153.

14. Cailliet R. *Hand Pain and Impairment.* 4th ed. Philadelphia: FA Davis Company; 1994.

15. Calandruccio JH, Jobe MT, Akin K. Rehabilitation of the hand and wrist. In: *Handbook of Orthopaedic Rehabilitation,* Brotzman SB, ed. St Louis: Mosby-Year Book; 1996.

16. McQueen MM, Michie M, Court-Brown CM. Hand and wrist function after external fixation of unstable distal radial fractures. *Clin Orthop.* 1992;285:200–204.

17. Warwick D, Field J, Prothero D, Gibson A, Bannister GC. Function ten years after Colles' fracture. *Clin Orthop.* 1993;295:270–274.

18. Yowell R. Scaphoid fractures: understanding the wrist's anatomy. *Sports Med Update.* 1997;12(4):4–6.

19. Shankman GA. *Fundamental Orthopedic Management for the Physical Therapist Assistant.* St Louis: Mosby-Year Book; 1997.

20. Glassman S. Injury can occur on the links—golfer's wrist. *Advance Magazine.* 1998;9(23):27–28.

21. Zablinski SJ. Investigating carpal injuries. *Sports Med Update.* 1997;12(4):7–10.

22. Sutin JA. Tissue and joint impairments in rheumatoid arthritis. In: *Rehabilitation of Persons with Rheumatoid Arthritis,* Chang RW, ed. Gaithersburg, MD: Aspen Publishers, Inc; 1996.

23. Shirley KD, Lowenstein KL. The hand. *Orthop Phys Ther Clin N Am.* 1997;6(3):283–304.

24. Steinberg DR, Szabo RM. Decision making in the upper extremity problems in the elderly. *Clin Orthop.* 1995;316:63–69.

25. Costi J, Krishan J, Pearcy M. Total wrist arthroplasty—a quantitative review of the last 30 years. *J Rheum.* 1998;25(3):451–458.

26. Wachtl SW, Guggenheim PR, Sennwald GR. Cemented and noncemented replacements of the trapeziometacarpal joint. *J Bone Joint Surg.* 1998;80-B(1):121–125.

27. Kirschenbaum D, Schneider LH, Adams DC, Cody RP. Arthroplasty of the metacarpophalangeal joints with use of silicon-rubber implants in patients who have rheumatoid arthritis. *J Bone Joint Surg.* 1993;75-A(1):3–12.

28. Philips CA. Rehabilitation of the patient with rheumatoid hand involvement. *Phys Ther.* 1989;69(12):1091–1098.

29. Feldmann SV. Exercise for the person with rheumatoid arthritis. In: *Rehabilitation of Persons with Rheumatoid Arthritis,* Chang RW, ed. Gaithersburg, MD: Aspen Publishers, Inc; 1996.

30. Saunders SR. Physical therapy management of hand fractures. *Phys Ther.* 1989;69(12):1065–1076.

31. Lam N, Thurston A. Association of obesity, gender, age and occupation with carpal-tunnel syndrome. *Austral and New Zealand J Surgery.* 1998;68(3):190–193.

32. Lewis RA, Shea OF, Shea KG. Acute carpal tunnel syndrome. *Physician Sportsmed.* 1993;21(7):103–108.

33. Awada A, Amene P, Abdulrazak M, Obeid T. Carpal-tunnel syndrome—a prospective clinical study of 100 cases. *Saudi Med Journal.* 1998;19(2):166–169.

34. Burke DT, Burke MM, Stewart GW, Cambre A. Splinting for carpal tunnel syndrome: in search of the optimal angle. *Arch Phys Med Rehabil.* 1994;75(11):1241–1244.

35. Wright PE. Carpal tunnel and ulnar tunnel syndromes and stenosing tenosynovitis. In: *Campbell's Operative Orthopaedics,* 9th ed, Canale ST, ed. St Louis: Mosby-Year Book; 1998.

36. Mullins PAT. Management of common chronic pain problems in the hand. *Phys Ther.* 1989;69(12):1050–1058.

37. Jobe MT, Wright PE. Peripheral nerve injuries. In: *Campbell's Operative Orthopaedics,* 9th ed, Canale ST, ed. St Louis: Mosby-Year Book; 1998.

38. Sorenson MK. The edematous hand. *Phys Ther.* 1989;69(12):1059–1064.

39. Calandruccio JH. Dupuytren contracture. In: *Campbell's Operative Orthopaedics,* 9th ed, Canale ST, ed. St Louis: Mosby-Year Book; 1998.

40. Travell JG, Simons DG. *Myofascial Pain and Dysfunction. The Trigger Point Manual.* Baltimore: Williams & Wilkins; 1983.

17

Balance Intervention for the Orthopaedic Patient

Jerline Carey

INTRODUCTION

Balance is defined as

- The ability to maintain the center of mass (COM) over the base of support (BOS).
- The ability to maintain equilibrium under a variety of internal disturbances created by our interaction with the environment. These internal perturbations can be of two types: (1) displacement caused by reaching, manipulating things, or turning the head and (2) displacement caused by changing postures and locomotion such as going from sitting to standing, getting out of bed, bending down to pick something up from the floor, and walking.
- The ability to maintain equilibrium during disturbances from outside forces such as slipping, tripping, or being bumped (external perturbations).

In everyday life the COM and BOS relationship are constantly varying in relation to postures and movements. Postures are lying down, sitting, and standing with transitions being made in, within, and out of each of these positions. Movements are eye-hand-related tasks and walking. Balance is a significant component of these everyday tasks. The importance of balance becomes apparent when considering how often a person turns over in bed, repositions on the couch, gets up and down from the dining room chair, or walks from room to room. All of these tasks require COM and BOS shifts performed without much, if any, conscious thought. The fundamental importance of balance is also apparent when considering the patient who walks slowly, staggers and stumbles often, uses an assistive device, cannot get up from a soft living room chair, or repeatedly falls. Therapists can make a significant difference in the functional abilities patients gain once balance is better understood and balance problems are treated appropriately. This chapter is intended to provide basic information necessary to understand the components of balance, and to outline evaluation and intervention approaches that will allow the therapist to remediate problems with balance more successfully.

BALANCE—THE COMPONENTS AND INFLUENCING FACTORS

Balance has been often classified as static (when the BOS does not move, as in standing

I would like to acknowledge Jim Aubert, who introduced me to Trudy. Also thanks to Pat and Katie, my family, who were thoughtfully supportive through this writing project.

or sitting) or dynamic (when the BOS moves, as in walking). One key element in controlling balance is the body maintaining a close relationship between the COM and BOS. If the COM and BOS become separated to too great a degree, a fall is imminent. For instance, if a person leans too far forward, a step forward is needed to prevent a fall. This step forward creates a new BOS under the COM and ensures the COM and BOS remain close. If the person does not take the step in time, the COM will tumble to the floor resulting in a loss of balance. Functional static balance involves the COM being able to move over a stable BOS or, in other words, the COM has a certain range of motion (ROM) it can safely exert over a steady BOS. If the COM does not have controlled range of motion over the BOS, the person standing or sitting will be very rigid and nonfunctional. This COM range of movement and its relationship to the BOS has been called the sway envelope (cone of stability) with the outer ranges being labeled as the limits of the cone of stability.[1(p7)] The therapist wishing to treat balance problems needs to evaluate for the COM's range of

movement capability over the BOS in the various functional postures. Figures 17–1 to 17–4 show the cone of stability for sitting and standing for the mature normal older adult.

Functional dynamic balance involves a person being able to have an unstable situation and maintain balance throughout. To walk, one must sacrifice some degree of stability to accomplish the desired forward mobility. The task of walking is inherently unstable, but the normal person easily stays balanced throughout. During walking, the COM is never directly over the BOS, and the relationship of the two is constantly changing. See Figure 17–5 for the BOS and COM relationship during normal walking. In the normal gait cycle there are predictable times (expressed as %) for single support, swing, and double support time for the lower extremities. Single support or single stance time is the most unstable, whereas double support times are the most stable. In comparison to quiet standing, all of walking is unstable. To some degree the faster one walks the easier it is to balance; the slower one walks, the more energy must be put into bal-

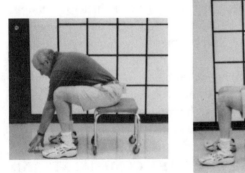
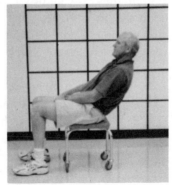
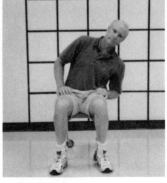

A   B   C

Figure 17–1 Sitting cone of stability. An individual's cone of stability forward (**A**), backward (**B**), and sideways (**C**) make up the full range the HAT (head, arms, and trunk) can move on the seated body.

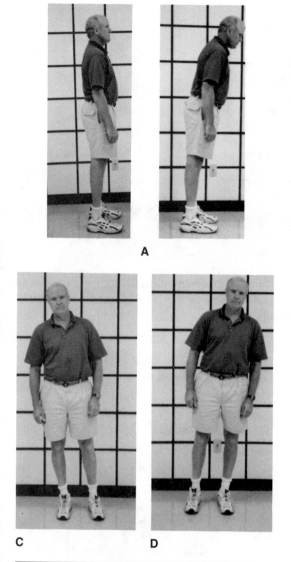

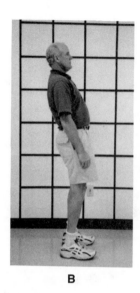

Figure 17–2 Standing cone of stability using the ankle strategy. When an individual stands holding the HAT upright, movement occurs at the ankle in the forward range of motion presented in **A**, the backward range presented in **B**, and the sideways or lateral ranges presented in **C** and **D**.

ancing while moving forward. Normal self-selected walking speed has been established for varying age groups and is available in Table 17–1. Balance problems are a major contributor to self-selected walking speed slowing down to below normal levels and for increased double support percentages.

Standing balance or postural control has been described as having multiple compo-

nents or factors influencing its success, and including the following:[2(p108),3(p240)]

- motor components (including biome-chanical considerations)
- sensory components
- other factors such as endurance capability, lifestyle related to physical fitness, cognition, confidence in balance ability

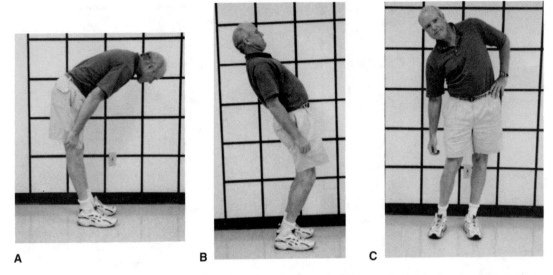

Figure 17–3 Standing cone of stability using the hip strategy. When an individual responds to balance disturbances by movement at the hip, the range of motion available forward can be seen in **A**, the backward range in picture **B**, and the sideways or lateral range in **C**.

and fear of falling, attention demands during standing and walking, medications and pathologies
• normal functional abilities related to balance

• age-related changes with our bodies
• falling and risk of falls

The therapist benefits from understanding these components and influential factors and

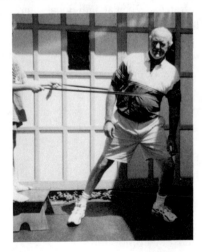
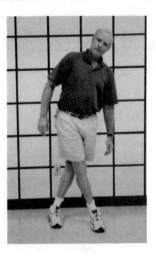

Figure 17–4 Standing cone of stability using the stepping strategy. When the COM exceeds the BOS limits, a step needs to be taken to stay upright. A sideways step can be taken as seen in picture **A** or a cross-over step can be used as seen in **B**.

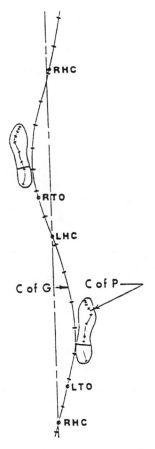

Figure 17–5 BOS/COM relationship. *Source:* Reprinted with permission from D. Winter, *ABC of Balance During Standing and Walking*, p. 41, © 1995, Waterloo Biomechanics.

uses them to outline assessment and treatment of balance problems. The following serves to provide an introductory background in each of these areas.

Motor Components

These can include

- motor strategies for standing: ankle, hip, and stepping (static balance).
- balance during walking (dynamic balance).

- balance (postural control) during internal perturbations during control of tasks such as reaching and head turning; and during transitions of posture such as getting up from sitting to standing.
- balance (postural control) during external perturbations such as tripping, slipping, or being shoved or bumped.
- muscle strength and flexibility.

Motor Strategies for Standing (Static Balance)

Horak first outlined the ankle, hip, and stepping motor strategies occurring in the normal adult. If absent or inappropriately used, an abnormally functioning balance system can be assumed to exist.[4(p1882)] The abnormality may not translate into dysfunction depending on the demand for balance throughout a person's day.

Ankle Strategy. This muscle-firing sequence develops during the person's first year of life as independent standing is experienced and learned.[5(p158)] The firing sequence that evolves uses muscles from the BOS (feet) up to the neck, all timed to fire appropriately to maintain upright posture during a desired manipulative task. Movement during use of the ankle strategy occurs primarily at the ankle; all other joints are stabilized. The firing sequence has anterior, posterior, and lateral patterns and involves the motor system, which responds to the displacement of the COM in relation to the BOS. If the COM is too far forward, the gastroc/soleus complex, the hamstrings, and the low back extensors will sequentially fire to pull the COM back; if the COM is too far back, the tibialis anterior, quadriceps, and abdominals sequentially activate to pull the COM more forward. The body has a 4° backward excursion, an 8° forward excursion, and 16° lateral excursion available for normal

Table 17–1 Age-Related Normative Values for Self-Selected Speeds for Walking

Age (ys)	Cm/Sec	Ft/Min	time to walk 10 ft
1	64 cm/sec[1]	126 ft/min	4.76 sec
1.5	71	139.8	4.34
2	72	141.7	4.23
2.5	81	162	3.80
3	86	168	3.54
3.5	99	195	3.08
4	100	197	3.05
5	108	210	2.86
6	109	3.6	2.80
7	114	224.4	2.67
6–12	116[2]	228.5	2.6
13–19	122.1	240	2.5
19–29	138.5[3]	272.4	2.2
39–49	139.2	274.2	2.19
55–66	133.2	262.2	2.29
Avg male adult	143.3[4]	282	2.13
Avg female	128.3	257.6	2.38
60–80	127.02[5]	250.2	2.4
60–70	110[6]	216.6	2.77
80–90	23.3–73.3	45.6–144	13.16–4.17

[1]cm/sec data from Sutherland (1988) The development of mature walking. Philadelphia, JB Lippincott Co.

[2]cm/sec data from Waters RL et al (1988) Energy-speed relationship of walking: standard tables. *Journal of Orthopaedic Research*, Vol 6, pp 215–222.

[3]cm/sec data from Cunningham DA et al (1982) *Journal of Gerontology*, Vol 37, pp 560–564.

[4]cm/sec data from Perry J (1992) *Gait Analysis: Normal and Pathological Function.* Slack Inc, New Jersey.

[5]cm/sec data from Ostrosdy KM et al (1994) A comparison of gait characteristics in young and old subjects. *Physical Therapy*, Vol 74, pp 637–643.

[6]cm/sec data from Scully RM & Barnes MR (1989) *Physical Therapy.* Philadelphia, JB Lippincott Co.

range of movement when using a "pure" ankle strategy (Figure 17–2). Body sway is constantly occurring at slow speed. The ankle strategy adequately controls the COM to BOS relationship for this particular speed. If the sway were faster, a different strategy would have to be utilized to maintain the COM to BOS relationship.

The sensory information from the ankles and feet is important input that allows a person to use the ankle strategy.[6(p170)] If a person has diabetic neuropathy that limits sensation in the feet, the ankle strategy is limited and the person instead uses other strategies to stand. This limitation may make standing and doing a task such as ironing or reaching above the head very difficult. Other essential elements for having an ankle strategy include having enough ROM at the ankle to allow the body to move on the feet and also adequate hip strength to stabilize the trunk.[7(p11)] Important to note also is the learning situation of the infant and child where the desire to be upright is acquired in relation to wanting to play. This situation provides the "unconscious" mode that balance plays when reaching, manipulating, and walking. It provides an example for the therapy principle of always learning balance and underlying postural control while doing functional tasks.

Hip Strategy. This strategy involves forward, backward, and lateral bending at the hips. Refer to Figure 17–3 for the cone of stability associated with the hip strategy. Hip strategy is used when the COM is moving at a fast rate over a static BOS. Balance is more likely to be maintained if the COM is lowered and has a greater area through which it can move. Also, the hip muscles are stronger than the ankle muscles so when the head, arms, and trunk (HAT) are moving quickly, larger muscles need to be called on to keep it upright. The hip strategy is readily called in when standing on a narrow beam or standing tandem. This strategy is closely associated with the balance system of being able to receive and interpret vestibular system information.[6(p173)]

Ankle and hip strategies try to keep the center of mass stabilized over a stationary BOS. Normal adults use combinations of ankle and hip strategies to remain standing while engaged in tasks such as washing the dishes, painting a wall, reaching for a coat, and various other everyday manipulations.

Stepping Strategy. Sometimes movement of the COM is too great to allow for maintenance of upright unless the BOS is reestablished under the falling COM. This is what the stepping strategy does. When the COM moves too far away from the BOS in an upright position, the foot is automatically placed out far enough to balance the falling center of mass and reestablish control (Figure 17–4). Falling risk has been found to relate to how fast and far a person can place the lower extremity sideways.[8(p488),9(pM81)] Walking is actually a controlled process of falling that uses the stepping strategy. To initiate movement for walking, the COM is moved to the edge of the cone of stability, and then the foot moves forward at the right time to prevent a fall. The normal adult has learned how to use the stepping strategy to allow stumbling while regaining control over the COM.

Balance during Walking (Dynamic Balance)

Balance discussion cannot be limited to the standing position, especially when most falls occur during walking.[10(p647)] Any treatment for balance must extend to locomotion-related dynamic balance. Information in the development of walking in infants and toddlers has identified the locomotor patterns for walking in place much earlier than the balance necessary to walk independently.[5(p270)] For pediatric therapy, emphasizing balance treatment rather than heel-to-toe progression may yield better outcomes with functional improvement. The same assumption can be made when treating adult gait problems. The importance of balance in successful walking is apparent when looking at the development of walking as presented in Exhibit 17–1. Gait deviations commonly noted in many of our patients may be voluntarily developed as a

Exhibit 17–1 Developmental Sequence for Walking

Initial Stage:	Difficulty maintaining upright posture
	Unpredictable loss of balance
	Rigid, halting short steps
	Flat foot contact
	Wide base of support with out-turned toes
	Flexed knee at contact and loading followed by a quick extension
	(immature action of the gastroc/soleus complex)
Middle Stage:	Increased step length
	Beginning heel to toe contact
	Reduced out-toeing and reducing base of support
	Increased pelvic motions involved with gait
Mature Stage:	Full arm swing used (reciprocal, automatic)
	Narrow, normal base of support
	COM is controlled to within the normal adult model of movement
	Better defined heel to toe contact

Source: Reprinted with permission from D.L. Gallahue, *Understanding Motor Development: Infants, Children, Adolescents,* p. 236, © 1989, The McGraw-Hill Companies.

necessary sacrifice of the locomotor pattern because of poor balance skills.

Winter, Gage, and Perry all have identified tasks the body should be able to perform to have normal gait: balance, holding the body upright against gravity, controlling forward momentum (energy absorption), generating energy at the appropriate times, handling the swinging foot and progressing the contact foot forward, and developing energy conservation methods for efficient gait.[11(p2),12,13(p22)] Exhibit 17–2 lists the essential components for each of these normal gait tasks with balance being the most fundamental element. By identifying the missing components of dysfunctional gait, the therapist may more accurately identify treatment needs.

Exhibit 17–3 provides a clearer description of the phases of gait and COM and BOS changes. Exhibit 17–4 provides a spatial view of the COM trajectory during walking as it relates to the phases of gait and the constantly changing BOS.

The BOS and COM relationships described in Exhibit 17–3 and seen in Figure 17–5 can be used to plan task specific dynamic balance activities directly related to walking. The above descriptions of gait provide cause-related information that can direct intervention approaches with more clarity than the typical kinematic (descriptive) gait assessments done in the past. The attention to balance as the task to train rather than working only with the specific locomotor movements of gait also is a change from traditional therapy approaches.

Balance during Internal Perturbations (Reaching, Postural Transitions)

Identifying the strategies associated with standing has been invaluable for therapy advances in assessment and treatment of standing balance problems. The concept

Exhibit 17–2 Essential Components for the Tasks of Gait

Balance:	Control over the BOS and COM relationships (refer back to the cone of stability information) Ability to move the trunk in slight flexion and extension movements in relation to the L/Es Ability to allow trunk to fall forward and eccentrically control its progression Ability to weight shift Hip strength to support head, arms, and trunk (HAT) actions
Upright against Gravity:	Timing the extension push upward (postural synergy) at midstance to raise the COM during midstance time Gastroc, quadriceps, and gluteus maximus timed to perform postural synergy
Energy Absorption:	Control the forward fall of the trunk (gluteus maximus and hamstrings) Control the fast swinging leg so foot contact is slowed (hamstrings) Control the fast forward progression of the tibia after initial contact (gastroc)
Energy Generation:	COM forward fall Manipulation of the COM in its up/down and lateral excursions so energy is transferred efficiently Push off can use gastroc contraction to increase energy Push off can include hip flexor pull off action to increase energy Energy needed to be used to start and stop gait, to turn
Energy Conservation:	Energy transfer methods from initial COM "fall" Pelvic actions to control the COM excursion (pelvic tilt, rotation, drop) Knee bend at initial contact that helps with shock absorption and energy transfer

Source: Copyright © 1998, Jerline Carey.

that balance for standing is dependent on the development of automatic easily accessible motor programs can be translated into treatment approaches that have the patient learning and practicing the ankle, hip, and stepping strategies. The breakdown of the motor strategies for standing has opened the door for use of information that breaks down essential components for functionally related tasks such as reaching, going from sitting to standing, rolling over in bed, and getting up from the floor. Shepherd provides analysis for essential components of reaching and going from sitting to standing.[14(p51)] An outline of these is provided in Exhibit 17–4.

Exhibit 17–3 COM/BOS Relationships for Observational Gait Assessment

Initial Contact:	Double support time (weight on the rear foot; front foot contacting the ground)
	BOS is shifting from behind the COM and will suddenly change to in front during LR
	COM moving forward, medially and downward
	HAT falling forward (trunk flexing, free fall time)
Loading Response:	Double support time (weight on front foot now, rear foot hasn't picked up yet)
	HAT is being decelerated (trunk extending or slowing forward falling action)
	COM is medial and will begin to rise with the loading and trunk deceleration
	COM is behind BOS
	Energy absorbed from slowing down the trunk and absorbing the loading will be sent up the LE and translated into swinging the other LE forward
Midstance:	Single leg support time (weight all on one side)
	COM inside of BOS (not directly over) and progressing from behind to over and then to in front of BOS; the first half COM moves toward weight bearing side; second half it is moving toward opposite side
	COM rises until over BOS and then begins falling forward as it goes in front of BOS
Terminal Stance:	Double support time (matches with initial contact and loading response on opposite side)
	COM is ahead of BOS; weight is on forefoot (heel is off) and swing leg is reaching to land the advancing foot and prepare for weight transfer
	COM is moving toward the other side and at its lowest point
Preswing:	COM continues its movement to the other side and push off is completed
Swing:	COM shift coupled with pelvic action creates a longer step/reach with the swing leg in end stages of swing
	Primary effort is to clear the swinging foot, which is accomplished by enough weight shift and knee flexion

Source: Copyright © 1998, Jerline Carey.

VanSant breaks down the task of getting from the floor to standing by outlining each body segment's possible role for normal functioning (Table 17–2).[15(p190)] The therapist is referred to the work by these researchers for more information. The examples given should assist the therapist in recognizing functional balance ability as made up of automatic motor programs acquired through practice and learning. If

Exhibit 17–4 Shepherd's Essential Components for Reaching and Transitional Posture for Sit to Stand

Essential elements of reaching:	Hold postural position of lying down, sitting, standing Flex shoulder, open hand, extend wrist in timed sequence Grasp action with timed sequence of finger extension, thumb abduction, hand & finger closure Manipulation skills involving opposition, release, movement of objects within the hand
Dysfunction of reaching occurs with:	Problems with postural support and dynamic stability Problems with the essential elements of reaching & grasp/manipulation skills
Essential elements of sit to stand:	Ability to bring the trunk forward with momentum and time this with an overall extension action from the lower extremities Lower extremity extensor abilities to bring the hips from flexion to extension, knee flexion to extension, ankle dorsiflexion to neutral or slight plantarflexion ROM in the ankle that allows for the foot to be positioned under the knee appropriately
Dysfunction of sit to stand occurs with:	Problems generating force with lower limb extensor muscles (hip, knee, ankle) Feet cannot be moved back far enough Not enough flexion can occur between the HAT and hips Not enough control over the momentum of the HAT movement Cannot time the activities correctly Muscle weakness Too much substitution with the hands Inability to control the lowering of the trunk (for stand to sit)

Source: Copyright © 1998, Jerline Carey.

the motor programs used for balance do not reach an automatic level but instead remain available only at a cognitive level (requiring a great deal of attention), then the person's functional level of performing the task is reduced. For instance, if a person is afraid to reach because balance underlying the action is not well developed, the speed and accuracy of the reaching will be reduced.

Table 17–2 VanSant's Common Forms for Coming to Standing

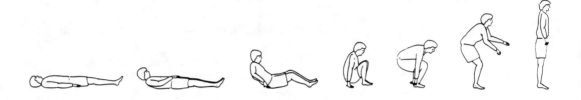

Fig. 1. Most common form of rising to a standing position: upper extremity component, symmetrical push; axial component, symmetrical; lower extremity component, symmetrical squat.

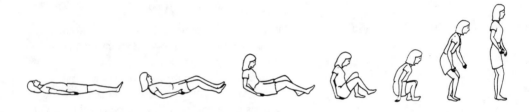

Fig. 2. Second most common form of rising to a standing position: upper extremity component, symmetrical push; axial component, symmetrical; lower extremity component, asymmetrical squat.

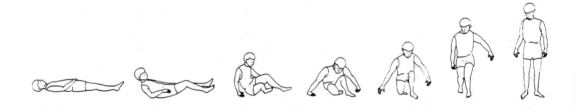

Fig. 3. Third most common form of rising to a standing position: upper extremity component, asymmetrical push and reach; axial component, partial rotation; lower extremity component, half kneel.

continues

Table 17–2 continued

% of Occurrence for UE Components Category	Description	Occurrence
Push and reach to symmetrical push	One hand placed on support surface beside pelvis; other UE reaches across body, hand is placed on support surface; both hands push against support surface to an extended elbow position; UEs are then lifted and used for balance	12.2% (N = 320)
Push and reach	One hand placed on support surface beside the pelvis; other UE reaches out to assist in balance throughout movement; supporting UE pushes into extension and is then lifted, assisting in balance	27.5%
Symmetrical push to push and reach	Both hands placed on support surface, one on each side of pelvis; both hands push against the support surface as trunk moves forward; one hand leaves the support surface before the other to assist in balance	10.6%
Symmetrical push	Both hands placed on support surface, one on each side of pelvis; both hands push against support surface before point when UEs are lifted simultaneously and used to assist in balance	46.6%
Symmetrical push	UEs reach forward, leading the trunk; used to assist in balance throughout the movement	3.1%

% of Occurrence for LE Components Category	Description	Occurrence
Half kneel	LEs are brought toward the trunk assuming an asymmetrical crossed-leg position with one foot, the opposite thigh contacting the support surface; body	15.9%

continues

Table 17–2 continued

% of Occurrence for LE Components Category	Description	Occurrence
	weight is transferred from the thigh to the knee of the same LE, as body is rotated over LEs into half-kneeling position; weight is then transferred to opposite foot as the LEs extend	
Asymmetrical squat	One or both LEs are brought toward trunk, assuming asymmetrical or crossed-leg position with soles of feet contacting the support surface; LEs pushed up to extended position; crossing or asymmetry may be corrected during extension phase by circumduction or stepping action	40.9%
Symmetrical squat with balance step	LEs are flexed synchronously and symmetrically, placing soles of feet on support surface; foot placement is adjusted before extension or at end of straightening by stepping or hopping	16.9%
Symmetrical squat	LEs are brought symmetrically into flexion with heels approximating buttocks; weight is transferred from buttocks to feet; LEs extend vertically	26.3%

Profiles Demonstrated by Normals UE	LE	Axial*
Symmetrical push	Symmetrical	Symmetrical squat
Symmetrical push	Symmetrical	Asymmetrical squat
Asymmetrical push and reach	Partial rotation	Half kneel
Symmetrical reach	Symmetrical	Asymmetrical squat

*Axial percentages of occurrences and component categories and descriptions not included in this figure.

Source: Adapted from A. VanSant, *Physical Therapy,* Alexandria, Virginia, American Physical Therapy Association, 1998, Vol. 68, pp. 188–191, with permission of the American Physical Therapy Association.

Balance during External Perturbations (Tripping, Slipping, and Shoving)

External disturbances related to balance have been clinically expressed with the therapist eliciting equilibrium responses from the patient while sitting or standing. The therapist wants to see head righting, trunk tilting, and quick acting protective extension in the extremities, which are fundamental motor responses to equilibrium problems. Practicing these alone, however, will not suffice in dealing with the external perturbation problems most adults face in everyday life. Environmental safety issues such as poor lighting, crowded rooms or hallways, or closely aligned furniture that does not allow ease or quickness of movement can increase the risk of slipping, tripping, or being unexpectedly bumped.[3(p239)] Exhibit 17–5 has an environmental safety checklist that is clinically useful.

Making the environment safe will not be enough to arm the older adult against risk of balance problems. Increasing age has been associated with decreased ability to slow the swing foot down for initial contact during walking.[16(p344)] This inability increases the likelihood of slipping and risking a fall during this phase of gait. Decreased ability to react to obstacles also occurs with increasing age.[17(pM227)] The older adult is less capable of tolerating attention demands during walking without risking a fall. Strategies to avoid or accommodate situations resulting in a slip or trip are not as easily activated and used by the older population. As a result, an older adult is more likely to slip on a loose rug, trip over an obstacle, or misjudge the needed response to stay balanced and, therefore, have increased risk of falling with advancing age. Practice at handling slipping and tripping surfaces (such as skating on the glide boards),

clearing obstacles, ducking or clearing unexpected flying obstacles, and stumbling and staggering but staying upright all are valuable experiences in maintaining reaction abilities to unexpected perturbations.

Muscle Strength and Flexibility

Muscle strength and flexibility remain fundamental to any motor skill. Functional ROM needs must be identified as differing from passive ROM. Gaining ROM and strength while in a functional position is more effective than simply lengthening the muscle in an unrelated position.[18(p153)] Strengthening to improve function means that the strengthening occurs within 10° of the position the muscle is in while doing a specific task. It is generally believed that the best way to get stronger at a specific task is to practice specifically that task. Using walking as a technique to improve walking is likely superior to any other approach. Component parts of walking can be isolated and practiced such as strengthening the knee during standing. Before the therapy session or episode of care is completed, the entire task with the newly learned component must be practiced in its entirety for the strength gain to become functional. The therapist is responsible for combining treatment for the select joint recovery with treatment for recovery of complex functional tasks of balance and gait. For example, to finally resolve a shoulder problem, reaching while standing and walking needs to be a part of the treatment program.

The major strength needed for improvement in balance is that muscular strength that will control the COM. This is related to eccentric and closed chain muscle action.[19(p23)] Any exercise program meant to improve balance-related flexibility and strength should have these components. For example:

Exhibit 17–5 Environmental Safety Checklist

I.   **Identify if person is at high risk for falling**

II. **Evaluate the environment for intent to "fall-proof" the inside of the home**
   A. Check floor coverings for slipperiness, loose rugs, transition areas that can be tripped over
   B. Check floor area for obstacles, cluttered areas, trip hazards
   C. Check patient's footwear
   D. Check patient's clothing type for robes that are long, clothes that can bind on the legs while walking
   E. Check the lighting that it is bright enough in comparison to patient's visual need; consider use of night lights
   F. Check for need for handrails (stairs, bath)
   G. Consider furniture placement so support to do transitional postures is available (i.e., a sturdy chair by bedside, a heavy table by the easy chair)
   H. Consider furniture that is easy to get in and out of; chairs with armrests; get rid of any furniture that is unsteady
   I. Consider raising the toilet seat (with a sturdy device)
   J. Consider a bath chair (extended one that allows the patient to sit down, then swing legs into the tub)
   K. Check the stairways for easily seen stair edges and firmly fitting carpeting or treads; always have the light on when walking the stairs and use the rail if needed
   L. Check the garbage and laundry storage areas as this task can be overly burdensome; consider smaller containers that are emptied more often; consider placement of the containers so that they are easily accessed for emptying
   M. Check where the phone is and plan out the speed of responding to it

III. **Evaluate for safety while entering and leaving the home**
   A. Check stairs for clear markings on the edges; check lighting
   B. Check stairs for firm, even distances (old porches, old sidewalks have cracks, unevenness, or wear that can be dangerous)
   C. If appropriate, check ramp for ease of use and steepness
   D. Check ability to get in/out of a car, public bus, or taxi. If using special transportation, work out the details so the patient can easily perform the transfers needed to be safe
   E. Check out safety in carrying out any outdoor home care tasks (lawn, garden, and other hobby areas) with the same scrutiny for safety as in the home.

Source: Copyright © 1998, Jerline Carey.

- To improve balance, strengthening the hips can be helpful. The balance-related hip strength is that which controls the HAT movement over the lower extremities. To control the HAT, the hip muscles act eccentrically to keep the trunk from falling forward as the COM is pulled into gravity. The muscles involved are the gluteus maximus and hamstrings, which slow forward flexion of the HAT, the gluteus medius and tensor fascia latae controlling lateral movement of the HAT, and the hip flexors and likely the iliopsoas and rectus femoris for controlling backward movement of the HAT.[11(p58)] Pendulum-type movements of the trunk on the hips (closed chain lower extremity) would provide this strengthening activity.

- Most strength gains are made first by improving central nervous system recruitment of necessary motor units and muscle sequences and later by overloading.[18(p57)] Many of the current therapy programs adhere to the overloading principle only.

- Muscles that cross two joints are considered to provide the balance-related muscle action—one part of the muscle crossing one joint stabilizes that joint, while the other part of the muscle crosses a second joint to provide controlled movement ability. Monoarticular muscles provide the strength that supports the above described action, but coordination and the final strength ability of a joint is compromised when the biarticular muscles lack appropriate length and strength.[19(p2)] Kendall and colleagues' work on standardization of testing for length and strength of the muscles that cross two joints is a useful guide for this work and the reader is referred to her resources.[20(pp27,131,177)]

- The interrelationship of muscles for postural control is not readily understood, but recent evidence in pediatric studies suggests that tibialis anterior dysfunction in the gait cycle is likely related to the gastroc/soleus complex not having adequate strength.[21(p105)] Strengthening the tibialis anterior may never benefit the person if the gastrocnemius remains weak. Gluteus medius strengthening to prevent Trendelenburg signs has also shown better outcome if the gluteus maximi (hip extensors) are

strengthened at the same time. The interrelationship of the lower extremity muscles in providing complex actions for postural support and a manipulative task is not fully understood, but relationships between muscles appear to be of significant importance in determining successful functional strengthening programs.

- The "use it or lose it" principle is important to consider when strengthening and flexibility needs are related to postural control. If a person does not use balance skills regularly, muscle strength and flexibility loss will occur. Loss of daily use or practice may account for loss of strength and flexibility and, eventually, of balance skills in many older adults. Studies indicating that reduction of fall risk and balance problems is associated with high levels of physical fitness and exercise done regularly support the notion that one needs to experience the "edges" of balance ability to retain balance throughout the older years[10(p658)] and that for any person to have an improvement in balance skills, the person needs to have balance challenged.

Although this information may appear significant in amount and content, the picture of balance remains only half completed without understanding the role that sensory information plays in developing and using the motor skills for successful balance.

Sensory Components

Quick access to the motor strategies developed for standing is important and can only be accomplished if the sensory components have developed appropriately. Sensory information important to successful motor performance has been connected or "mapped" to the motor plan and programs specific to standing (ankle, hip, and stepping strategies). In the mature adult, this connection allows for quick assessment of a current situation (sensory-wise) followed by choosing and executing a movement that is automatic, skilled, and efficient. These movements are adaptable and variable so they can be used in multiple situations. Standing is functional for many position variations, and walking is functional over multiple types of surfaces.

Sensory information related to a motor task is gathered from the body and environment to help plan and carry out the movements needed to perform the desired task. The more automatic a motor task, the less reliant the motor system is on incoming sensory information; but the newer a task or the more varied a task is, the more the motor system relies on sensory information to help execute a successful program.[5(p31)] The person wanting to accomplish something that is "everyday" such as getting out of bed only thinks "get out of bed." Beneath that cognitive goal is a sensorimotor system that kicks into action, collecting necessary relevant sensory information and calling on motor memory of what accomplished the task before. To get out of bed, the sensorimotor system has to register what position the body is in to start with, where the body is to move to, what force and speed are needed to get out of bed. Then, finally, the motor plans need to be set into motion.

DiFabio and Emasithi discuss three frames of reference relevant to postural control: exocentric, egocentric, and geocentric perceptions.[22(p460)] The exocentric reference provides information about the body in relation to the environment—such as recognizing the person is sitting, standing, or lying down. The egocentric reference informs us about body segment positions such as the head in

relation to the arm. The geocentric reference deals with upright in relation to gravity demand and in general keeps tabs on where the COM is in relation to the BOS. These classifications explain how the sensorimotor system transforms simple sensory information into spatial perception. To form these sophisticated frames of reference (that essentially tell us where our body is at all times), the balance system has had to use information from three primary sensory systems: proprioception, visual, and vestibular. The information from each of these senses has then been connected to motor strategies for various postures in a multitude of complexity that allow us to practice and be able to do complex movements such as skating, basketball, football, gymnastics, or ballet dancing.

Each sense contributes information to the balance system, but the organization of this multiple, seemingly redundant information appears to be fundamental to developing the ability to perform high-level coordinated skills. Any deterioration of these systems or the organizational abilities of information from these systems results in deterioration of balance ability. Trauma, disuse, and even age-related changes in each of these systems may be in part responsible for the increasing risk of falls seen in the aging population. The following information will outline known sensory contributions to the task of standing and is the most developed sensorimotor balance information available currently.

Proprioceptive Information

Proprioceptive information is collected from the weight-bearing surface of the feet and joints (joint proprioception and kinesthesia). When standing on a solid surface, collection of information from the weight-bearing joints is consistent. The motor task of standing, once established at a motor program level between 7 to 18 months of age, is an easy task for the normal mature person. If the supporting surface becomes noncompliant or dynamic (such as with a tilt board or when walking on an inflatable mattress), the balance system will listen a lot closer to the incoming proprioceptive information because it is not predictable. The balance system will also turn to other sensory systems to provide the necessary information to make the task of staying upright as easy as possible.

Evidence exists that in adults proprioceptive information is most often used by the balance system during easy tasks.[5(p133)] Proprioceptive information is thought to be mapped to ankle strategy. As mentioned earlier in the text, with proprioceptive damage such as with diabetic neuropathy, the person may not be able to access ankle strategy easily and will depend on the hip and the stepping strategies instead. Reliance on proprioceptive information is probably primarily undertaken by the visually impaired population. Although successful balance is present, learning to balance for complex tasks such as skiing becomes much more difficult because of limited sensory information available for motor learning.

Fingertip contact has been recently indicated as strongly related to helping learn or accomplish improved balance.[23(p478)] Improvement in balance capability has been demonstrated with only light fingertip contact and may lead to revisions in assistive devices and training methods for those with proprioceptive impairment in the feet. Proprioceptive information from body parts other than the weight-bearing surface are likely important to the development of the frames of reference. What those relationships are and how the information translates into treatment approaches is not yet well un-

derstood. The proprioceptive system clearly plays a role in the balance system being able to know where the COM is.

Visual Information

Visual information's role in postural control is less well understood than that of the other two senses. Focal or central vision (related to visual acuity) can be used to orient oneself to a point in the environment. The mature balance system uses what is termed ambient vision (or optical flow) to supply the relevant information. This is the information that is passing through the peripheral visual field that records the speed of images.[24(p622)] This information can be used to indicate speed and direction of movement but, interestingly, the eye cannot tell the balance system what is moving—the world or the body.

Our visual memory includes what the movement of the environment (on the ambient visual area) is in relation to a particular speed of sway. The ankle strategy involves a particular speed of sway and results in a particular ambient visual pattern being produced. The hip strategy produces a different speed and pattern of ambient flow of information. The motor system learns to respond to ambient visual flow information and execute a motor strategy meant to keep the person upright.

An example of the motor system being tricked to fire an inappropriate motor response occurs when a person is standing on a dock looking at rippling water. That person may experience a rocking feeling because the motor system is firing the ankle strategy in response to the moving water. In actuality, the person is standing on solid ground and the motor system executions result in the person truly swaying more instead. Moving wall studies have demonstrated that 4-

month-old infants already have motor programs for balancing the head in response to ambient visual flow.[5(p154)] In the dock example, the body feels unstable based on the visual input, and the balance system responds as though the body were moving (not the water as was the case). The motor response then produces movement to counter what was a perceived tipping, and the discovery is made by the balance system that indeed the body is not tipping. This is the point when the person no longer feels "woozy" looking at the water because the balance system turns off the visual input as it discovers the inaccuracy.

The balance system is not intended to rely on visual information alone. As the demand of the world causes a person to turn and look at things, track objects through space, or quickly look from one side to another, the balance system must learn to suppress some of the visual information in relation to planning for balance. The balance system must know when to release itself from visual stimuli and turn to other sensory informants so it is not fooled by following visual information that will lead to a fall. Releasing the eyes from being balance informants is interconnected with a vestibular ocular system not well understood in relation to balance. The ability to turn and track objects, stare at objects not directly ahead, glance between objects (saccadic movements), and close our eyes without losing balance requires a balance system that knows how to prioritize visual information. Vestibular rehabilitation programs have gaze stabilization exercises that are meant to free the balance system from inappropriate reliance on visual input for balance.[5(p298)]

The balance system also uses visual information labeled as feedforward information, which tells us what is in front of us.[5(p131)] Feedforward visual information tells a person about obstacles, upcoming disturbances, or assures someone that there are no concerns ahead related to balance. Visual feedforward information is important to collect so motor planning can be appropriate. Think of the toddler who learns to go around objects rather than through and realize what a valuable lesson it is for learning obstacle avoidance or accommodation merely by seeing it.

Vision's role is multiple and varied in relation to postural control. Reliance on this system alone can cause serious disturbances in postural control with the turn of the head or the closing of the eyes. Gaze stabilization during movement, executing saccadic movements, tracking objects, turning the head, and using head and hand movement while walking or running all require the visual system's sophisticated integration. The patient who does not turn her head while walking is probably overly reliant on the visual system for balance-related information, and is a patient who needs to learn to listen to other sensory systems to improve balance.

Vestibular Information

The vestibular system comprises signals sent from the inner ear. This information is used to determine the speed and direction the head is traveling. After this information is interpreted by the balance system, motor responses that balance the person or reach out and protect him or her from a fall are executed in response to the perceived information.

The vestibular system is responsible for providing eye stabilization (gaze stabilization) from 2 months of age through adulthood while the head is moving.[5(p154)] The vestibular ocular reflex is a necessary component to our visual world remaining stable and not bouncing with each body movement. There are established vestibular rehabilitation programs that have been successful in reducing dizziness from practicing quick changes of position, quick head movements, gaze stabilization, gaze shift, and head turning exercises. These exercises are also useful to improve abilities to integrate sensory information for standing and walking so persons can turn the head, reach for an object, and shake the head, all while walking and staying upright. Many times a "normal" vestibular system is not being attended to by the balance system, and simple exercises done for 3 weeks can change that.

The vestibular system originally was believed to offer input for balance only if the proprioceptive and visual systems were in conflict.[6(p168)] This appears to be the case when postural demand is low, such as with quiet standing; however, when movement is complex, it is more likely that all three systems contribute information so the motor system can provide sufficient postural support. If a football player is sprinting at 20 mph and turning his head to catch the ball while executing a sideways leap, efforts such as gaze stabilization, head turning, and running where there is no foot-to-ground support occurring. This complex situation would demand multiple sensory inputs. The availability of all three senses likely allows the successful completion of complex coordinated motor tasks. If one system is not available, a compromise in end skill potential would be the result.

Sensory Integration

Each sense listed above is important to the final development of the frames of reference. If any one sense is missing, the balance system is left with fewer resources to analyze the task ahead. A reduction in the sensory resources is thought to compromise the final level of coordination that a person can achieve. If someone depends solely on visual input to stand, he or she can be at high risk for falling while walking, with the simple turning of the head. The ability of the body to use these multiple inputs quickly and readily is in part what allows variations with movement. Walking on thick carpet, crossing bumpy lawns, and walking on uneven or graveled surfaces without fear of falling are easily done if the sensory systems are all contributing information and it is being processed appropriately.

A sensory organization test, commonly called the foam and dome, is a very useful clinical tool for identifying sensory contributions and motor strategies used under altered sensory conditions while standing.[4(p1885)] It is a test that takes 10 to 15 minutes to perform after the therapist is familiar with it; it can indicate the necessary sensory-related treatment that will improve balance. Age-related studies indicate that people 60 and older can do all six subtests successfully in an average of 20 seconds, while the younger adults should be able to perform each subtest for 30 seconds.[26(pM264)] Bohanan has demonstrated a relationship between function and standing balance[27(p995)]; therefore, the therapist can assume that if the sensory testing done in standing indicates problems, the patient has problems with sensory information while walking as well. A person can pass the standing test and still have difficulties with walking balance. The Dynamic Gait Index test, a test devised by Shumway-Cook, can be used to identify and score some of the sensory-related problems for walking.[5(p323)] More work is needed to understand sensory contributions for walking, and more factors than these three senses are likely involved. Research in fall prevention is well funded currently, and clinical progressions for better testing should become available soon. In the meantime, several very adequate tools are available.

Other Factors

Endurance ability, level of physical fitness, amount of exercise done on a regular basis, cognition, need for assistive devices, fear of falling and confidence in balance skills, and toleration of attention demands during walking or standing all are influential in the success or interruption of balance.[3(p243),10(p647),28(p16)] These factors will not be discussed further in this chapter, but they are presented for the therapist to recognize the complexity of identifying the cause of balance difficulties. Several assessments available collect information in relation to these factors.

Medications and Pathologies

Many medications interfere with balance.[29(p178)] Because pharmacological intervention is a common treatment approach, overmedication is a significant problem in the elderly. A screening of medications the person is taking and an understanding of their impact on balance are necessary for a comprehensive review of balance problems. Exhibit 17–6 has common clinical complaints and possible medications that could be related to the complaint.

Normal Functional Abilities Related to Balance

Another way to ensure that balance abilities are supporting functional movement is to see if the patient can walk the necessary speed to cover an appropriate distance to cross the street in the time a light stays green or to walk far and fast enough to do community activities such as grocery shopping, banking, or department store shopping.[30(p37)] Timing a task, whatever it is, and relating that to reasonable time to perform is an easy and underutilized functional measure. One of the easiest measures to take is the velocity a person selects to walk and call normal pace (Table 17–1).

To stand from a sitting position in under 2 seconds is related to being able to walk at a functional speed.[31(p90)] Another easily done functionally related task is timing how long it takes to do ten sit-to-stands. The assessment section has age-related information for this repetition task.

A last recommendation for functional understanding of balance is to review the activities of daily living (ADL) tasks for basic and community level abilities and recognize that balance is a large part of each task listed. Using successful performance and being sure a patient can do each one is a reasonable measure of functional abilities. Goldstein provides the information that helped create Table 17–3, which consists of a checklist for basic and instrumental ADL motor tasks.[31(p19)]

Age-Related Changes That Can Lead to Balance Problems

The following is a list of age-related changes that could lead to balance problems.[5(p172),32(p221)] It is not a complete list but does relate to the components previously discussed. Age-related changes in the body are inevitable, although research has not clearly identified which of these are age- or pathology-related. The interaction of the components of the balance system and the ability of some functions to remediate for lost functions can explain why there is little change in functional ability overall in balance and walking related to basic ADL requirements. What can be seen as degraded with aging is the ability to perform complex demanding tasks easily.

- visual acuity loss
- peripheral vision loss
- depth perception loss

Exhibit 17–6 Examples of Medications That Affect Balance

Common side effects of drugs that influence balance:	Postural hypotension, fatigue & weakness, dizziness
Examples of drugs that cause postural hypotension:	Antidepressants, antipsychotics, antihypertensive drugs, diuretics, opiate narcotics, vasodilator drugs, Parkinson's drugs (i.e., levodopa)
Examples of drugs that cause fatigue and weakness:	*Cardiovascular drugs:* beta blockers, Ca channel blockers, digitalis, diuretics, drugs that prolong depolarization, organic nitrates, vasodilators *Antidepressants* *Most of the drugs used for diabetes mellitus for insulin absorption* *Parkinson's drugs* *Pain and Inflammation related drugs:* corticosteroids *Most of the cancer related drugs*
Drugs that cause dizziness:	*Cardiovascular drugs:* alpha-blockers, beta-blockers, Ca channel blockers, digitalis, diuretics, drugs that prolong repolarization, organic nitrates, sodium channel blockers *Peripheral neuropathy drugs:* ethambutol, isoniazid, metronidazole, nitrofurantoin, phenytoin, vinblastine *Parkinson's disease drugs:* dopaminergic agents, anticholinergics, antidepressants, antihistamines *Pain and Inflammation related drugs:* narcotic analgesics, NSAIDs, corticosteroids *Cancer drugs:* alkylating agents, antimetabolites, zinterferons

Source: Data from C. Ciccone, Geriatric Pharmacology in *Geriatric Physical Therapy*, A. Guccione, ed., © 1993, Mosby Year-Book, Inc. and L. Eddy, *Physical Therapy Pharmacology*, © 1992, Mosby Year-Book, Inc., B. Hodgson, R. Kizior, and R. Kingdom, *Nurse's Drug Handbook*, WB Saunders, Inc.

- reduced receptors in the vestibular system
- reduced proprioceptive input from the ankles
- slowed central nervous system processing
- increased reaction time
- changed sequencing of muscle firing patterns
- loss of strength
- joint stiffness

Each change related to age listed above may not occur in every individual or the change that does occur may not result in a change in balance ability. At what point age-related changes impact function remains an unanswered question and the complexity of balance makes the identification of the change agent causing the balance problems difficult at best.

Table 17–3 Checklist for BADL and IADL Motor Tasks

	BADL-Related Activities			
Bed Activities	*Self Care/Hygiene*	*Eating*	*Dressing*	*Mobility*
Moving in bed	Brushing teeth	Using utensils	Undergarments	Transfers:
Moving pillow	Bathing/	Managing glass	Shirt/slacks	Bed to chair
Moving blankets	showering	Managing cup	Skirts/dresses	Bed to stand/
Reaching for	Combing hair	Cutting meat	Socks/panty-	to toilet
objects	Toileting		hose	Chair to stand
Getting up	Shaving		Shoes	Stand to bath
	Putting on		Coats/sweaters	Stand to bed
	makeup			Into car
				Gait:
				Walk on level
				surfaces
				room to room
				Transporting
				items as
				needed
				Stairs
				Getting in/out
				of the house

	IADL-Related Activities				
Meal Preparation	*Light Housework*	*Home Business*	*Sexually Related*	*Getting In/Out of the House*	*Transportation*
Cutting up	Dusting	Check writing	Determined by	Handling	Transferring
vegetables	Washing	Telephone	individual	doors	in/out of
Carrying/mea-	dishes	use		Getting on	car
suring	Mopping	Getting the		outside	Transferring
things	floors	mail		clothes	in/out of
Oven use	Cleaning	Computer		Stairs, curbs,	public
Preparing a	sinks	use		sidewalks	transport
meal	Vacuuming				Getting
Mixing things					to/from
					appts

continues

Table 17–3 continued

Shopping	Banking	Yard Work	Leisure Activities	Work/ School	General Fitness/Other
Walking Pushing a cart Reaching Carrying items/bags Handling money	Managing check- book & accounts Walking Standing in line	Raking Mowing Watering lawn Leaf bags? Gardening	Determined by individ- ual	Determined by individual Walking needs? Standing needs? Transfer needs?	Determined by individual

Source: Copyright © 1998, Jerline Carey.

Falling and Risk of Falls[3(p238),9(pM75),25(pM264),33(p447),34(p735),35(p1146),36(p327),37(p1108)]

At any given time, 30 to 70% of community dwellers are at risk for falls. Falls are a problem in the hospital setting for geriatric patients with acute illnesses. 28 to 45% of nursing home residents have falls. The risk for fall increases with each decade past 60. Age- and pathology-related changes are thought to lead to balance impairment related to falls. Some studies have demonstrated that a decline in function can easily follow these traumatic events. A significant number of hip fractures are the result of falls. Fear of falling is a major problem that can result in deconditioning, muscle weakness, and increased immobility. Measuring for risk of fall and concern about prevention of falls becomes a significant part of any physical therapist's caseload, regardless of the work setting. Identifying who is at risk and using prevention strategies have been demonstrated as effective in decreasing the incidence of falls.

Falling—What Are the Risk Factors?

Falls are a multifaceted problem caused sometimes by extrinsic factors such as trip-ping because of poor lighting and sometimes by intrinsic factors such as pathologies, medications, or a degradation of the sensory or motor system necessary for successful balance. Prevention is not a single answer that can be applied to everyone, but instead demands an evaluative approach to identify extrinsic and intrinsic cause of a fall or multiple falling episodes; then treatment is done in response to the identified problem areas.

History of a Fall

If a fall occurs, a history describing the onset, probable cause, and activities at the time of fall should be done. Checking for dizziness or lightheadedness, taking a medication history, and clearly describing the fall are also important. Exhibit 17–7 is an example of a fall history form that would be helpful in the clinical setting.

Intrinsic Causes for Falls

An evaluation that involves checking the sensory and motor systems and functional abilities would be appropriate to identify internally related problems contributing to the fall. The entire section outlining balance identifies all the factors to be considered for intrinsically related falls. The evaluation sec-

Exhibit 17–7 Example of a Fall History Form

How many falls have occurred in the past week? _____ past month?_____ past year? _____
When was your last fall? _____
Describe the recovery from the fall incident: _____

Describe how the fall occurred:
  Sudden/gradual _____

  _____

  Activities at the time of fall _____

  Direction of fall _____

  Recovery attempts _____

  Patient description of cause _____

Categorize fall as extrinsic cause/intrinsic cause/both:

Extrinsic: Trip/slip/bump/environmental hazard (see list in Exhibit 17–5)
Intrinsic: Dizziness/weakness or fatigue/other (see list in Table 17–5)

Source: Data from J. Chandler and P. Duncan, Balance and Falls in the Elderly: Issues in Evaluation and Treatment in *Geriatric Physical Therapy*, A. Guccione, ed., pp. 237–251, © 1993, Mosby Year-Book, Inc.

---

tion of this chapter outlines how to go about this process.

Extrinsic Causes for Falls

Falling is not a problem exclusive to the older adult. Small children fall often, as do all age groups. A full regimen improving the body's functions for balancing may do nothing to prevent that fall caused by tripping over an obstacle or slipping on an ice patch. Nevertheless some environmental analysis to check for general safety can go a long way in fall prevention. Dimly lit rooms, overcrowded rooms, slippery rugs, uneven stairs, and stairs without a railing are all environmental factors that can be easily modified to reduce the risk of tripping and falling. A fall risk assessment would include environmental checklists to find the hazards. See Exhibit 17–5 for a safety checklist that can be used

for evaluation of fall risk due to extrinsic factors. The SAFE AT HOME assessment given in Appendix 1–A is also a useful tool for evaluating extrinsic factors.

Anyone presenting for medical treatment because of problems from a fall should have an assessment for prevention of future recurrences. Also, those at risk in the community, nursing homes, and hospitals should be identified and the actual fall prevented where possible. Intrinsic-related causes should be considered for remediation through therapeutic intervention. The following balance assessment recommendations include these considerations for the various groups.

BALANCE ASSESSMENT

Assessment is performed for multiple reasons. Assessment helps determine

- the extent of a presenting problem in relation to function
- the impairment-related problems so treatment can be directed appropriately
- prognosis and diagnosis so the potential for improvement can be identified and goals established for changing the situation
- if treatment goals and final outcome expectations were met.

Many reliable and valid testing tools related to balance ability are available to therapists, although these tests all represent bits and pieces of balance. The therapist is left to establish the minimal comprehensive testing requirements needed for evaluating balance problems since no common approach yet exists. New information will likely be available on an ongoing basis over the next few years, and the following information is presented to give the interested clinician a starting point to begin evaluating and planning intervention for balance problems.

Functional Assessment

The fundamental purpose and ideal outcome for rehabilitation therapy is to improve functionally related abilities of a patient for the achievement of independence in all aspects of life. It makes sense then to identify first the functionally related balance problems a patient is having. This can be done by identifying where the patient has difficulties with ADL or safety-related problems with balance that may result in a fall. Once the particular problem tasks are identified, then evaluating for the related balance and gait problems while doing that task is helpful for treatment planning purposes. For instance, if a person cannot walk from the bed to the bathroom in a timely safe manner, improving balance and speed of walking in that particu-

lar environment become the necessary task to work on.

Other easily done measures closely related to carrying out the ADL successfully include normal walking velocity, normal temporal distance measures of walking (e.g., cadence, BOS, stride length, velocity over distance), timed tests for coming to standing, or timed walking over distance. Five easy-to-use fall risk assessments include the Berg Balance Test, the Tinetti, timed Get Up and Go, the Dynamic Gait Index, and the GARS. The scores from these assessments indicate risk for falls; retesting can indicate improvement toward decreasing the risk for a fall that translates into improved safety. The "Fast Evaluation of Mobility, Balance, and Fear" appears to be a comprehensive screening tool.[38(p904)] Use of all of these tests at one time is not recommended; instead, the therapist needs to choose the most appropriate test or tests from this list for a particular individual. There is a learning time needed to become proficient and reliable with these tests, and the therapist is encouraged to practice administering these tests before using them clinically. These tests yield quantitative information in the functional realm and are well received by third-party payers looking for evidence of need for and effectiveness of physical therapy interventions.

ADL Checklist

Checking to see if a person can or cannot do each of the listed tasks clearly indicates ADL abilities or problem areas. Refer back to Table 17–3 as a qualitative testing tool is recommended.

Walking Velocity. This is easily measured by videotaping a person walking over a 10-foot distance and establishing a feet/minute measure. This can be compared to the norms presented in Table 17–1. If a person scores below normal, then ADL compromise can be assumed in relation to instrumental or basic ADL (IADL or BADL). The studies involving community walking demands have helped identify the distances and velocities needed for gait to be at an IADL level.

Walking over Time and Distance.[39(p1607)] Measuring how far a person can walk in 2, 6, or 12 minutes is an endurance-related walking test that can tell the therapist if a person has the capability to walk a block or walk long enough to shop for groceries. Having a measured course of 100 feet or longer with a chair to rest as needed allows easy administration of this test. The test findings can be reviewed against normal walking speeds people use for walking crosswalks, walking for shopping, or other speeds used to carry out other IADL.

Temporal Distance Measures of Walking.[40(p21)] A footprint test can give objective measures for BOS, stride length, cadence, and velocity. This author's experience with her standardized footprint test is that it takes about three to four practices to get the testing time to 10 minutes and the scoring time to about 12 minutes.

Timed Tests for Coming to Standing.[41(p77)] The number of repetitions a person can go from sit to stand in a given amount of time has been associated with age as well as the ability to control descent speed used to go from stand to sit positions. Table 17–4 indicates the normative values to expect for each decade of life. Another quickly done measure is to record the time it takes a person to go from sit to stand. Under 2 seconds is normal.[31] This therapist has had numerous patients take 6 to 8 seconds or longer to get from sit to stand at the initial evaluation.

Berg Balance Test.[42(p242),43(p576),44(p306),45(p466)] This is a 56-point test with 14 items in which

a score of 40 or less indicates a high risk for falls. A normal person can easily pass all items, so any scoring less than 56 indicates a problem with balance but does not indicate a risk for falls unless the score is 40 or under. Exhibit 17–8 has the score sheet for this test. This is a standing balance test and may not reflect a balance problem during walking. The sensitivity of the Berg is improved with measuring gait velocity; if both scores are reduced from normal, the fall risk problem is more clearly identified. The Berg has been shown to be most sensitive when used with the nursing home population. After several practices the Berg takes about 12 to 15 minutes to administer to most patients. The items are practical, functionally related, and provide qualitative information about balance with narrowed base of support, balance during turning and reaching, and the capability of postural control during transitions in positions.

Tinetti.[46(p9),47(p604)] This is a well-researched risk test for falls assessment tool that takes about 15 minutes to administer. It has a standing and walking section with a combined score of less than 19 to 24 of the 28 indicating a high risk for falls. This test has been shown to be most sensitive to the community dwelling population. The scoring forms for this test are in Exhibit 17–9.

Timed Get Up and Go.[48(p387)] For this test, the person stands up from a chair, walks 10 feet, turns, and then returns. The normal person can do this in less than 10 seconds. The patient is scored qualitatively on a five-point ordinal scale for quality of balance. This test has been shown to indicate risk for falls reliably. Videotaping is recommended and scoring from the video produces the best reliability.

Dynamic Gait Index.[5(p323)] This is an easily done eight-item, 24-point test where a

Table 17–4 Age-Related Normative Values for 10 Repetitions Sit-to-Stand

Age (years)	Women (time in seconds)	Men
20	10.9	8.8
25	11.8	9.8
30	12.6	10.8
35	13.4	11.7
40	14.3	12.7
45	15.1	13.7
50	15.9	14.7
55	16.8	15.6
60	17.6	16.6
65	18.4	17.6
70	19.3	18.5
75	20.1	19.5
80	20.9	20.5
85	21.8	21.5

Source: Reprinted from *The American Journal of Medicine,* Vol. 78, Cuska & McCarty, Simple Method for Measurement of Lower Extremity Muscle Strength, pp. 77–81, Copyright 1985, with permission from Excerpta Media Inc.

normal person should score 24 of 24 of the points. The items include: walking at a normal pace for 20 feet; changing walking speeds without difficulty; walking in a straight line while turning the head from side to side, then looking up and down; performing a quick stop and turn without problems; walking over and then around obstacles while maintaining a steady walking pace; and ascending and descending a flight of stairs without difficulty. The items are scored from normal to mild, moderate, or severe impairment on a scale of 3 to 0. This test applies some of the sensory integration components of gait not covered by the other tests and has been useful with those patients who have balance problems while walking. Another advantage of this test content is that it provides internal perturbations-related information that the other tests do not. The reader is referred to the resource for a copy of this test.

GARS.[49(pM14)] This is an easily done test that has a shorter version available called the m-GARS (modified GARS). The original test, which this author has found useful for treatment planning as well as functional assessment, requires videotaping a person walking 10 feet and turning. Scoring from the videotape results in a possible perfect and normal score of 0. Scoring 18 or above indicates a high risk for falls. This test is available in Exhibit 17–10.

General Recommendations for the Functional Testing

This author most commonly uses the ADL checklist, walking velocity, sit to stand timed tests, and the Berg for the initial evaluation. If

Exhibit 17–8 Berg Score Sheet

EQUIPMENT:
Stop Watch
Ruler
Regular chair with armrest
Slipper
Wall dot
Stool without armrests (optional) or low mat

1. **Sitting to Standing (Use Regular Chair with Armrests)**
   Instructions: Please stand up. Try not to use your hands for support.
   (   ) 4 able to stand without using hands and stabilize independently
   (   ) 3 able to stand independently using hands
   (   ) 2 able to stand using hands after several tries
   (   ) 1 needs minimal aid to stand or to stabilize
   (   ) 0 needs moderate or maximal assist to stand

2. **Standing Unsupported**
   Instructions: Please stand for two minutes without holding.
   (   ) 4 able to stand safely 2 minutes
   (   ) 3 able to stand 2 minutes with supervision
   (   ) 2 able to stand 30 seconds unsupported
   (   ) 1 needs several tries to stand 30 seconds unsupported
   (   ) 0 unable to stand 30 seconds unassisted

   If a subject is able to stand 2 minutes unsupported, score full points for sitting unsupported. Proceed to item #4.

3. **Sitting with Back Unsupported but Feet Supported on Floor or on a Stool**
   Instructions: Please sit with arms folded for 2 minutes.
   (   ) 4 able to sit safely and securely 2 minutes
   (   ) 3 able to sit 2 minutes under supervision
   (   ) 2 able to sit 30 seconds
   (   ) 1 able to sit 10 seconds
   (   ) 0 unable to sit without support 10 seconds

4. **Standing to Sitting**
   Instructions: Please sit down.
   (   ) 4 sits safely with minimal use of hands
   (   ) 3 controls descent by using hands
   (   ) 2 uses back of legs against chair to control descent
   (   ) 1 sits independently but has uncontrolled descent
   (   ) 0 needs assistance to sit

5. **Transfers (Use Regular Chair to Mat or Chair to Stool)**
   Instructions: Arrange chair(s) for a pivot transfer. Ask subject to transfer one way toward a seat with armrests and one way toward a seat without armrests. You may use two chairs (one with and one without armrests) or a bed and a chair.

continues

Exhibit 17–8 continued

( ) 4 able to transfer safely with minor use of hands
( ) 3 able to transfer safely with definite needs of hands
( ) 2 able to transfer with verbal cuing and/or supervision
( ) 1 needs one person to assist
( ) 0 needs two people to assist or supervise to be safe

6. **Standing Unsupported with Eyes Closed**
Instructions: Please close your eyes and stand still for 10 seconds.
( ) 4 able to stand 10 seconds safely
( ) 3 able to stand 10 seconds with supervision
( ) 2 able to stand 3 seconds
( ) 1 unable to keep eyes closed 3 seconds but stands safely
( ) 0 needs help to keep from falling

7. **Standing Unsupported with Feet Together**
Instructions: Place your feet together and stand without holding.
( ) 4 able to place feet together independently and stand 1 minute safely
( ) 3 able to place feet together independently and stand for 1 minute with supervision
( ) 2 able to place feet together independently but unable to hold for 30 seconds
( ) 1 needs help to attain position but able to stand 15 seconds feet together
( ) 0 needs help to attain position and unable to hold for 15 seconds

8. **Reaching Forward with Outstretched Arm while Standing**
Instructions: Lift arm to 90 degrees. Stretch out your fingers and reach forward as far as you can. (Examiner places a ruler at end of fingertips when arm is at 90 degrees. Fingers should not touch the ruler while reaching forward. The recorded measure is the distance forward that the fingers reach while the subject is in the most forward lean position. When possible, ask subject to use both arms when reaching to avoid rotation of the trunk.)
( ) 4 can reach forward confidently 25 cm (10 inches)
( ) 3 can reach forward 12 cm safely (5 inches)
( ) 2 can reach forward 5 cm safely (2 inches)
( ) 1 reaches forward but needs supervision
( ) 0 loses balance while trying/requires external support

9. **Pick Up Object from the Floor from a Standing Position (Use Slipper)**
Instructions: Pick up the shoe/slipper that is placed in front of your feet.
( ) 4 able to pick up slipper safely and easily
( ) 3 able to pick up slipper but needs supervision
( ) 2 unable to pick up but reaches 2–5 cm (1–2 inches) from slipper and keeps balance independently
( ) 1 unable to pick up and needs supervision while trying
( ) 0 unable to try/needs assist to keep from losing balance or falling

10. **Turning To Look Behind over Left and Right Shoulders while Standing (If Needed, Use Dot on the Wall)**
Instructions: Turn to look directly behind you over toward left shoulder. Repeat to the right. Examiner may pick an object to look at directly behind the subject to encourage a better twist turn.

continues

Exhibit 17–8 continued

(   ) 4 looks behind from both sides and weight shifts well
(   ) 3 looks behind one side only, other side shows less weight shift
(   ) 2 turns sideways only but maintains balance
(   ) 1 needs supervision when turning
(   ) 0 needs assist to keep from losing balance or falling

11. **Turn 360 Degrees**
    Instructions: Turn completely around in a full circle. Pause. Then turn a full circle in the other direction.
    (   ) 4 able to turn 360 degrees safely in 4 seconds or less
    (   ) 3 able to turn 360 degrees safely one side only 4 seconds or less
    (   ) 2 able to turn 360 degrees safely but slowly
    (   ) 1 needs close supervision or verbal cuing
    (   ) 0 needs assistance while turning

12. **Place Alternate Foot on Step or Stool while Standing Unsupported (Use 4″ Platform Stool)**
    Instructions: Place each foot alternately on the step/stool. Continue until each foot has touched the step/stool four times.
    (   ) 4 able to stand independently and safely and complete 8 steps in 20 seconds
    (   ) 3 able to stand independently and complete 8 steps > 20 seconds
    (   ) 2 able to complete 4 steps without aid with supervision
    (   ) 1 able to complete > 2 steps needs minimal assist
    (   ) 0 needs assistance to keep from falling/unable to try

13. **Standing Unsupported One Foot in Front**
    Instructions: (DEMONSTRATE TO SUBJECT) Place one foot directly in front of the other. If you feel that you cannot place your foot directly in front, try to step far enough ahead that the heel of your forward foot is ahead of the toes of the other foot. (To score 3 points, the length of the step should exceed the length of the other foot and the width of the stance should approximate the subject's normal stride width.)
    (   ) 4 able to place foot tandem independently and hold 30 seconds
    (   ) 3 able to place foot ahead of other independently and hold 30 seconds
    (   ) 2 able to take small step independently and hold 30 seconds
    (   ) 1 needs help to step but can hold 15 seconds
    (   ) 0 loses balance while stepping or standing

14. **Standing on One Leg**
    Instructions: Stand on one leg as long as you can without holding.
    (   ) 4 able to lift leg independently and hold >10 seconds
    (   ) 3 able to lift leg independently and hold 5–10 seconds
    (   ) 2 able to lift leg independently and hold = or > 3 seconds
    (   ) 1 tries to lift leg unable to hold 3 seconds but remains standing independently
    (   ) 0 unable to try or needs assist to prevent fall

    (   ) **TOTAL SCORE** (*Maximum = 56*) *40 or lower at risk for fall

Source: Reprinted with permission from K. Berg, S. Wood-Dauphinee, J. Williams, and D. Gayton, Measuring Balance in the Elderly: Preliminary Development of an Instrument. *Physiotherapy Canada*, Vol. 41, No. 6, p. 306, © 1989, Canadian Physiotherapy Association

the patient has problems with the Berg, an intervention program is started at the standing level. As the patient progresses, then either the Dynamic Gait Index, the Tinetti, or GARS is used to indicate advanced balance problems. If the patient is going to be independent in the home, the Berg and Dynamic Gait Index tests, once passed, correlate with the ability for safe gait. The community dwellers, people who are functioning outside the home and need community-related mobility, benefit from the timed walking tests and the footprint tests. These recommendations are not a research-based approach yet, but this author has found this approach works well for identifying the functional problems in the various settings of hospital, nursing home, home health care, and outpatient care.

Impairment Assessment

For the practicing therapist, the most appreciated assessment is one that can indicate the most efficient and effective intervention. For balance problems, the therapist needs to use tests and measures that assess the component parts of balance and indicate where the treatment-related problems exist. While there are objective tests that can be used, qualitative evaluation remains a large part of impairment testing for balance problems. Table 17–5 outlines the component parts of balance as discussed in the previous section of this chapter and lists several testing methods related to each component.

The following tests or procedures are reviewed for consideration by the therapist for use in the impairment-related testing.

Foam and Dome (Sensory Components and Standing Motor Strategies)[4(p1885),25(p1550)]

This is by far one of the most underused tests that is easy to perform and yields useful intervention planning information. This test consists of six subtests, each having altered sensory conditions. Each subtest is a 30-second test with the first three tests done on a firm surface (the floor) first with eyes open, then eyes closed, and finally wearing a visual conflict dome. The dome is a specially constructed dome that causes visual misinformation to be registered during standing and results in the patient having to solve a sensory conflict of information. The last three subtests are done with the patient standing on a noncompliant foam that is specially ordered. Again the tests are done with eyes open, closed, and then with the visual conflict dome. The therapist notes the strategies the patient uses to remain standing, records the time, and protects the patient from a fall should one occur during testing. The full test takes about 10 minutes to administer. The score sheet this author uses is in Exhibit 17–11, and the interpretive information is in Exhibit 17–12. The intervention section of this chapter has treatment plans for the test in relation to the interpretative findings.

Observational Gait Assessment

Enough cannot be said in support of videotaping several gait cycles over a known distance for analyzing at a later time. Double support time, velocity, and the qualitative information listed in the tables on observational gait assessment are much more reliably identified on video rather than using the naked eye.[50(p1031)] Balance problems in walking are related to reduced velocity, altered swing/stance ratios, and COM/BOS relationship changes. The increased evaluation time invested is often rewarded with an improved focus with treatment.

Kendall's Strength and Length Testing (Strength and ROM)

A comprehensive presentation of this information is beyond the scope of this chapter

Exhibit 17–9 Tinetti Score Sheet

TINETTI ASSESSMENT TOOL
BALANCE TESTS

Initial Instructions: Subject is seated in hard, armless chair; the following maneuvers are tested:

1. Sitting balance	Leans or slides in chair	= 0
	Steady, safe	= 1____
2. Arises	Unable to without help	= 0
	Able, uses arms to help	= 1
	Able without use of arms	= 2
3. Attempts to rise	Unable without help	= 0
	Able, requires > 1 attempt	= 1
	Able to arise, 1 attempt	= 2____

4. Immediate standing balance (first 5 seconds)

Unsteady (swaggers, moves feet, trunk sway)	= 0
Steady but uses walker or other support	= 1
Steady without walker or other support	= 2____

5. Standing balance

Unsteady	= 0
Steady but wide stance (medial heels > 4″ apart)	
and uses cane or other support	= 1
Narrow stance without support	= 2____

6. Nudged (subject at maximum position with feet as close together as possible, examiner pushes lightly on sternum with palm of hand 3 times)

Begins to fall	= 0
Staggers, grabs, catches self	= 1
Steady	= 2 ____

7. Eyes closed

Unsteady	= 0
Steady	= 1____

8. Turning 360 degrees

Discontinuous steps	= 0
Continuous	= 1
Unsteady (grabs, staggers)	= 0
Steady	= 1____

9. Sitting down

Unsafe (misjudged distance, falls into chair)	= 0
Uses arms or not a smooth motion	= 1
Safe, smooth motion	= 2____
BALANCE SCORE	/16

continues

Exhibit 17–9 continued

GAIT TESTS

Initial instructions: Subject stands with examiner, walks down hallway or across room, first at "usual" pace, then back at "rapid, but safe" pace (using usual walking aids)

10. **Initiation of gait** (immediately after told to "go")
    Any hesitancy or multiple attempts to start   = 0
    No hesitancy   = 1

11. **Step length and height**
    a. Right swing foot
       Does not pass left stance foot with step   = 0
       Passes left stance foot   = 1
       Right foot does not clear floor completely with step   = 0
       Right foot completely clears floor   = 1
    b. Does not pass right stance foot with step   = 0
       Passes right stance foot   = 1
       Left foot does not clear floor completely with step   = 0
       Left foot completely clears floor   = 1____

12. **Step symmetry**
    Right and left step length not equal (estimate)   = 0
    Right and left step appear equal   = 1____

13. **Step continuity**
    Stopping or discontinuity between steps   = 0
    Steps appear continuous   = 1____

14. **Path** (estimated in relation to floor tiles, 12″ diameter; observe excursion of 1 foot over about 10-foot course)
    Marked deviation   = 0
    Mild/moderate deviation or uses walking aid   = 1
    Straight without walking aid   = 2____

15. **Trunk**
    Marked sway or uses walking aid   = 0
    No sway but flexion of knees or back or spreads arms out while walking   = 1
    No sway, no flexion, no use of arms, and no use of walking aid   = 2____

16. **Walking time**
    Heels apart   = 0
    Heels almost touching while walking   = 1____

        GAIT SCORE: /12

TOTAL SCORE: BALANCE + GAIT SCORE =   /28

Source: Reprinted with permission from *Journal of American Geriatric Society.* Vol. 34, pp. 119–126, © 1986, Williams & Wilkins.

and the reader is referred to Kendall, Mc-Creary, and Provance's text for these testing and treatment techniques.[20(pp27,131,177)] Biarticular (two joint) muscles appear to be the most significant to gain the appropriate length and strength within that correct length, and each is closely associated with monoarticular muscles. The muscle list to consider for specific length and strength testing for improving balance includes:

- tensor fascia latae and gluteus medius
- hamstrings and gluteus maximus
- rectus femoris
- gastrocnemius
- tibialis anterior
- peroneus longus

Goal Writing

The therapist can write long-term goals in relation to expected changes in the tests and measures used with the functional goals. An example would be an expected improvement on the Berg Balance Test score after three or six weeks time following balance training. Another example could be writing a goal for improving the speed with which the person can walk around the house and complete identified self-care tasks. Short-term or treatment-related goals can then be written in relation to improvement in the impairment-related areas. For example, an improvement in the length and strength measures or the Foam and Dome score should be expected as treatment progresses.

Overall, evaluation is intended to help guide appropriate treatment planning and to show effectiveness of therapy. Using both quantitative and qualitative testing will help the therapist in the treatment planning process and qualifying the need for treatment.

TREATMENT FOR BALANCE DYSFUNCTION

Many balance dysfunctions can be remediated; however, orthopaedic geriatric patients are often discharged from physical therapy before the balance problems have been sufficiently evaluated and treated. Safety standards related to normal balance and gait are evaluation areas left undone by therapists unfamiliar with the new information on balance. Much of the balance work can be done by adding 5 to 10 minutes of treatment time during the subacute phase of recovery. Follow-up can be two to three times a week or as little as one to two times a month with balance training advanced as the patient practices independently. Many geriatric patients with balance deficits can likely reach functional safety levels within a short time if the cause is accurately identified and treatment targeted appropriately.

Assessment (by examination, testing, measuring, and evaluating) is the important first step in alleviating balance dysfunction. A second important step is to match the intervention to the problem. A single balance treatment protocol would be impossible to develop because the balance system is complex and the possible problems are numerous. In this next section a brief introduction is provided for the therapist wanting to begin balance treatment. The therapist is recommended to continue pursuit of information in balance intervention approaches beyond the very limited introduction provided in this chapter. The information provided does not present a balance protocol but instead provides an introductory summary of possible interventions for multiple problems areas. The evaluating therapist has to identify cause and plan a related treatment program for the individual patient.

Exhibit 17–10 Gait Abnormality Rating Scale (GARS) Score Sheet

---

A. **General Categories**

1. **Variability**—a measure of inconsistency and arrhythmicity of stepping and of arm movements
   0 = fluid and predictably paced limb movements;
   1 = occasional interruptions (changes in velocity), approximately < 25% of time;
   2 = unpredictability of rhythm, approximately 25–75% of time;
   3 = random timing of limb movements.

2. **Guardedness**—hesitancy, slowness, diminished propulsion and lack of commitment in stepping and arm swing
   0 = good forward momentum and lack of apprehension in propulsion;
   1 = center of gravity of head, arms, and trunk (HAT) projects only slightly in front of push-off, but still good arm-leg coordination;
   2 = HAT held over anterior aspect of foot, and some moderate loss of smooth reciprocation;
   3 = HAT held over rear aspect of stance phase foot and great tentativity in stepping.

3. **Weaving**—an irregular and wavering line of progression
   0 = straight line of progression on frontal viewing;
   1 = a single deviation from straight (line of best fit) line of progression;
   2 = two to three deviations from line of progression;
   3 = four or more deviations from line of progression.

4. **Waddling**—a broad-based gait characterized by excessive truncal crossing of the midline and side-bending
   0 = narrow base of support and body held nearly vertically over feet;
   1 = slight separation of medial aspects of feet and just perceptible lateral movement of head and trunk;
   2 = 3–4″ separation feet and obvious bending of trunk to side so COG of head lies well over ipsilateral stance foot;
   3 = extreme pendular deviations of head and trunk (head passes lateral to ipsilateral stance foot) and further widening of base of support.

5. **Staggering**—sudden and unexpected laterally directed partial losses of balance
   0 = no losses of balance to side;
   1 = a single lurch to side;
   2 = two lurches to side;
   3 = three or more lurches to side.

B. **Lower Extremity Categories**

1. **% Time in Swing**—a loss in the percentage of the gait cycle constituted by the swing phase

---

continues

Exhibit 17–10 continued

> 0 = approximately 3:2 ratio of duration of stance to swing phase;
> 1 = a 1:1 or slightly less ratio of stance to swing;
> 2 = markedly prolonged stance phase, but with some obvious swing time remaining;
> 3 = barely perceptible portion of cycle spent in swing.
>
> 2. **Foot Contact**—the degree to which heel strikes the ground before the forefoot
>   0 = very obvious angle of impact of heel on ground;
>   1 = barely visible contact of heel before forefoot;
>   2 = entire foot lands flat on ground;
>   3 = anterior aspect of foot strikes ground before heel.
>
> 3. **Hip ROM**—the degree to which heel strikes the ground before the forefoot
>   0 = obvious angulation of thigh backward during double support (10 degrees);
>   1 = just barely visible angulation backward from vertical;
>   2 = thigh in line with vertical projection from ground;
>   3 = thigh angled forward from vertical at maximum posterior excursion.
>
> 4. **Knee ROM**—the degree of loss of knee range of motion seen during a gait cycle
>   0 = knee moves from complete extension at heel-strike (and late stance) to almost 90° (to 70°) during swing phase;
>   1 = slight bend in knee seen at heel-strike and late stance and maximal flexion at midswing is closer to 45° than 90°;
>   2 = knee flexion at late stance more obvious than at heel-strike, very little clearance seen for toe during swing;
>   3 = toe appears to touch ground during swing, knee flexion appears constant during stance, and knee angle during stance, and knee angle during swing appears 45° or less.
>
> C. **Trunk, Head, and Upper Extremities Categories**
>
> 1. **Elbow Extension**—a measure of the decrease of elbow range of motion
>   0 = large peak-to-peak excursion of forearm (approximately 20°), with distinct maximal flexion at end of anterior trajectory;
>   1 = 25% decrement of extension during maximal posterior excursion of upper extremity;
>   2 = almost no change in elbow angle;
>   3 = no apparent change in elbow angle (held in flexion).
>
> 2. **Shoulder Extension**—a measure of the decrease of shoulder range of motion
>   0 = clearly seen movement of upper arm anterior (15°) and posterior (20°) to vertical axis of trunk;
>   1 = shoulder flexes slightly anterior to vertical axis;
>   2 = shoulder comes only to vertical axis or slightly posterior to it during flexion;
>   3 = shoulder stays well behind vertical axis during entire excursion.
>
> 3. **Shoulder Abduction**—a measure of pathological increase in shoulder ROM laterally
>   0 = shoulders held almost parallel to trunk;
>   1 = shoulders held 5–10° to side;

continues

Exhibit 17–10 continued

    2 = shoulders held 10–20° to side;

    3 = shoulders held greater than 20° to side.

4. **Arm Heel-strike Synchrony**—the extent to which the contralateral movements of an arm and leg are out of phase

    0 = good temporal conjunction of arm and contralateral leg at apex of shoulder and hip excursions all of the time;

    1 = arm and leg slightly out of phase 25% of the time;

    2 = arm and leg moderately out of phase 25–50% of the time;

    3 = little or no temporal coherence of arm and leg.

5. **Head Held Forward**—a measure of the pathological forward projection of the head relative to the trunk

    0 = ear lobe vertically aligned with shoulder tip;

    1 = ear lobe vertical projection falls 1″ anterior to shoulder tip;

    2 = ear lobe vertical projection falls 2″ anterior to shoulder tip;

    3 = ear lobe vertical projection falls 3″ or more anterior to shoulder tip.

6. **Shoulders Held Elevated**—the degree to which the scapular girdle is held higher than normal

    0 = tip of shoulder (acromion) markedly below level of chin (1–2″);

    1 = tip of shoulder slightly below level of chin;

    2 = tip of shoulder at level of chin;

    3 = tip of shoulder above level of chin.

7. **Upper Trunk Flexed Forward**—a measure of kyphotic involvement of the trunk

    0 = very gentle thoracic convexity, cervical spine flat, or almost flat;

    1 = emerging cervical curve, more distant thoracic convexity;

    2 = anterior concavity at mid-chest level apparent;

    3 = anterior concavity at mid-chest level very obvious.

Source: Reprinted with permission from L. Wolfson et al., Gait Assessment in the Elderly: A Gait Abnormality Rating Scale and Its Relation to Falls, *Journal of Gerontology*, Vol. 45, No. 1, p. M14–M15, © 1990, The Gerontological Society of America.

COM Movement over the BOS, Motor Strategies

Balance cannot improve if it is not challenged. Most balance problems result in the patient locking up the COM movement over the BOS, so treatment to improve the ability to move the COM again is helpful. Practicing body sway using the ankle and hip strategy actions are examples of COM movement over the BOS. Weight shifting over the entire surface of the feet, from right to left, from the edges of the cone of stability in different postures of sitting, and standing all are COM and BOS movements. Following are several examples of exercises for encouraging the various movement strategies:

- ankle strategy can be practiced by having the person lock up the body except for the ankles and sway back and forth, sideways, and circular; placing a flashlight at the waist (a ski headlight) and

Table 17–5 Components of Balance and Related Impairment Testing

Component Part	Testing
Cone of Stability: sitting, standing	Qualitative testing, videotape ROM for cone of stability
Motor Components:	
Ankle, Hip, Stepping Strategies	Foam and Dome
Static Balance Abilities	Berg, Balance Section on the Tinetti Romberg
Dynamic Balance Abilities	OGA using Exhibits 1, 2, & 3 as a guide
	Dynamic Gait Index
	Gait Section on the Tinetti
GARS	
Get Up and Go	
Essential Elements for Reaching and Sit to Stand	
	Observational, qualitative testing using Shepherd's table
External Perturbations	Equilibrium testing in sitting and standing
	Qualitative evaluation of reaching effect on balance
	Qualitative evaluation of effect of tripping, obstacles, stepping over things
	Dynamic Gait Index
Muscle Strength and Flexibility	Kendall's approach to testing biarticular muscles
Sensory Components:	Foam and Dome
Other Factors:	
Endurance	Timed walking tests over distance
	VO_2 max
Confidence/Fear Issues	Tinetti's Confidence Scale
Medications/Pathologies	History taking

Source: Copyright © 1998, Jerline Carey.

having the person move the light in a directed pattern (such as lines on the wall, or following a light the therapist is directing).

- hip strategy can be practiced by placing a temporary brace that locks the ankle and then have the patient do reaching tasks in the standing position; the patient can progress from feet apart to tandem standing positions while moving the HAT in various planes.

- step strategy can be practiced by braiding actions while standing, lateral walking, lunges, and backwards stepping.

The exercises mentioned so far represent static balance COM to BOS relationships where the BOS remains steady and the COM moves. Exercises and activities that work with moving the BOS while maintaining a static COM, and with moving the BOS and the COM both are a logical progression that

Exhibit 17–11 Foam and Dome Score Sheet (Sensory Organization Test)

General Testing Conditions: use a quiet, well-lit room
barefoot; when using foam, flip it between each test and allow it to regain its form before proceeding with the next test; hands on opposite elbows; arms crossing; place hands above elbows

Instructions: stand erect but not rigid, without moving your feet, looking straight ahead at an x that has been placed on the wall; eyes closed, or looking at the x in the dome from the time I say "go" to "stop," which will be 30 seconds or however long you can successfully stand.
criteria for stopping: arms become uncrossed, feet move away from position, fall or loss of position occurs (spotters will not allow fall)
criteria for scoring: **time** person stands successfully; 3 trials are allowed to reach 30 seconds; if 30 seconds is reached in Trial One; immediately score all remaining trials as 30 seconds and go to the next test; **strategies person uses to stand; sway amount; sway speed**

Indicate foam type used for this test: blue   green   other (describe)

Indicate if any of the following conditions exist that may indicate "not normal" subject:
history of ankle sprains, chronic, more than 1 at grade 2
neurological soft signs (tremors, slowed reflexes, c/o clumsiness)
cold at time of testing
hearing deficits
visual deficits (myopia, cannot see without glasses or contacts, blindness)
known vestibular diagnosis
    other:

Condition 1: feet shoulder width apart

Test:	1 (eyes open) floor	2 (eyes closed) floor	3 (dome) floor	4 (eyes open) foam	5 (eyes closed) foam	6 (dome) foam
Time: Tr 1:	_____ sec	_____ sec	_____ sec	_____ sec	_____ sec	_____ sec
Tr 2:	_____ sec	_____ sec	_____ sec	_____ sec	_____ sec	_____ sec
Tr 3:	_____ sec	_____ sec	_____ sec	_____ sec	_____ sec	_____ sec
Total	_____	_____	_____	_____	_____	_____

Strategy
Comments:
(hip, ankle,
combination,
rotation) lockup _____

Sway amount:
(little, moderate,
excessive)_____

Speed of sway:
(slow, normal,
fast) _____

continues

Exhibit 17–11 continued

Condition 2: standing with malleoli touching, feet together, side-by-side

Test:	1 (eyes open) floor	2 (eyes closed) floor	3 (dome) floor	4 (eyes open) foam	5 (eyes closed) foam	6 (dome) foam
Time: Tr 1:	_____ sec	_____ sec	_____ sec	_____ sec	_____ sec	_____ sec
Tr 2:	_____ sec	_____ sec	_____ sec	_____ sec	_____ sec	_____ sec
Tr 3:	_____ sec	_____ sec	_____ sec	_____ sec	_____ sec	_____ sec
Total	_____	_____	_____	_____	_____	_____

Strategy
Comments:
(hip, ankle,
combination,
rotation) lockup _____

Sway amount:
(little, moderate,
excessive) _____

Speed of sway:
(slow, normal,
fast) _____

Condition 3: tandem standing with dominant LE behind (check dominance by having them imitate kicking a ball—kicking leg is dominant leg)

Test:	1 (eyes open) floor	2 (eyes closed) floor	3 (dome) floor	4 (eyes open) foam	5 (eyes closed) foam	6 (dome) foam
Time: Tr 1:	_____ sec	_____ sec	_____ sec	_____ sec	_____ sec	_____ sec
Tr 2:	_____ sec	_____ sec	_____ sec	_____ sec	_____ sec	_____ sec
Tr 3:	_____ sec	_____ sec	_____ sec	_____ sec	_____ sec	_____ sec
Total	_____	_____	_____	_____	_____	_____

Strategy
Comments:
(hip, ankle,
combination,
rotation) lockup _____

Sway amount:
(little, moderate,
excessive) _____

Speed of sway:
(slow, normal,
fast) _____

Source: Adapted from F. Horak, *Physical Therapy*, Alexandria, Virginia, American Physical Therapy Association, 1987, p. 1885, with permission from the American Physical Therapy Association.

Exhibit 17–12 Interpretation Guide for the Foam and Dome

Normal performance would be scoring the full time on the test within three trials on all six conditions. **Abnormal performance** then would not be scoring the full time within three trials on all six conditions. **Each subtest represents the following specific sensory conditions:**

Subtest 1: central vision is able to maintain standing (may have help from other senses)

Subtest 2: proprioception is able to maintain standing on a firm surface (vision occluded)

Subtest 3: conflict for vision exists, standing must be maintained by proprioception after conflict discovered and responded to (some vestibular likely involved)

Subtest 4: central vision with unreliable proprioception is used to maintain standing

Subtest 5: unreliable proprioception is all that is available for standing

Subtest 6: vestibular information is all that is available for standing

- Visual dependency would occur with poor or abnormal scoring on subtests 3, 5, and 6 or only poor performance on conditions 3 and 6.
- Proprioceptive difficulty would be suspected with poor or abnormal scoring on subtests 2, 3, 4, 5, and 6 or 5 and 6 or only poor performance on 4, 5, and 6.
- Vestibular problems would be suspected with poor performance on 5 and 6 or 6 alone.

Source: Copyright © 1998, Jerline Carey.

allows the patient to experience static to dynamic situations. Examples of a moving BOS with a static COM can include working with a noncompliant surface under the feet while engaged in a hand task (such as piling cones) and sitting. Another example is to be working with a noncompliant surface under the feet while engaged in a hand task and standing in the parallel bars. The idea is to provide weight-shifting experiences while in a stable position, to have an occupying task, and to have a noncompliant surface under one or both feet. Examples of a noncompliant surface would be a rocker board, noncompliant foam, or a flat-shaped inflatable.

Examples of working with a moving BOS and moving COM could involve progressive challenges from sitting on a large ball and tapping the feet while doing hand activities, standing on a wobbleboard while stretching a piece of Theraband™ or shaking a Body blade, and finally—the most difficult—

walking across multiple noncompliant surfaces. The complexity of movement can be challenged with mazes that involve walking through sand, water, thick carpeting, or uneven terrain. Obstacles to go around or step over also present appropriate challenge to some. Goldstein in her functional exercise progression provides balance and gait basic, intermediate, and advanced exercise list; these are outlined in Exhibit 17–13.[31(p70)]

When considering COM/BOS relationships during standing and walking, the therapist also needs to consider which assistive device will protect that relationship and yet allow functional mobility. The choice of a rear walker or crutches instead of a front supporting walker, or the type of gait training done for use of the assistive device all become important treatment approaches that can minimize or maximize the loss of COM movement over the BOS. The type of assistive device and the pattern of walking a per-

Exhibit 17–13 Goldstein's Basic, Intermediate, and Advanced Standing and Walking Treatment Ideas

Standing Basic Level:
Vary the BOS the client uses
Vary the sensory input used to stand
Vary the floor texture
Vary the environment from quiet to noisy

Standing Intermediate Level:
Squat, crouch, and lunge
Throw a ball, catch a ball
Lift an object from the floor or varying heights
Reach overhead
Hit a foam ball with hand or paddle

Standing Advanced Level:
Real-life situations
Standing in line at the grocery store
Standing to get dressed
Standing to prepare meals
Standing to putt (golf)

Walking Basic Level:
Work with the gait deviation at the joint problem areas
Increase the step size on purpose
Add resistance to gait with theratubing, pulling something
Change the levels of the surface
Change velocity demands
Change environments; use simple mazes
Side-step, backward walking
Lunge and lunges with resistance
Cross-over stepping
Circular and figure-of-eight walking
Shuttle drills: walk and do quick turns
Easy plyometrics (stepping over objects, hopping over small objects, skipping)
Treadmill walking that is constant; preset speed with handrails

Walking Intermediate Level:
Obstacle courses
Pushing open doors, pushing grocery carts, moving furniture, pulling a golf cart
Carrying things
Dribbling a ball
Stepping up to hit a foam ball
Closed chain exercise series

Walking Advanced Level:
The real environment

Source: Copyright © 1998, Jerline Carey.

son uses with that device can improve or reduce balance abilities. The therapist is encouraged to maintain and improve balance abilities as much as possible as soon as possible. Prevention of balance loss is a better approach than trying to regain that lost from unnecessary disuse.

The new unweighting systems can be very helpful in separating the demand of doing the locomotor skill of walking from the demand of balancing.[51(p69)] The individual tasks and components of gait can be worked on in an unweighted (nonposturally demanding) environment so quality of the locomotion can be improved and strengthened while the postural control demands are minimized. Then over time, the person is given graded increases in having to handle the postural control (balance) along with the locomotor task of walking so dynamic balance and locomotor skills of walking are both improved over the treatment time. The studies regarding this treatment seem to indicate a very effective method of working with improving gait and dynamic balance. The reader is referred to those for further information.

Muscle Strength and Length Treatment

Biarticular muscles and hip muscles appear to be the targeted muscles for length and strength training related to improving control of the HAT on the lower extremities. Open chain approaches for strengthening the individual muscles can be a helpful start for gaining strength in the first week of treatment, but the use of closed chain approaches is likely more functionally based. The closed chain approach would involve having the person move the HAT over the BOS in varied ways to maximize full length and strength of the biarticular muscles related to holding the HAT. Some closed chain hip exercise examples are presented in Figures 17–6 to 17–10.

Therapy involving the motor system that works with balance and coordination exercises represents only partial treatment. The sensory aspects of therapy also need close consideration.

Sensory Integration Training[5(p230),31(p57),52,53(p36)]

Foam and dome assessment results can indicate if a patient has sensory dependency (visual, proprioceptive, or vestibular) or sensory selection/integration issues in relation to balance abilities. Suggestion lists for each problem area follow. The reader is again reminded that the following represents an introductory approach to this treatment area with much of the information compiled for this author's clinical applications.

Visual Dependency

With visual dependency problems, the person is relying only on visual information to determine the motor patterns needed to stay upright. Visual information is less available for a task such as reading, or sewing when a person is reliant on visual information for the postural control or balance needed for standing. The motor abilities used for balancing would also likely benefit from the balance system listening to proprioception and vestibular information more while reducing or eliminating the need for visual input. To promote this pattern of better use of sensory information, the therapist should have the patient practice various forms of manipulating visual input. These can be elimination of vision entirely, distorting vision, creating distracting vision (called "visual noise"), and finally by creating situations where the eyes, head, and hands are required to function through various posturally changing situations. All of these forms of visual manipulations can be done in static

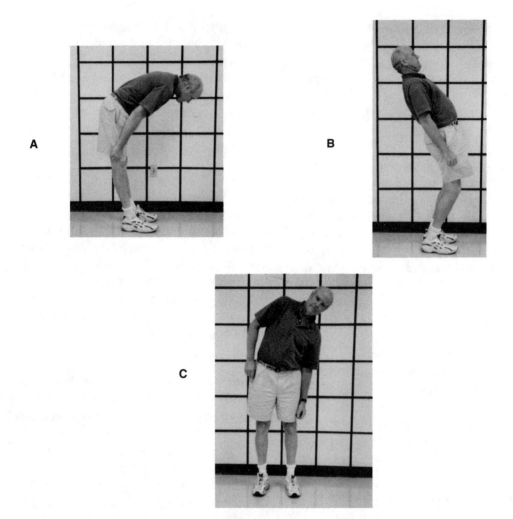

Figure 17–6 Closed Chain Exercise: Pendulum Exercises for the HAT. Strengthening the hip extensors to control movement of the HAT forward (**A**), the hip flexors to control movement of the HAT backward (**B**), and/or the hip abductors and adductors to control movement laterally (**C**) are important for learning control for balancing the HAT.

balance positions (sitting or standing on a solid surface) and can progress to being done in dynamic situations where the BOS is unstable or moving. The following are examples of each visual manipulation:

- eliminate vision by closing the eyes during movements (or wear a blindfold). The movements can be performed in sit-

ting and standing positions while doing a hand task. Short distances of walking using the hands as a guide or walking with eyes closed while holding onto a rope encourage attention to the proprioceptive system instead. Another idea for eliminating vision is to have the person do walking activities in a dimly lit setting.

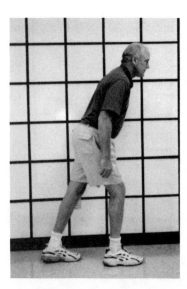

Figure 17–7 Closed Chain Exercise: Standing on one leg while stepping out with the other. The supporting leg needs hip stabilization and control of the HAT while the open chain lower extremity moves into position. For the hip fracture patient, the closed chain activity of the involved lower extremity is more functional than the open chain ability in relation to balance.

- distort vision by wearing swim goggles while performing tasks; head coverings that allow very narrow visual fields also help reduce the use of vision for balance.
- create visual "noise" around the person as activities are performed in sitting and standing positions at first and then progress to having the "noise" in the peripheral visual field while walking. Examples of this are having busy scenes on large panels that can be moved while the person is seated nearby, patterned shower curtains that have a fan blowing behind them causing significant movement and having the person walk by this visually moving scene.

- create situations where the eyes and head are turning and moving while the person is required to remain balanced. A progression of this type of activity could be to practice balancing while doing gaze stabilization exercises, saccadic movements of the eyes, tracking objects through various visual field areas, doing eye tracking and reaching with the hands to touch moving objects, and lastly, to move the head (shake it side to side) while trying to reach and touch objects accurately in various places. One could progress the patient from doing this sequence of eye exercises while sitting, then standing, then walking.

All of the above activities serve to make the balance system turn to sensory information other than from the visual system for staying upright and balanced. The sequence of events occurring in terms of dissociation of the eyes from the balance system seem to be first freeing eye movement from that of the head, then adding hand activity coupled with the eye movement. Next, letting the head move while the eyes practice stable visual information collection and coupling that action with hand activity; lastly to do both of those visually differing tasks while the body is in varying static positions (sit, stand) and eventually while walking. Some of the above information has been more traditionally included in vestibular rehabilitation programs, but this author believes the vestibular and visual systems to be integrated to the point that to treat one is to treat the other. Vestibular programs are briefly referred to later.

Proprioceptive Dependency

With proprioceptive dependency problems, the patient appears unable to tolerate unreliability in the proprioceptive informa-

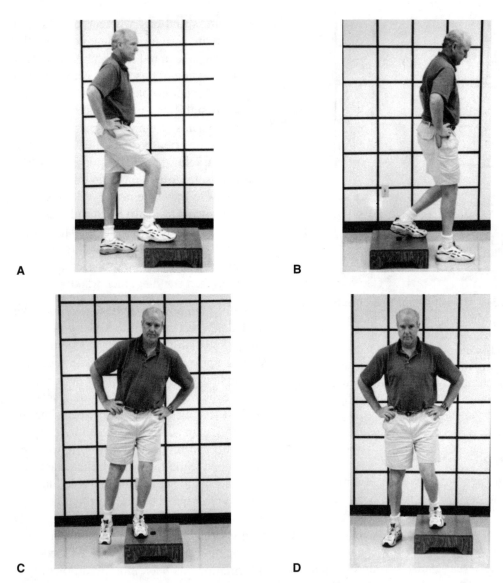

Figure 17–8 Closed Chain Exercise: Stepping Up and Down. The closed chain aspect of this exercise involves the supporting lower extremity. Balance of the HAT becomes the postural challenge. Movement or open chain strength is minimal compared to the closed chain and eccentric action controlling the body as it ascends or descends. Forward (**A** and **B**) and lateral (**C** and **D**) stepping are helpful exercises.

tion. If the person is standing on a firm solid surface, the information coming from the proprioceptive system is consistent and predictable. However, if that person stands or walks on a surface such as thick carpeting or grass, the motor system doesn't seem able to plan a response that allows balance to be accomplished easily. To be able to walk on uneven surfaces that have some unpredictability, one must be able to adjust to varying proprioceptive information. The following activities seem to promote this capability:

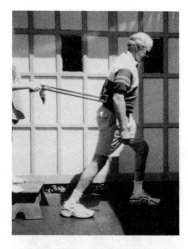

A

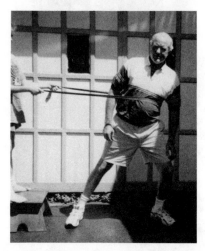

B

Figure 17–9 Closed Chain Exercise: Walking with Theraband Resistance at the HAT. Control of the HAT and hip stabilization ability are enhanced with resistance placed at the COM area **A**, presents resistance to forward movement and **B**, presents resistance to sideways movement. Backward movement can also be done.

- working with varying BOS and a variety of terrain in sitting, standing, and walking. The BOS can be varied by foot arrangement changes (one foot on a stool, feet more tandem than side to side, etc.) or by placing a foot or both feet on dynamic surfaces such as inflat- ables or noncompliant foam. Examples of these are doing hand tasks while sitting and having the patient's feet on a wobbleboard; sitting on a large inflated ball and doing hand activities while keeping the ball stable; standing in the parallel bars with one foot on the wobbleboard and doing hand activities; walking across a large inflatable (such as a camping mattress).

- setting up obstacle courses that require standing on and progressing to walking on inflatables, unstable surfaces, and varying surfaces. This can involve having to walk around or over obstacles also.

Vestibular Problems

There are entire texts devoted to treating problems with this system, and the reader is referred to these for more complete information. Most balance problems the therapist encounters with musculoskeletal system problems are likely going to be in underuse of this system for balance information. Vestibular rehabilitation programs generally use practice of fast movements and changing positions, eye exercises to improve saccadic movement control, tracking abilities, and gaze stabilization skills. Gait with head movements and surface orientation (proprioceptive attending) exercises are also included. This cursory review does not do justice to the vast amount of information available to the therapist, but hopefully it helps place it in perspective.

Sensory Selection Problems

With sensory selection exercises, the driving concept is to have the person improve choice made for balance-related problem-solving situations. A simplistic approach for treatment for this problem is to make sure the

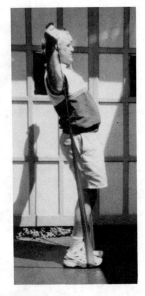

A

B

C

Figure 17–10 Closed Chain Exercise: Maintaining Standing while Doing Upper Extremity Resistance Exercises. Any action of the upper extremities presents internal perturbation problems and balance of the HAT becomes necessary. To prepare for multiple task demand, the patient could exercise with upward arm pulls along with a backwards movement as in **A**, with upward arm pulls and maintaining a neutral position as in **B**, or **C**, waist level arm pulls while bending sideways. These are only a few examples of possibilities of upper extremity movement with resistance while holding or transitioning with postures.

patient has to use the balance skills present and be challenged safely and regularly throughout the day. If a person only has hip strategy available for a motor response to balance problems, effort to teach more motor strategies and activities promoting that choice need to be experienced by the patient. Shumway-Cook and Woollacott's motor control text is recommended reading for the therapist wishing more information in this area.

Perturbation Training

Perturbations are basically of two kinds: internally generated from reaching or moving the body and externally generated from being bumped, tripping, or slipping. Practicing both types of perturbations that will occur in a patient's everyday life is warranted along with grading the practice so balance is successfully accomplished by the patient. Activities for each type of perturbation are listed below:

- reaching practice at various levels; start with sitting, then standing, then while taking a step, bending, squatting, or walking
- practicing transitional movement: going from sitting to standing, sitting to the floor, standing to the floor, practicing a slow controlled falling action
- walking with resistance at the HAT area (walking with Theraband™ resistance)
- walking through constructed mazes with objects that need to be stepped over, avoided, or gone around at various heights
- practicing quick turns
- receiving unexpected disturbances in the various static and dynamic positions
- performing higher level coordination tasks such as working on side gliding motions or low level plyometrics would

also allow the patient to deal with perturbations.

ADL-Related Training

To improve a task, the best therapeutic technique can be to practice the task itself. Stepping in and out of a tub, getting to a bathroom quickly, and standing while undoing clothing are examples of tasks that can be practiced to improve balance. The ADL checklist in Table 17–3 can be used as a guide for activities to be practiced for independence in BADL and IADL areas. Transitional posturing, reaching at all levels for all positions, and velocity of gait maintained over time and distance are also tasks that with practice improve a person's balance abilities, endurance, and functional skills.

Safety of the Environment

Exhibit 17–5, mentioned earlier, provides a list that can help eliminate barriers to safety. Teaching attention to task if the environment is treacherous also can be helpful to the patient. The SAFE AT HOME assessment in Appendix 1-A (Chapter 1) is another comprehensive home evaluation that includes safety considerations in multiple areas.

CLINICAL APPLICATIONS

Several examples are provided to indicate clinical use of this chapter's information. See Exhibit 17–14 for a Hip fracture/THA patient example.

Another example would be for the acute hospital patient admitted for acute episode of illness (i.e., gallbladder surgery, pneumonia). This therapist has found that most elderly patients who have had 1 to 2 weeks of lessened activity are in need of balance training. The same assessment recommendations made for

Exhibit 17–14 Hip Fracture/THA Patient Example

Acute Stage of Recovery
- History of fall (if appropriate)
- Muscle length & strength assessment and intervention
- ADL training for BADL using assistive device and assistance as needed
- Treatment considerations would involve promoting as little loss of muscle length, strength, and ADL-related use of standing and walking (preservation of COM/BOS, cone of stability, gait skills as able).

Subacute Stage of Recovery
- ADL checklist—basic; then progress to instrumental levels, being sure to indicate previous condition prior to injury
- Berg; progress to Dynamic Gait Index (other options include Tinetti, GARS, Get up and Go); do weekly if needed to demonstrate progress and need
- Walking velocity & OGA
- Continue with muscle length and strength
- Environmental Safety Checklists; SAFE AT HOME
- Foam and Dome
- Confidence and Fear Scale if appropriate
- Treatment considerations would involve being sure balance (both static and dynamic) is above risk for fall levels or better. Emphasis would be placed on strengthening functional balance and gait abilities in addition to the joint specific treatment needed.

---

the hip fracture patient at the subacute stage could be used for those elders admitted to the hospital for acute episodes of illness with additional emphasis placed on pharmacology screening. There is a significant amount of literature supporting ADL and balance training for the hospitalized geriatric patient.[36(p325),54]

A last example could be the long-term nursing home patient who has had numerous falls this year. This is an interesting and varied group for which to begin investigating and planning treatment. These patients often have limited potential in the intrinsic balance system and therefore have a moderate to high risk of falls even when functioning at their potential. This author has found many have difficulty with getting regular exercise and walks that would decrease the risk for falls. Also cognitive impairment, restraint issues, and the plans of care that can be devised for the pa-

tients relate to having a thorough balance assessment and treatment approach. Teaching the nursing staff to keep the halls clear, using lowered beds, and modifying the environment are often identified as needed changes along with an improvement in general exercise for the patient. The application to this type of patient again is beyond the scope of this chapter and book, but the therapist can easily plan a balance assessment approach using this chapter's information. General considerations should include looking at the history of falls to determine cause(s), establishing a clear risk of falls using Berg or Tinetti, medication-related check, particularly an environmental modification and safety check, and finally, checks for intrinsically related problems (i.e., secondary deficits, muscle strength and length, general fitness, and endurance). Staff education can be a significant part of the plan of care for this chronic risk for falls patient.

SUMMARY

This chapter was written to assist the therapist in reviewing balance and its component aspects so as to be able to better include balance training as a part of all treatment. Balance and gait changes occur with any significant injury to the body or any episode of illness requiring excessive rest. The significantly high number of falls occurring that result in serious problems for the older adults alone indicate the need to include balance assessment and treatment as a usual and customary part of all treatments. The information presented here should help the therapist more successfully assess and treat the balance system.

REFERENCES

1. Nashner L. Sensory, neuromuscular, and biomechanical contributions to human balance. In: Duncan P, ed. *Balance: Proceedings of the APTA Forum*. American Physical Therapy Association; 1989:5–12.

2. Horak F, Shumway-Cook A. Clinical implications of postural control research. In: Duncan P, ed. *Balance: Proceedings of the APTA Forum*. American Physical Therapy Association; 1989:105–111.

3. Chandler J, Duncan P. Balance and falls in the elderly: issues in evaluation and treatment. In: Guccione A, ed. *Geriatric Physical Therapy*. St Louis: Mosby-Year Book; 1993, 237–251.

4. Horak F. Clinical measurement of postural control in adults. *Phys Ther*. 1987;67:1881–1885.

5. Shumway-Cook A, Woollacott M. *Motor Control: Theory and Applications*. Baltimore, MD: Williams & Wilkins; 1995.

6. Horak F, Nashner L, Diener H. Postural strategies associated with somatosensory and vestibular loss. *Exp Brain Res*. 1990;82:167–177.

7. Winter D. *ABCs of Balance during Standing and Walking*. Waterloo, Ontario: Waterloo Biomechanics; 1995.

8. Maki B, McIlroy W. The role of limb movements in maintaining upright stance: the "change-in-support" strategy. *Phys Ther*. May 1997;77:488–507.

9. Maki B, Holliday P, Topper A. A prospective study of postural balance and risk of falling in an ambulatory and independent elderly population. *J Geriatr*. 1994;49:M72-M84.

10. Woollacott M, Tang P. Balance control during walking in the older adult: research and its implications. *Phys Ther*. 1997;77:646–660.

11. Winter D. *The Biomechanics and Motor Control of Human Gait: Normal, Elderly, and Pathological*. 2nd ed. Waterloo, Ontario: University of Waterloo Press; 1991.

12. Gage J. *Normal Walking*. St Paul, MN: Gillette Children's Hospital; 1993.

13. Perry J. *Gait Analysis: Normal and Pathological Function*. Thorofare, NJ: Slack Inc; 1992.

14. Shepherd R. *Physiotherapy in Paediatrics*. 3rd ed. Jordon Hill, Oxford, UK: Butterworth-Heinemann Ltd.; 1995, 43–88.

15. VanSant A. Rising from supine position to erect stance: description of adult movement and a developmental hypothesis. *Phys Ther*. 1988;68:185–192.

16. Winter D, Patla A, Frank J, Wait S. Biomechanical walking pattern changes in the fit and health elderly. *Phys Ther*. 1990;70:340–347.

17. Chen H, Ashton-Miller J, Alexander N, Schultz A. Effects of age and available response time on ability to step over an obstacle. *J Gerontol*. 1994;49: M227–233.

18. Kisner C, Colby L. *Therapeutic Exercise: Foundations and Techniques*. Philadelphia: FA Davis Co; 1995.

19. Friesen K, Carey J. The role of the bi-articular muscles in human movement: implications for gait analysis. Unpublished paper. Physical Therapy Department, College of St. Scholastica. Duluth, MN; 1997.

20. Kendall F, McCreary E, Provance P. *Muscles: Testing and Function*. 4th ed. Baltimore, MD: Williams & Wilkins; 1993.

21. Comeaux P, Patterson N, Rubin M, Meiner R. Effect of neuromuscular electrical stimulation during gait in children with cerebral palsy. *Ped Phys Ther*. 1997;9:103–109.

22. DiFabio R, Emasithi A. Aging and the mechanisms underlying head and postural control during voluntary motion. *Phys Ther.* May 1997;77:458–475.

23. Jeka J. Light touch contact as a balance aid. *Phys Ther.* May 1997;77:476–487.

24. Wade M, Jones G. The role of vision and spatial orientation in the maintenance of posture. *Phys Ther.* 1997;77:619–628.

25. Shumway-Cook A, Horak F. Assessing the influence of sensory interaction on balance. *Phys Ther.* October 1986;10:1548–1550.

26. Judge J, King M, Whipple R, Clive J, Wolfson L. Dynamic balance in older persons: effects of reduced visual and proprioceptive input. *J Gerontol.* 1995; 50A:M263–270.

27. Bohannon R. Standing balance and function over the course of acute rehabilitation. *Arch Phys Med Rehabil.* 1995;76:994–996.

28. Bach J, Carey J. Dynamic Balance. Unpublished paper. Department of Physical Therapy,. College of St. Scholastica. Duluth, MN; 1998.

29. Ciccone C. Geriatric pharmacology. In: Guccione A, ed. *Geriatric Physical Therapy.* St Louis: Mosby-Year Book; 1993, 171–197.

30. Robinett C, Vondran M. Functional ambulation/velocity and distance requirements in rural and urban communities. *Phys Ther.* 1988;68:1371–1373.

31. Goldstein T. *Functional Rehabilitation in Orthopaedics.* Gaithersburg, MD: Aspen Publishers, Inc; 1995.

32. Guccione A, ed. *Geriatric Physical Therapy.* St Louis: Mosby-Year Book; 1993.

33. Feltner M, MacRae P, McNitt-Gray J. Quantitative gait assessment as a predictor of prospective and retrospective falls in community-dwelling women. *Arch Phys Med Rehabil.* 1994;75:447–453.

34. Gehlsen G, Whaley M. Falls in the elderly: part I, gait. *Arch of Phys Med Rehabil.* 1990;71:735–741.

35. King M, Tinetti M. Falls in community-dwelling older persons. *J Am Geriatr Soc.* 1995;43:1146–1154.

36. Salgado R, Lord S, Packer J, Ehrlich F. Factors associated with falling in elderly hospital patients. *Gerontol.* 1994;40:325–331.

37. Norton R, Campbell A. Circumstances of falls resulting in hip fractures among older people. *J Am Geriatr Soc.* 1997;45:1108–1112.

38. DiFabio R, Seay R. Use of the "fast evaluation of mobility, balance, and fear" in elderly community dwellers: validity and reliability. *Phys Ther.* 1997; 77:904–917.

39. Butland R, Pang J, Gross E, Woodcock A, Geddes D. Two-, six-, and 12-minute walking tests in respiratory disease. *Brit Med J.* 1982;284:1607–1608.

40. Kennedy K. Gait assessment using footprint analysis. Unpublished paper. Physical Therapy Department, College of St. Scholastica. Duluth, MN; 1995.

41. Csuka M, McCarty D. Simple method for measurement of lower extremity muscle strength. *Am J Med.* 1985;78:77–81.

42. Berg K. Balance and its measure in the elderly: a review. *Physiotherapy Canada.* 1989;41:240–246.

43. Thorbahn L, Newton R. Use of the Berg balance test to predict falls in elderly persons. *Phys Ther.* 1996;76:576–583.

44. Berg K, Wood-Dauphinee S, Williams J, Gayton D. Measuring balance in the elderly: preliminary development of an instrument. *Physiotherapy Canada.* 1989;41:304–311.

45. Haarda N, Chiu V, Damron-Rodriguez J, et al. Screening for balance and mobility impairment in elderly individuals living in residential care facilities. *Phys Ther.* 1995;75:462–469.

46. Lewis C. Balance, gait test proves simple yet useful. *PT Bulletin.* 1993;Feb 10:9,40.

47. Gill T, Williams C, Tinetti M. Assessing risk for the onset of functional dependence among older adults: the role of physical performance. *J Am Geriatr Soc.* 1995;43:603–609.

48. Mathias S, Nayak U, Isaacs B. Balance in elderly patients: the "get up and go" test. *Arch Phys Med Rehabil.* 1986;67:387–389.

49. Wolfson L, Whipple R, Amerman P, Tobin J. Gait assessment in the elderly: a gait abnormality and its relation to falls. *J Gerontol.* 1990;45:M12–M19.

50. Krebs D, Edelstein J, Fishman S. Reliability of observational kinematic gait analysis. *Phys Ther.* 1985; 65:1027–1033.

51. Henderson K. The investigation and implementation of comprehensive gait evaluation measures. Unpublished paper. Physical Therapy Department, College of St. Scholastica. Duluth, MN; 1996.

52. Carey J. Workshop notes: Sensory aspects of postural control and gait. November 13 and 14, 1997. Continuing Education Resources, Chicago, IL.

53. Altewelt L, Carey J. Sensory organization testing: the foam and dome. Unpublished paper. Physical Therapy Department, College of St. Scholastica. Duluth, MN; 1998.

54. University of Wisconsin Hospital and Clinics: Workshop. Functional consequences of hospitalization of the elderly. February 26–27, 1993.

Index

Page numbers in *italics* denote figures and exhibits; those followed by "t" denote tables.

Balance dysfunction treatment—*continued*
    total hip arthroplasty, 80, *81*
  environmental safety, 377
  matching protocol to problem, 362
  motor strategies related to center of mass movement
    over base of support, 362–371, *370*
  muscle length and strength treatment, 371, *372–376*
  perturbation training, 377
  sensory integration training, 371–377
    proprioceptive dependency, 373–375
    sensory selection problems, 375–377
    vestibular problems, 375
    visual dependency, 371–373
  time required for, 362
Barton's fracture, 311
Base of support (BOS), 327–328. *See also* Balance
Berg Balance Test, 353, 354, *356–358*
Bicep curl, *292*
Blood pressure, 3, *21*
Bone effects
  of aging, 2–3
  of hypokinetics, 7
Bone mineral density, 2. *See also* Osteoporosis
Bony palpation, 15
BOS. *See* Base of support
Boutonniere deformity, 314
Braces, patellar, 151–152, *152,* 161
Breathing, 3, 20, *21*
Broomstick curl up, *292*
Bunion, 182, 184t, 191, 192t
Bursa(e)
  around hip, 32, *33*
  iliopectineal, 32
  infrapatellar, 100, 142
  ischiogluteal, 32
  around knee, 100–101, *101*
  medial gastrocnemius, 101
  pes anserine, 101
  popliteal, 101
  prepatellar, 100, 142
  around shoulder, 234
  subdeltoid, 234, *236*
  suprapatellar, 100–101
  trochanteric, 32
Bursitis
  of hip, 82–83
    iliopectineal, 83
    ischiogluteal, 83
    treatment of, 83
    trochanteric, 83
  of knee, 142–143
    Baker's cyst, 142

    infrapatellar, 142
    prepatellar, 142
    treatment of, 142–143
  subacromial, 262
Buzzwords for documenting patient care, 293, 294t

C

Calcaneus, *165*
  fracture of, 176
"Calf pump," 169
Calluses, 194
Capitate, 298
Cardiac output, 3
Cardiac warning signs and interventions, *21*
Cardiopulmonary reconditioning, 20, 20t
Cardiopulmonary screening, 14–15
Cardiopulmonary system
  effects of aging on, 3
  effects of hypokinetics on, 7–8
  exercise-induced changes in, 9
Carpal bones, 297–298, *299, 318*
  fractures of, 313–314
Carpal tunnel syndrome (CTS), 318–320
  anatomy and, 318, *319*
  after Colles' fracture, 312–313
  definition of, 318
  risk factors for, 318
  signs and symptoms of, 318–319
  treatment of, *319,* 319–320
Carpometacarpal (CMC) joints, 298
  immobilization orthosis for, 317, *317*
  osteoarthritis of, 316–317
"Carrying angle," 279
Cartilage, articular
  aging effects on, 2
  of knee, 97
Causalgia, 320
Center of mass (COM), 327–328. *See also* Balance
Cerebral atrophy, 3
Cerebrovascular accident (CVA), 271
Cervical arthritis, 218–219
Cervical radiculopathy, 218, 219t
Chondroitin sulfate, 2
Claudication, neurogenic vs. vascular, 220, 221t
Clavicle, 233, *234*
Claw fist exercise, 316, *317*
Claw toe deformity, 182, 185t, 191, 193t
CMC. *See* Carpometacarpal joints
Cognitive status evaluation, 17
Collagen, 2, 3
Colles' fracture, 311–313, *312*